Bronchial Asthma

CURRENT CLINICAL PRACTICE

Bronchial Asthma

*A Guide for Practical Understanding
and Treatment*

FIFTH EDITION

Edited by

M. Eric Gershwin, MD

*Division of Rheumatology/Allergy and Clinical Immunology
Department of Medicine
School of Medicine
University of California at Davis
Davis, CA*

Timothy E. Albertson, MD, MPH, PhD

*Division of Pulmonary and Critical Care Medicine
Department of Medicine
School of Medicine
University of California at Davis
Davis, CA
and
Veterans Administration Northern California Health Care System
Mather, CA*

HUMANA PRESS ✳ TOTOWA, NEW JERSEY

This publication is printed on acid-free paper. ∞
ANSI Z39.48-1984 (American Standards Institute) Permanence of Paper for Printed Library Materials.

Cover Illustration: Figure 1, Chapter 13, "Allergic Bronchopulmonary Aspergillosis: *An Evolving Challenge in Asthma*," by Brian M. Morrissey and Samuel Louie.

Cover design by Patricia F. Cleary

Production Editor: Amy Thau

For additional copies, pricing for bulk purchases, and/or information about other Humana titles, contact Humana at the above address or at any of the following numbers: Tel.: 973-256-1699; Fax: 973-256-8314; E-mail: orders@humanapr.com, or visit our Website: http://humanapress.com

Printed in the United States of America. 10 9 8 7 6 5 4 3 2 1
eISBN: 1-59745-014-6
Library of Congress Cataloging in Publication Data
Bronchial asthma : a guide for practical understanding and treatment/
edited by M. Eric Gershwin, Timothy E. Albertson.-- 5th ed.
     p. ; cm. -- (Current clinical practice)
  Includes bibliographical references and index.
  ISBN 1-58829-604-0 (alk. paper)
  1. Asthma--Diagnosis. 2. Asthma--Treatment.
  [DNLM: 1. Asthma--diagnosis. 2. Asthma--therapy. WF 553 B8683
2006] I. Gershwin, M. Eric, 1946- II. Albertson, Timothy Eugene.
III. Series.
  RC591.B753 2006
  616.2'38--dc22
                        2005017322

Dedication

They asked if the sneezles
Came after *the wheezles,*
Or if the first sneezle came first.[1]

This text is dedicated to helping the many millions of people who suffer from asthma.

[1]From "Sneezles," by A.A. Milne, in *Now We are Six*. New York, E.P. Dutton and Co., 1927.

Series Editor's Introduction

Usually a chronic asthmatic has some favorite substance to inhale or to smoke...ordinary tobacco cigarettes are sometimes helpful.
—William Osler, *The Principles and Practice of Medicine*,
9th edition, 1922

The science of diagnosing and treating asthma has advanced dramatically. *Bronchial Asthma: A Guide for Practical Understanding and Treatment, 5th Edition* is an important resource for primary care physicians who want a concise yet comprehensive overview of the diagnosis and treatment of asthma. Asthma is common, with a prevalence of more than 11%, and as such, it is a condition that primary care physicians encounter daily. Because most asthma care is provided by family physicians, internists, and pediatricians, it is important for those of us in primary care to be experts in the care of asthma. In *Bronchial Asthma: A Guide for Practical Understanding and Treatment, 5th Edition*, Drs. Gershwin and Albertson provide the information we need to have a high level of expertise in the care of pediatric and adult patients with asthma.

Bronchial Asthma: A Guide for Practical Understanding and Treatment, 5th Edition reviews diagnostic approaches including the use of radioallergosorbent assay testing and pulmonary function testing. It also covers environmental and occupational influences on asthma—important but often underemphasized topics in many texts—that are covered in detail here. Finally, the book discusses in detail both acute and ongoing management of asthma. Internists, family doctors, and pediatricians can be confident that by understanding the material in *Bronchial Asthma: A Guide for Practical Understanding and Treatment, 5th Edition*, and by having this book as a reference on their shelf, they will have the knowledge to provide high-quality care to their patients with asthma.

Neil S. Skolnik, MD
Abington Memorial Hospital
Abington, PA
and
Temple University School of Medicine
Philadelphia, PA

Preface

The prevalence and socioeconomic impact of bronchial asthma continue to escalate. Thirty years ago, when the first edition of *Bronchial Asthma: A Guide for Practical Understanding* was published, nearly every patient with chronic asthma was seen by a specialist. Now the number of asthma sufferers simply makes the latter practice an anachronism, and the vast majority of patients is cared for by primary care physicians in internal medicine, pediatrics, and family practice. In fact, asthma remains the most common chronic childhood illness, and is among the most common chronic adult diseases. Despite improved medications, increased awareness, and a better understanding of the pathophysiology of this disease, mortality and morbidity continue to rise. Both national and international consensus positions that offer guidance as to treatment approaches have been published.

The importance of the primary care physician and provider in the appropriate diagnosis and management of this disease cannot be overestimated. The management options in asthma are changing rapidly with the advent of new drugs and approaches. The recent introduction of dry powder inhalers, as well as combinatorial therapies with steroids/long-acting β-agonists, have gone a long way toward improving patient compliance and response. The introduction of Xolair® and the likelihood that other biological modifiers will appear open up exciting vistas for patients with asthma.

Bronchial Asthma: A Guide for Practical Understanding and Treatment, Fifth Edition will discuss these newer treatments, but its emphasis remains on, and directed at, primary care providers, who must be able to face the challenge of diagnosis and the management of asthma in a variety of patient subpopulations. We will continue to emphasize the definition, medications, and the use of asthma treatment plans. However, we will also provide definitive focus on the special needs patient, including the pediatric patient, the pregnant patient, and the patient undergoing surgery, as well as the common issues of exercise and asthma, pulmonary aspergillosis, occupation, recreational drug use, and psychological/social issues. The care of patients with asthma needs to be individualized and we need to reduce the toxicity of the drugs we use. There is increasing concern about the role of systemic and oral corticosteroids in inducing osteoporosis and, especially, avascular necrosis.

The goal of *Bronchial Asthma: A Guide for Practical Understanding and Treatment, Fifth Edition* is to provide a basic framework upon which a successful treatment option can be built. We will likewise emphasize the need for patient education because this is an essential element to good asthma care. Finally, the editors and authors are particularly grateful to Nikki Phipps who has contributed enormously not only to the fifth edition, but also to the first through fourth editions.

M. Eric Gershwin, MD
Timothy E. Albertson, MD, MPH, PhD

Contents

xi

Contributors

RAHMAT AFRASIABI, MD • Division of Rheumatology/Allergy and Clinical Immunology, Department of Medicine, School of Medicine, University of California at Davis, Davis, CA

TIMOTHY E. ALBERTSON, PhD, MD, MPH • Division of Pulmonary and Critical Care Medicine, Department of Medicine, School of Medicine, University of California at Davis, Davis, CA and Veterans Administration Northern California Health Care System, Mather, CA

CHARLES BOND, JD • Charles Bond and Associates, Berkeley, CA

ANDREA BORCHERS, PhD • Division of Rheumatology/Allergy and Clinical Immunology, Department of Medicine, School of Medicine, University of California at Davis, Davis, CA

CHRISTOPHER CHANG, MD, PhD • Division of Rheumatology/Allergy and Clinical Immunology, Department of Medicine, School of Medicine, University of California at Davis, Davis, CA

DENNIS L. FUNG, MD • Department of Anesthesiology, School of Medicine, University of California at Davis, Davis, CA

M. ERIC GERSHWIN, MD • Division of Rheumatology/Allergy and Clinical Immunology, Department of Medicine, School of Medicine, University of California at Davis, Davis, CA

LAUREL J. GERSHWIN, DVM, PhD • Department of Pathology, Microbiology, and Immunology, School of Veterinary Medicine, University of California at Davis, Davis, CA

KIMBERLY A. HARDIN, MD • Division of Pulmonary and Critical Care Medicine, Department of Medicine, School of Medicine, University of California at Davis, Davis, CA

RUSSELL J. HOPP, DO • Department of Pediatrics and Medicine, University of Utah School of Medicine, Salt Lake City, UT

RICHARD E. KANNER, MD • Division of Respiratory, Critical Care and Occupational Medicine, Department of Medicine, University of Utah School of Medicine, Salt Lake City, UT

CARL L. KEEN, PhD • Departments of Medicine and Nutrition, School of Medicine, University of California at Davis, Davis, CA

NICHOLAS J. KENYON, MD • Division of Pulmonary and Critical Care Medicine, Department of Medicine, School of Medicine, University of California at Davis, Davis, CA

GERALD L. KLEIN, MD • Vice President of Medical Affairs and Clinical Research, Dey Laboratories, Napa, CA

DONNA KINSER, MD • Department of Emergency Medicine, School of Medicine, University of California at Davis, Davis, CA

ARVIND KUMAR, MD • Division of Rheumatology/Allergy and Clinical Immunology, Department of Medicine, School of Medicine, University of California at Davis, Davis, CA

ALBIN B. LEONG, MD • Department of Pediatric Pulmonology and Allergy, Kaiser Permanente Medical Group, Sacramento, CA

THEODORE G. LIOU, MD • Division of Respiratory, Critical Care and Occupational Medicine, Department of Medicine, University of Utah School of Medicine, Salt Lake City, UT

SAMUEL LOUIE, MD • Division of Pulmonary and Critical Care Medicine, Department of Medicine, School of Medicine, University of California at Davis, Davis, CA

BRIAN M. MORRISSEY, MD • Division of Pulmonary and Critical Care Medicine, Department of Medicine, School of Medicine, University of California at Davis, Davis, CA

STEVE OFFERMAN, MD • Department of Emergency Medicine, School of Medicine, University of California at Davis, Sacramento, CA

ARIF M. SEYAL, MD • Division of Rheumatology/Allergy and Clinical Immunology, Department of Medicine, School of Medicine, University of California at Davis, Davis, CA

SUZANNE S. TEUBER, MD • Division of Rheumatology/Allergy and Clinical Immunology, Department of Medicine, School of Medicine, University of California at Davis, Davis, CA

ROBERT G. TOWNLEY, MD • Department of Pediatrics, Creighton University School of Medicine, Omaha, NE

KEN Y. YONEDA, MD • Division of Pulmonary and Critical Care Medicine, Department of Medicine, School of Medicine, University of California at Davis, Davis, CA

I DEFINITIONS AND HOST RESPONSES TO BRONCHOSPASM

1

The Origins and Characteristics of Asthma

Russell J. Hopp, DO, and Robert G. Townley, MD

KEY POINTS

- Asthma has become a common medical problem in the United States, especially among blacks.
- Wheezing is a frequently encountered pediatric problem. When wheezing is recurrent, asthma is an important consideration.
- Risk factors for pediatric asthma are strongly associated with genetics (parental) and being atopic.
- Adult-onset asthma is more common in females, but other risk factors, as seen in children, are not as strongly associative.
- Asthma many relapse after years of quiescence.
- Asthma is characterized by bronchoconstriction, bronchial hyperresponsiveness, β-adrenergic blockade, and inflammation.
- Pulmonary eosinophilia is a common feature of asthma.
- Increased exhaled nitric oxide is a marker of inflammation.
- Specific T-cell cytokines are unique to asthma, including interleukin (IL)-4, IL-5, and IL-13.
- IL-13 may play an important role in asthma pathogenesis.

INTRODUCTION

It is widely accepted that asthma has greatly increased in the United States during the past 20 yr. Acute asthma is among the leading causes of hospitalization in pediatric

From: *Current Clinical Practice: Bronchial Asthma:*
A Guide for Practical Understanding and Treatment, 5th ed.
Edited by: M. E. Gershwin and T. E. Albertson © Humana Press Inc., Totowa, NJ

hospitals throughout the country. If we accept the premise that asthma has a strong familial basis, a fact long recognized, it is difficult to explain the rapid rise of asthma on any substantial shift in genetic tendencies.

In this introductory chapter, the epidemiology of asthma in children and adults during the past two decades is reviewed, factors currently known to influence the development of asthma across various age ranges are explored, what is intrinsic to the phenomenon of the active person with asthma is defined, as are what changes when asthma remits.

The authors recognize the incompleteness of the knowledge of what "makes an asthmatic an asthmatic," and the indistinction, especially in children, of wheezing and being an "asthmatic." However, the magnitude of this illness in our society and its impact on the medical dollar compels continued and aggressive research into the cause and treatment of this disease. The authors hope to provide an overview of the asthmatic constitution.

WHEEZING: WHAT IT IS AND WHAT IT ISN'T

The presence of wheezing is not synonymous with a diagnosis of asthma. Wheezing is, however, used in epidemiological studies as a "marker" of a pulmonary symptom that is well recognized by an individual, parents, and health care providers. In fact, wheezing is used as a surrogate for asthma in the International Study of Asthma and Allergies in Childhood (ISAAC), and was also used in the May 2004 Global Initiative for Asthma (GINA) survey of the current prevalence of asthma in the world. An overview of the prevalence of wheezing and the risk factors for wheezing in children and adults provides insight for the asthma discussion.

Infants and Young Children

In infants and young children, the usual precipitating event for the first wheezing episode is a viral respiratory illness. Even without laboratory confirmation, the initial event is usually labeled as "bronchiolitis" and treated accordingly. The dilemma presents itself when the young child returns with subsequent episode(s) of wheezing.

Martinez et al.'s 1995 study (1) provides epidemiological evidence into the patterns of recurrently wheezing infants. A group of 826 infants, enrolled in a health maintenance organization, were prospectively followed for 6 yr. During this time, 49% of the enrolled subjects had a wheezing episode. The authors retrospectively divided the wheezing children into three groups: transient early wheezers, late-onset wheezers, or persistent wheezers.

Using odds-ratio analysis, the characteristic of these three groups of wheezers was defined and compared with the 425 children who had not wheezed by age 6. Transient early wheezers had wheezing within the first 3 yr, but not at 6 yr of age. In these children, maternal smoking was significantly associated with wheezing. These children also had lower length-adjusted pulmonary function, suggesting a negative effect of the passive smoke exposure. The children who developed wheezing after age 3 yr (late-onset wheezers) were more likely to have mothers with asthma, to be male, and to have had rhinitis in the first year of life. (Although not stated, these would be common characteristics of young patients with asthma.) Children who wheezed throughout the 6 yr of the study (persistent wheezers) had a significant incidence of maternal asthma, wheezing often or very often, wheezing without colds, eczema, Hispanic background, and maternal smoking. Of these children, 25% had been labeled asthmatic by age 6 yr.

Multiple studies have identified intrauterine and (extrauterine) smoke exposure and small airway caliber as additional causes for wheezing in young infants and possibly younger children. An emerging body of literature has also recognized the role of respiratory syncytial virus (RSV) as a factor contributing to recurrent wheezing, possibly into adolescence. These facts question the epidemiological use of recurrent wheezing as a "true" surrogate for asthma.

A review of wheezing-related cofactors obtained from an English-literature Medline search (wheezing/wheeze and childhood/children) for 2002–2004 yielded various statistically associated risk factors (excluding RSV, tobacco smoke exposure, and low infantile lung function), and a representative sample is summarized in Table 1. Because the authors accept that some of the wheezing children are truly asthmatic (or developing asthma), the risk factors have applicability to this review.

Adults

The authors also reviewed the current literature for the association of wheezing in adults and the risk factors statistically associated with this respiratory symptom (*see* Table 2). As a reference, the National Health and Nutrition Examination III Survey (NHANES) (1988–1994) revealed that 16.4% of adult Americans reported wheezing in the previous year *(2)*.

CURRENT ASTHMA PREVALENCE

In May 2004, GINA released a comprehensive survey of the current prevalence of asthma in the majority of regions of the world *(3)*. The United States was included in the North American region. Using various methodologies *(3)*, the estimate of patients with asthma in the United States and Canada is 35.5 million, with a mean prevalence of 11.2% (United States 10.9%).

The asthma prevalence in adults, divided by race/ethnicity was assessed by the Centers for Disease Control and Prevention (CDC), using the Behavioral Risk Factor Surveillance System (BRFSS) *(4)*. This standardized survey randomly calls US civilians over 18 yr old. Lifetime asthma is defined as a "yes" to the question: Have you ever been told by a doctor, nurse, or other health professional that you have asthma? Current asthma is defined as a "yes" response to the first question, and an affirmative response to: Do you still have asthma?

The BRFSS response rate for 2002 reported a lifetime prevalence of 11.9%. The prevalence of current asthma in 2002 was 7.6% (50 states, Washington, DC, Guam, Puerto Rico, and the US Virgin Islands). In the 50 states and Washington, DC, the current asthma rate was 7.5%. Asthma prevalence rates were higher among black, non-Hispanic, multiracial, non-Hispanic, Native American/Alaska Native, and non-Hispanic. Overall, the 2002 survey revealed higher adult lifetime prevalence rates than the 2000 and 2001 surveys. In the same 2002 survey, the rates for current asthma in adult males was 5.5%, whereas the adult female rate was nearly doubled at 9.4%.

In pediatric patients, the CDC uses data from the National Health Interview Survey *(5)*. In 1997, the National Health Interview Survey changed the asthma current prevalence questions to: "Has a doctor or other health care professional ever told you that

Table 1
Risk Factors for Wheezing in Children

Characteristics of wheezing children	Factor (significantly statistically associated)	Odds-ratio, if reported	Country of study	Mean age of studied subjects	Likely related to an asthma phenotype[a]
Hospitalized children 3 to 18 yr	Rhinovirus if not winter months		United States	Children less than 3 yr	No
Hospitalized children 3 to 18 yr	Atopic characteristics		United States	Children 3–18 yr	Yes
Older than 3 mo with three wheezing events	Signs of dampness	1.5	Sweden	Less than 2 yr	No
	New painted surfaces	1.6			
Body mass index greater than 95%	Obesity		Israel		
Children at ages 1, 2, and 4 yr	Male (ages to 4 yr)	1.4–1.5	Sweden		Yes
	Maternal allergy (to age 4 yr)	2.2			Yes
	Male × parental allergy (wheeze age 4 yr)	2.9			Yes
Any wheeze (no asthma Dx) in previous year	Ear infections	1.55	United States (National Health and Nutrition Examination Survey [NHANES])	Ages 2–11 yr	No
Children in Texas with wheeze previous year	Urban living		United States	16 yr or younger	Yes
	Highest bodymass quartile	2.45			?
Children to age 1 yr with wheeze	Day care	Both enhanced Rhinovirus wheeze	Childhood Origins of Asthma Study	Birth to age 1 yr	No
	Older sibling				
Children who are nonatopic	Maternal asthma	2.1	Isle of Wight birth cohort	Age 10 yr	Yes
	Recurrent chest infections	3.99			No

6

Risk factor	Odds ratio	Location	Age	Modifiable[a]
Children who are atopic		Isle of Wight birth cohort	Age 10 yr	
Sibling asthma	2.10			Yes
Eczema at 1 yr	2.80			Yes
Rhinitis at age 4 yr	4.74			Yes
Male	2.73			Yes
Recurrent wheeze		Germany	By age 2 yr	
Cesarean birth	1.41			No
Wheezing (viral isolation negative)		New Haven, CT	By age 5 yr	
Human metapneumovirus plus reverse transcriptase				No
Birthweight less than 1501 g		Finland	By age 10 yr	
Lifetime prevalence of wheeze	3.71			No
Diet		Italy (International Study of Asthma and Allergies in Childhood [ISAAC] questionnaire)	Ages 6 and 7 yr	
Bread and margarine	2.52			?
Butter for cooking	2.19			?
Early infant wheeze		Germany (Lifestyle-Related Factors on the Immune System and the Development of Allergies in Childhood [LISA] study group)	By age 2 yr	
Endotoxin levels in mattress dust	1.52 for high quartile			No

[a]Authors opinion.

7

Table 2
Risk Factors for Wheezing in Adults

Characteristics of adult	Factor (significantly statistically associated)	Odds-ratio, if reported	Country of study	Age of studied subjects	Likely related to an asthma phenotype[a]
Wheeze in previous 12 mo	Below poverty	1.35	United States (National Health and Nutrition Examination Survey [NHANES] III)	Older than 20 yr	Yes
	Lower education	1.18			Yes
	Current smoker	3.48			Yes
	Ever smoker	1.38			Yes
	Ever hay fever	2.11			Yes
	Body mass index (BMI) >30	1.30			?
		1.45			
	Use oven/stove	(crude OR)			?
Report of gastroeso- phageal reflux	Wheezing	2.5	Iceland, Belgium, Sweden	20–48 yr	No
Report of passive smoke exposure in workplace	Wheezing	2.12	Germany European Community Respiratory Health Survey (ECRHS)	Adults	?
Wheeze in past year without an asthma diagnosis	Men		England	Older than 11 yr	No
	Older age groups				?
	Lower social class				Yes
Wheeze	Female		Canada (ECRHS)	20–44 yr	Yes
Wheeze in adults	BMI >30	1.85 men	ECRHS	20–44 yr	?
		2.03 women			?

[a]In the authors' opinion.

your child has asthma?" *and* "During the past 12 mo has your child had an episode of asthma or an asthma attack?" This has been termed asthma attack prevalence. The rates (per 1000) in the United States before and since the change in the questions are presented in Fig. 1.

WHAT IS THE RISK OF DEVELOPING ASTHMA?

Pediatric-Age Subjects

In the United States, the dramatic increase in asthma in children occurred between 1980 and 1995. A change in asthma definition criteria for current asthma in 1997 (Fig. 1) suggests a stable rate in white and Hispanic children, with persisting higher rates in black children. Following are the known risk factors for developing asthma in the pediatric age group.

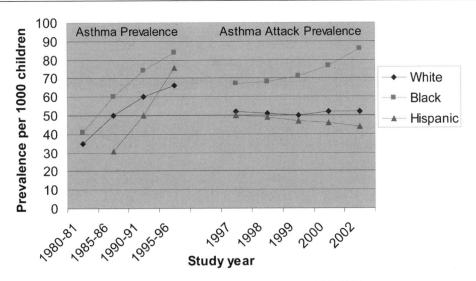

Fig. 1. Asthma prevalence for children 1980–2002.

AGE- AND GENDER-ASSOCIATED RISKS

Children are more likely to develop asthma before the age of 10 yr, compared with ages 11–21 yr. This is especially true for male children, whereas females are predominate in the adolescent years, with, essentially, equivalent prevalence by gender by the onset of adulthood.

RACE

A self-reported asthma prevalence survey by CDC in the United States since 1980 has shown a consistently higher rate (reports per 1000 population) for current asthma among individuals identifying themselves as black (white, black, or other) (Fig. 1). A review of National Health sources in the United Kingdom suggests a greater use of physician encounters in black groups compared with whites (6). Possible explanations for differences in ethnic groups, especially in the United States, include genetic and socioeconomic distinctions. A limited number of genome-wide searches have shown some differences in linkage to specific gene loci in ethnically distinct populations. Other studies have suggested that ethnic differences are associated with household income and urban residence. A review of the NHANES (1993–1996) data for race and income differences in asthma showed a complexity of socioeconomic interactions (7).

ATOPY

Having a positive allergy skin test(s) is a hallmark of most children with asthma. Current evidence suggests a strong likelihood for separate gene sets controlling asthma and atopy but with some common, yet unrecognized, link. In general, being atopic and or having a clinical diagnosis of allergic rhinitis confers an increased risk for developing asthma. In addition, an increased total serum immunoglobulin (Ig) E level may also predict the development of asthma.

Numerous studies have shown that elevated specific IgE to an individual allergen, largely indoor or perennial, has significant statistical association with asthma and, in theory, the risk (resulting from exposure) of developing asthma. These have included house dust mite, cockroach, mouse dander, and Alternaria.

FAMILY HISTORY AND GENETICS

Children with asthma have a strong familial association with atopic family histories and, in many situations, asthma. Maternal asthma has special consideration as a risk factor *(8)*. Because of the intense interest in finding the genetic cause of asthma, studies identifying statistical associations for asthma, phenotypic markers for asthma, biochemical or clinical presence of atopy, and specific genetic loci are regularly reported in the literature. Many of the associations have strong linkage to an atopy parameter and, therefore, a secondary association with asthma, or at least to the atopic asthma phenotype. By inference, the existence of a loci association with active asthma may, in the future, identify children (or adults) with a genetic susceptibility profile for developing asthma. A recent review has identified association studies for asthma and atopic disease *(9)*.

ENVIRONMENTAL TOBACCO SMOKE EXPOSURE

Independent of the concern for lower lung volumes that are associated with environmental tobacco smoke, most studies support a modest increased risk for asthma in children exposed to intrauterine and/or postuterine tobacco smoke exposure *(10)*.

RESPIRATORY INFECTIONS

It is universally accepted that viral illnesses are the paramount cause of an acute exacerbation of asthma. In many children, the first wheezing event is associated with a viral infection, often RSV. When new wheezing events subsequently develop, a diagnosis of asthma is entertained. The critical question to establishing risks for "developing asthma" is the role of the original infection. RSV takes center stage in the question of assigning risk. RSV carries numerous "asthmagenic" properties, including the induction of acute wheezing and the association of postbronchiolitic wheezing. Several studies have redirected the connection between RSV and asthma, with strong epidemiological support for a separate post-RSV wheezing syndrome that has a potential to last into adolescence *(11,12)*.

SOCIOECONOMIC FACTORS

Although asthma rates worldwide follow an increasing trend in higher income countries, a substantial body of literature, particularly in the United States, shows there is an increase in asthma in individuals of lower financial means. This fact is likely a surrogate for several interacting circumstances, including substandard housing, cumulative allergen load in older homes, urban crowding, education level, occupation, ethnicity, and specific air pollutants, including ozone and petroleum byproducts. Lower personal and family income also has a greater disparity of tobacco smoking, and obesity, which adds additional confounders to the story of asthma prevalence and financial status.

ALLERGIC DISEASE

Having another allergic disease confers additional risk for developing asthma. A child with allergic rhinitis with positive skin tests is of particular concern. Atopic dermatitis (AD), often seen in younger children, has traditionally been considered as the initial presentation of the atopic march. A recent study of the risk for asthma in children with AD suggests a concomitant pattern rather than a subsequent onset for asthma *(13)*.

OBESITY

The increase of asthma rates among children since 1980 has largely paralleled the increase in overweight and obese children. Numerous studies have now shown increased asthma rates in children with higher body mass index *(14)*. Associative factors of obesity and asthma prevalence likely include physical activity levels and dietary factors, especially fat intake, deficiencies of fruits and vegetables, and sodium intake. The decrease in breast-feeding, especially in the United States and other developed countries, may also have a role in the increasing prevalence of asthma.

HYGIENE HYPOTHESIS FACTORS

In Westernized countries, asthma prevalence has increased during the last 20 yr. This suggests change(s) in environmental factors. Critical to this theory is the concept of changing societal tolerance for common infectious agents, immunization practices, and a shift in America family childcare practices.

Central to the concept of the hygiene hypothesis is the lymphocyte type 1 helper (Th1) and type 2 (Th2) CD4+ T-cells. Th1 cells are responsible for thwarting serious infectious agents, whereas Th2 cells are seemingly involved with atopic responses. If children are more vigorously using their Th1 T-cells, less stimulation of Th2 cells occurs.

If the "hygiene hypothesis" has merit, it probably has more validity in highly developed nations, but it may also play a role in rural vs urban differences in developing nations.

Although not always specific for asthma risk, the hygiene hypothesis factors that may have relevance for asthma regarding enhancing or protecting against asthma (or atopy) are presented in Table 3.

BRONCHIAL HYPERRESPONSIVENESS

Bronchial (airway) hyperresponsiveness (BHR), as determined by a direct airway challenge using methacholine or histamine, is a characteristic of all patients with asthma (*see* Asthma section). By inference, the preexistence of BHR may be a risk for developing asthma. Children have increased BHR, as compared with adults, possibly being permissive for an enhanced onset of asthma in childhood. The authors have reported the presence of BHR before the onset of asthma in a population study of asthma in families *(15)*. Approximately 25% of the patients with allergic rhinitis exhibit BHR. This may add to their asthma risk.

NEONATAL FACTORS

A recent study from the United Kingdom included 173,319 births, among which 2230 infants were diagnosed with respiratory distress syndrome or transient tachypnea of the newborn. Those infants who experienced respiratory morbidity at term were at increased risk of being hospitalized for asthma (hazard ratio [HR] = 1.7, $p < 0.001$). For those born vaginally, the HR was 1.5, whereas for those born by cesarean section, the HR was 2.2. Delivery by cesarean section, without neonatal respiratory problems, was weakly associated with the risk of asthma in childhood (HR = 1.1) *(16)*.

Table 3
Hygiene Hypothesis Factors

Factor	Increases asthma risk (in theory or actual)
Birth order: first	↑ More relevant for allergy
Birth order: second or more	↓ More relevant for allergy
Day care early in life	↓
Day care late	↑
Immunizations	?
Antibiotic use	Possibly ↑
Frequent ear infections	↑
Higher endotoxin exposure	↓
Cesarean section birth	↑

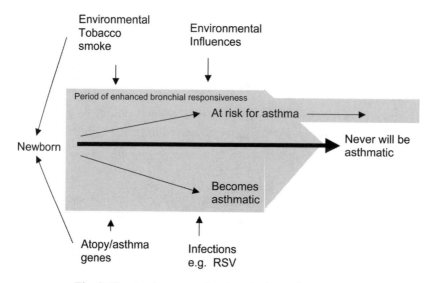

Fig. 2. The development of asthma in the pediatric years.

In summary, asthma risk in pediatrics is multifactorial. A depiction of many of the factors is presented in Fig. 2.

Adults

OVERVIEW

There are numerous ways an adult can "develop" asthma.

1. Children with asthma can maintain their disease into their adult years.
2. Asthma can develop as a new diagnosis in a young adult.
3. An adult can reactive his or her quiescent pediatric asthma (relapse asthma).
4. Asthma can start in older adults.

5. Adult-onset asthma may be hidden with other respiratory illnesses, often associated with chronic smoking, and the symptoms of wheezing, shortness of breath, and chest tightness are attributed to "chronic bronchitis" or "emphysema."

6. Adults can develop occupational asthma.

Relapse asthma is covered in a subsequent section. The authors treat adult asthma as a disease process that starts after age 21 yr. There is general support to the concept that asthma that occurs for the first time in a young adult has somewhat different characteristics in comparison to that that occurs in the senior years. When delineated in published reports, the authors separate these subtypes of adult-onset asthma.

The 2002 BFRSS (17) reported that for the United States and the District of Columbia, the rate of adult (>18 yr) current asthma was 7.5%, with male prevalence of 5.5% and female of 9.4%. Specific age-range prevalence was 8.3% for 18–24 yr, 7.4% for 25–34 yr, 7.1% for 35–44 yr, 7.7% for 45–54 yr, 7.8% for 55–64 yr and 7.1% for 65 yr and older.

The authors review the factors that often contribute to the development of asthma in adults.

GENDER

The 2002 Adult Self-Reported Lifetime Asthma Prevalence Rate (Percent) by sex, obtained using BRFSS showed in the 50 states, Washington, DC, and three US territories, a rate of 5.5% for current asthma and 9.9% lifetime asthma in adult males 18 yr or older. For adult females, current asthma was 9.4% and lifetime asthma was 13.6% (17). An analysis of the NHANES III data also reported a significant association of current asthma in adults older than 20 yr and female sex (2).

GENETICS

The adult asthma phenotype is not as well established as its pediatric counterpart. Therefore, virtually all genetic associative studies use an atopic, asthma (largely pediatric) phenotype. The limited published studies in adults demonstrate some atopic associations. Detailed studies in nonatopic, older-onset adult asthmatic are virtually unknown. Because adult-onset, nonatopic asthma is a distinct phenotype, its genetic background must be examined separately.

An analysis of adults with asthma 20–48 yr old from the European Community Respiratory Health Survey (ECRHS) showed that extrinsic asthma (asthma plus an allergic disease) in a parent was a higher risk factor for extrinsic asthma in the offspring compared to intrinsic asthma (asthma without an allergic disease) in the offspring. Intrinsic asthma in the parent was a risk for intrinsic asthma in a child but less than for a person with extrinsic asthma having an extrinsic offspring (18).

A recent review of 18,156 subjects from 0 to 44 yr from the ECRHS determined asthma HR for ages 0–10 yr, 10–20 yr, and 20–44 yr for asthma onset. The adults who were 20–44 yr had an equivalent or greater HR for asthma onset when parental history for asthma or allergies was the control variable (19).

BRONCHIAL HYPERRESPONSIVENESS

Increased BHR in childhood may allow for asthma onset in pediatrics. Likewise, it has been reported that young adults with new asthma had enhanced histamine hyperresponsiveness as children (20). Although it may be difficult to suggest that a 50-yr-old with new asthma had persisting BHR from childhood that only expresses itself after four or more decades, it is not inconceivable to consider a lifetime subclinical asthma "potential," with some lingering degree of BHR that is eventually redirected by environmental factors back to a BHR level that is associated with being asthmatic.

ATOPY AND ALLERGIC DISEASES

Having a preexisting allergic disease, either allergic rhinitis or AD, carries an increased risk for the development of asthma during a person's lifetime. Having positive allergy skin test or an elevated total IgE has similar predilection. This is especially evident in young adults. The onset of asthma in older adults often appears to be largely independent of a clinical allergic background, although an association with IgE levels is not totally excluded *(21)*.

TOBACCO SMOKE

Studies of the effects of passive smoke exposure and adult-onset asthma are limited. Exposure likely enhances the development of asthma. Given the clinical overlap of obstructive lung disease in adults, active smoking plays an important role in the development (or worsening) of adult-onset asthma and progression to chronic obstructive pulmonary disease *(22)*.

INFECTION

A viral infection is often the preliminary cause of wheezing in children, with subsequent recurrent wheezing and eventually an asthma diagnosis. A similar experience in adults is sketchy.

The ECRHS study *(19)* showed that early respiratory infections were a strong risk factor for the onset of asthma before age 20 yr but not significant for ages 20–44 yr. Some evidence exists for the development and severity of asthma with *Mycoplasma* and *Chlamydia pneumoniae* infection.

OBESITY

Paralleling the pediatric experience *(23)*, the average weight of American adults has increased since 1960. Likewise, studies are emerging that suggest an association of increased BMI in both asthma and asthma symptoms in adults.

OTHER

Additional epidemiological studies have linked risk for asthma onset in adults to indoor dampness, prolonged furry pet exposure, Alternaria exposure, chronic rhinitis, and a low education level.

The onset of asthma in the early adult years likely has strong pediatric risk-factor overlap. Those patients with asthma in older age groups have less defined risk factors and are understudied as a group, although they will undoubtedly comprise a greater percentage of the total asthma population in the United States because of the changes in age demographics. A pictorial summary of risk factors in adults is shown in Fig. 3.

Relapse Asthma

In discussing the long-term course of any patient with asthma, the most reasonable statement that can be made is that once a patient is diagnosed with asthma, he or she will forever either be an asthmatic or an former asthmatic, and never a nonasthmatic. In actuality, a third alternative exists: a former asthmatic can relapse and become a current

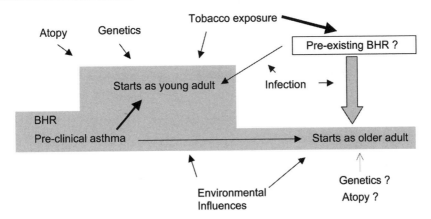

Fig. 3. The development of asthma in adult years.

Table 4
Risks for Relapsed Asthma

Characteristics of the patient with relapse asthma	Factors associated with relapsed asthma
Asthma before age 12 yr	Male
Remission before age 18 yr	More frequent asthma attacks
No symptoms for 5 yr	Lower spirometric values
Relapse between ages 20 and 42 yr	Allergy triggers
	Allergic
	Mite, dog, grass, and tree allergy
	Maternal atopic dermatitis
	Allergic rhinitis

asthmatic. There have been a few studies looking specifically at this entity. It can happen in several ways: childhood relapsing, childhood asthma relapsing as an adult, and adult relapsing. In the scope of this discussion, a review of the known risk factors associated with becoming a "relapsed" asthmatic are most pertinent.

Two recent studies are relevant to the risk of having relapse asthma *(24,25)* and are summarized in Table 4.

The authors also suggest that airway hyperresponsiveness (AHR) does not quickly diminish after he remission of asthma symptoms (*see* "Former Asthmatics") and BHR persistence may be an additional factor in the reoccurrence of asthma. The have also reviewed the older literature on this topic *(26)*. Previous studies emphasized the presence of increased serum eosinophils counts, higher IgE levels, atopy, and increased AHR in those individuals whose asthma relapsed.

CHARACTERISTICS OF CURRENT ASTHMA

Overview

HISTORICAL PERSPECTIVE

William Osler described asthma in his textbook, *The Principles and Practice of Medicine 1892,* as follows: "Bronchial asthma is a neurotic condition characterized by

Table 5
Asthma Pathogenesis

- Bronchoconstriction
- Bronchial hyperresponsiveness
- β-adrenergic blockade
- Inflammation

---

hyperemia and tumescence of the mucosa of the smaller bronchial tubes in a peculiar exudative mucin." In the 1940s, Osler's "neurosis" became "bronchospasm or reversible airway obstruction." Reversible airway obstruction has remained the hallmark of asthma in the sense that it either improves spontaneously over time or the pulmonary function improves with the use of a bronchodilator over a period of minutes to hours. However, in the 1960s, asthma became "hyperreactive airway disease," and the methacholine bronchial challenge test became standardized in 1975.

SYMPTOMS OF CURRENT ASTHMA

The characteristic symptoms of asthma are cough, a sensation of tightness in the chest, a sensation of dyspnea or shortness of breath either at rest or exertion, and wheezing, which may be audible across the room or only with careful auscultation. Of these, the most characteristic or the most specific is the sensation of tightness. Wheezing, cough, and dyspnea can be the result of several other maladies, such as chronic bronchitis or acute bronchitis. The cough is typically a chest cough as opposed to a throat cough and often productive of only a scant amount of sticky sputum even after severe coughing, which at times, can result in cough syncope or even breaking a rib. The sputum is characterized by tight spirals of mucous that emanate from the small bronchioles or sometimes large mucous plugs, which is characteristic of bronchopulmonary aspergillosis. In either case, the sputum is often loaded with eosinophils. The constellation of these clinical and pathological findings is associated with bronchial obstruction and bronchoconstriction.

Asthma Pathogenesis

Please *see* Table 5 for asthma pathogenesis.

BRONCHOCONSTRICTION AND AUTONOMIC DYSREGULATION IN ASTHMA

Patients with asthma will bronchoconstrict to a variety of pharmacological agents. There is evidence that bronchoconstriction in asthma is an autonomic dysfunction, with a decreased response to β-adrenergic bronchodilators and, to a much lesser extent, increased α-adrenergic agonist activity. This is exemplified at the human bronchus or trachea when suspended in a muscle tissue bath relaxes with epinephrine but will contract with epinephrine in the presence of propranolol. This autonomic dysfunction is further characterized by studies that show a decreased fall in diastolic pressure to intravenous isoproterenol *(27)*. Subsequently, Kaliner et al. reported a decreased pulse pressure and decreased cyclic adenosine monophosphate (cAMP) response to intravenous isoproterenol in patients with asthma *(28)*.

BHR IN VIVO AND IN VITRO

BHR to histamine and methacholine is *sine-qua-non* of asthma. However, BHR does not prove asthma, because numerous subjects without asthma may respond to methacholine (albeit usually to higher concentrations than most patients with asthma). Nonatopic patients without asthma rarely show any significant response to bronchial challenge with methacholine or histamine, but up to 30% of subjects with allergic rhinitis may respond, and it is these subjects who are at greater risk for subsequent development of asthma. BHR is a phenotypic marker for asthma as described in studies in twins in 1984 that demonstrated that monozygotic twins have a significantly higher correlation coefficient of their BHR to methacholine (as well as their serum IgE levels) as compared to dizygotic twins (29). The specificity and sensitivity to methacholine in normal subjects and subjects with asthma was described in 1984 with a best sensitivity and specificity at 200 breath units of methacholine in adults (30) and 100 breath units in children (31). The genetics of AHR was further studied in families with asthma, which demonstrated a bimodal distribution of BHR. This bimodal distribution suggested a possibility of asthma resulting from a single gene. Subsequently, the authors' group reported a segregation analysis to methacholine response in families with and without asthma, which showed that it was not the result of a single gene (32). It is still not entirely clear why normal subjects do not react to methacholine and histamine.

Airways from normal individuals who are nonatopic in a muscle bath contract to methacholine and histamine with essentially the same sensitivity and degree of contraction that patients with asthma do. However, in vitro the patients with asthma show a decreased relaxation response to β-agonists compared to the normal subjects. In vitro, the airways of subjects with asthma show a decreased cAMP response to β-agonist.

When β-adrenergic blocking agents became available in the 1960s for therapeutic use, agents such as propranolol, which block both β-1 and β-2 receptors resulted in increased morbidity and mortality in subjects with asthma. Subsequently, the authors demonstrated that certain genetic strains of mice and guinea pigs showed increased sensitivity to histamine, methacholine, and serotonin after blockade of the β-adrenergic receptors. These effects were more pronounced with the potent β-blocking agent propranolol. In mice and guinea pigs sensitized to an allergen and then challenged, there was a high mortality in guinea pigs in the presence of a β-adrenergic blocking agents (33). In these studies, it was clear that the increased bronchial response to allergen was greater than the increased bronchial response to methacholine, serotonin, and histamine, because β-receptors on mast cells inhibit mediator release. However, this was not true in the strains of mice and guinea pigs that do not show increased intrinsic sensitivity to allergens or to histamine, methacholine, and serotonin. It still remains to be determined what the genetic differences are in these strains of mice and guinea pigs that develop BHR after β-adrenergic blockade. However, the authors now know that the strains of mice that can be sensitized by β-adrenergic blockade are the ones that can also be sensitized by pertussis-toxin. In fact, it was the study of pertussis-toxin and the subsequent demonstration that β-adrenergic blocking agents mimicked many of the effect of pertussis-toxin that led to the β-adrenergic blockade theory of asthma as published by Szentivanyi (34).

β-BLOCKADE THEORY OF ASTHMA

It is now known that β-adrenergic blocking agents, especially those that block β-2 adrenergic receptors, are contraindicated in patients with asthma and in patients undergoing allergy skin testing or immunotherapy. The major tenets of the β-adrenergic blockade theory of asthma are included in Table 6.

Table 6
β-Blockade Theory of Asthma

- Bronchial obstruction (smooth muscle spasm, edema, mucous hypersecretion, etc.)
- The pharmacological abnormality
- The immunological abnormality
- Primary involvement of bronchial tissue
- Close association with respiratory infection
- Eosinophilia is a common occurrence
- Increased tolerance to epinephrine
- Effectiveness of agents that are capable of restoring adrenergic action

Although the β-adrenergic blockade theory was published nearly four decades ago, it is still yet to be proven or disproved. Persons with asthma have an abnormal reactivity to otherwise nontoxic concentrations of endogenously released or exogenously administered pharmacological mediators (e.g., histamine or leukotrienes). Recent studies involving certain cytokines have, however, thrown new light on this theory.

Pharmacological Abnormality

Even before the development of β-adrenergic blocking agents and the observation of their contraindication in asthma, *Bordetella pertussis* organisms injected into certain strains of mice and rats modified the normal response of the animals to numerous stimuli. This included hypersensitivity to endogenous released or exogenously administered histamine, serotonin, bradykinin, and, at least in some strains, acetylcholine. This also included hypersensitivity to less specific stimuli, such as cold air, changes in atmospheric pressure, and respiratory irritants. *B. pertussis* injections reduced sensitivity to catecholamines, enhanced antibody formation (particularly reaginic antibody), and induced marked eosinophilia. These changes are analogous to the situation in bronchial asthma. These findings in the pertussis-sensitized mouse also are associated with a reduced functioning of the β-adrenergic component of the autonomic nervous system. Regardless of whether the bronchi or the symptoms of asthma are triggered by an immunological response to an allergen or an infectious agent, the neurotransmitters released (and the accompanying diminished β-adrenergic response) results in an adrenergic imbalance. This deprives the bronchial tissue from its normal counter regulatory adjustment. In addition to animal studies, it is now well demonstrated that β-adrenergic blockade enhances BHR to inhaled allergens or methacholine in patients with seasonal allergic rhinitis (but without a previous history of bronchial asthma *(35)*.

Immunological Abnormality

B. pertussis not only causes a pharmacological hypersensitivity but also alters immune response both quantitatively and qualitatively, including production of reaginic antibody. Pertussis-toxin (histamine-sensitizing factor) is identical to the immunological adjuvant that produces increased levels of reaginic antibody. Furthermore, pertussis-toxin, like whooping cough, results in increased formation of lymphocytes.

Primary Involvement of Bronchial Tissue

The primary involvement of the bronchial tissue is exemplified by the fact that in patients with asthma, a low dose of histamine induces wheezing but not hives. In contrast to individuals with chronic urticaria, it has been reported that histamine will produce hives but not wheezing. In subjects with allergic rhinitis, a nasal allergen challenge with a specific allergen will reduce the airway lumen and result in nasal congestion and obstruction. This only rarely has an effect on the lower respiratory tract. In subjects with asthma, nasal allergen challenge rarely produces lower airway symptoms; however, the same amount of allergen introduced into the lower airways will result in obstructive pulmonary dysfunction.

The Close Association of Respiratory Infection and BHR

It has been known for many years that a common rhinovirus infection in normal people may result in increased airway reactivity to methacholine for up to 4–6 wk, long after the symptoms of the respiratory infection have cleared. Some virus infections in a patient with asthma not only results in increased BHR to methacholine but also is frequently the cause of severe exacerbation.

Eosinophilia

The eosinophilia that occurs in asthma is consistent with the observation that epinephrine and isoproterenol produce eosinopenia, and this catecholamine effect is blocked by propranolol. It has been demonstrated that the eosinopenic effect of epinephrine on circulating eosinophils is significantly reduced in patients with asthma as compared to normal subjects *(36)*. These same investigators also observed that pertussis vaccine and propranolol markedly impaired the eosinopenic effect of epinephrine in rats *(36)*. This further supports the observation that β-adrenergic mechanisms are impaired in patients with asthma. These observations were known long before the known effect of various cytokines (e.g., interleukin [IL]-5) and chemokines (e.g., eotaxin) on producing eosinophilia.

Increased Tolerance to Epinephrine

The increased tolerance to epinephrine is an important tenet exemplified by epinephrine-fast asthma and status asthmaticus, where epinephrine is either ineffective or much less effective than in the patient who is having only a mild asthma episode. This decreased response to epinephrine is consistent with a β-adrenergic blockade mechanism. The restoration of epinephrine responsiveness by corticosteroids (CSs), which increase the density and number of β-adrenergic receptors, is also consistent with this concept *(37)*. It is well recognized that CSs increase β-receptors in airway mucosa and airway smooth muscle, as well as on the lymphocytes of patients with asthma.

Restoration of Adrenergic Activity

Another tenet of the β-blockade theory is the therapeutic effectiveness of agents that are capable of restoring the effect of β-adrenergic activity. The principle components of this are (1) bypassing the biochemical site of the β-adrenergic receptor adenylates cyclase site of action by the use of theophylline and, more recently, more potent phosphodiesterase inhibitors, and (2) by sensitizing the β-receptor and lowering the receptor threshold to catecholamine action by the use of CSs. The current use of the combination of β-agonists and inhaled steroids showing greater efficacy than just doubling the amount of corticosteroids is reminiscent of prior observation in animals.

The authors have demonstrated that in strains of mice and rats that normally are quite resistant to histamine after β-adrenergic blockade or bilateral adrenalectomy there is increased histamine sensitivity and histamine-induced lethality *(38)*. When the authors administered increasing concentrations of epinephrine or isoproterenol, they could provide only a modest degree of protection. Similarly, when they gave increasing concentrations of CSs, they demonstrated only a modest degree of protection against histamine lethality. However, when they combine even low doses of catecholamine and CSs, the rodents demonstrated complete resistance to death. This indicates that gluco-corticoids are capable of sensitizing adrenergic target cells to the action of cate-cholamines.

Susceptibility to Other Precipitating Factors

The final tenet of the β-blockade theory is a susceptibility of the airways to various unrelated precipitating factors. Asthma may be triggered by numerous stimuli, such as infection, mast cell mediators, muscarinic neurotransmitters, changes in the tempera-ture of inhaled air, or nonantigenic dust or fumes and other irritants. The theory appears to necessitate that the primary defect in asthma be connected through a final common pathway. This is consistent with the observation that β-adrenergic agonists (albuterol) in the patient with asthma, when challenged with several bronchoconstrictors, will result in protection to against the bronchoconstriction. These agents include leukotrienes, histamine, methacholine, serotonin, or nonspecific agents, such as exer-cise or cold air challenge or osmotic challenges, such as hypertonic saline or sterile water. This supports the concept of a common mechanism.

INFLAMMATION

In the 1980s, inflammation became an obvious component of asthma.

Eosinophils

Eosinophils and the major basic protein of eosinophils can damage and denude air-way mucosa. This can result in a decreased bronchodilating effect as demonstrated in guinea pigs airway smooth muscle. Furthermore, eosinophils and major basic protein can damage the muscarinic-2 receptors in the pulmonary ganglia, which result in less feedback inhibition in the muscarinic-2 receptors and increased methacholine response on the muscarinic-3 receptors of the airways. When airways are denuded, exposure of the sensory nerves in the airway mucosa and resultant release of neuropeptides occur, such as Substance P and neurokinin A, and constriction of airway smooth muscle and edema along with vasodilatation. In the 1990s, the story of inflammation was further advanced by the understanding of the role mast cells, eosinophils, and lymphocytes in the airway mucosa.

Mast Cells

The mast cells' release of mediators, particularly leukotrienes, along with histamine and prostaglandins, induces bronchoconstriction in people with asthma. Mast cells, eosinophils, and lymphocytes produce several cytokines, which are currently undergo-ing intense investigation in asthma. The role of the mast cell may be important in terms of induction of AHR because of its interaction with airway smooth muscle. It is now recognized that the airways of people with asthma are infiltrated with mast cells. On the other hand, the role of the eosinophil is still not entirely clear. Although the eosinophil is (almost) universally present in asthma, it is not entirely clear whether its presence is only guilty by association rather then causally a factor. For example, in patients with eosinophilic bronchitis, the airways have a marked increase in eosinophils but not mast cells or AHR. Mast cells and basophils can produce lipid mediators, such as platelet-activating factor and leukotrienes, along with chemokines and cytokines that may cause AHR. Furthermore, activated mast cells can produce stem cell factor, chemokines, and cytokines that recruit more mast cells *(39)*. That CSs can reduce the number of mast cells in both the upper and the lower airways is consistent with the new guidelines for treatment of asthma.

Pharmacotherapy of Inflammation

Inhaled steroid are now first-line treatment for all levels of persistent asthma, and the combination with a bronchodilator therapy is recommended in patients who are not adequately controlled on low- to moderate-dose inhaled steroids. An additional advantage of a single inhaler delivering both drugs is the adherence with a glucocorticoid component is greater owing to a better secondary adherence rate with an inhaled bronchodilator because patients experience immediate relief in contrast to inhaled CSs. Furthermore, inhaled glucocorticoids used in combination have a sparing affect; therefore, fewer glucocorticoids are needed in combination. The fear regarding long-acting β-agonists masking underlying inflammation is no longer an issue when they are used in combination with a β-agonist. It is now demonstrated that the combination of inhaled fluticasone and salmeterol gives markedly greater improvement in forced expiratory volume in 1 s than either agent alone and also results in much greater asthma control than when either agent alone is administered.

Agents such as roflumilast are specific phosphodiesterase 4 inhibitors, which bypass the β-receptor and increase cAMP by preventing the metabolism of cAMP. These phosphodiesterase 4 inhibitors are anti-inflammatory drugs because they increase cAMP and block the proliferation of lymphocytes and smooth muscle cells and inhibit proinflammatory mediator release, such as tumor necrosis factor (TNF)-α, and augment the release of anti-inflammatory mediators, such as IL-10 and TNF receptor. Roflumilast has been demonstrated to block the allergen challenge, particularly the late reaction, although it modestly inhibits the early reaction; these effects on the late reaction are reminiscent of the effect of CSs, which also inhibit the late reaction. In phase 3 double-blind placebo-controlled trials, roflumilast showed significantly greater improvement in the forced expiratory volume in 1 s in patients with mild to moderate asthma and showed similar effects to montelukast in decreasing asthma symptoms and decreasing the need for rescue medication. Similarly, in a 12-wk comparative trial with beclomethasone, roflumilast showed a similar improvement in pulmonary function, as well as a similar improvement in asthma symptoms scores and similar decrease in the need for rescue medication. Furthermore, it showed lower incidence of adverse events and excellent tolerability during long-term treatment.

Nitric Oxide: An Inflammatory Marker

Exhaled nitric oxide (NO) is now recognized as a noninvasive marker of airway inflammation. Exhaled NO is easily measured and can be performed either online of offline even in young children. Previously, the authors had to rely on bronchial biopsies or bronchial lavage to demonstrate airway inflammation, but now they can simply measure the level of NO in the exhaled air. This is totally noninvasive because all the subject has to do is to exhale normally into an NO analyzer or into a bag that can subsequently be taken to an NO analyzer and measured. It is now recognized that anti-inflammatory agents, such as inhaled CSs or leukotriene antagonist or phosphodiesterase inhibitors, can lower the level of NO in the exhaled air. In a study by Covar *(40)*, the normal control children had levels of exhaled NO of approx 10–15 ppb, whereas in the patient with asthma it was approx 60 ppb in the placebo-treated group and approx 25 ppb in patients with asthma after budesonide treatment. In a separate study of 251 adults with suspected asthma where 160 were diagnosed with asthma based on their response to β-adrenergic agonists or methacholine challenge, the exhaled NO was 25 ppb in asthma vs 11 ppb in patients without asthma *(41)*. From these studies, one can conclude that exhaled NO can be used as a diagnostic tool for screening patients with suspected asthma. To diagnose asthma, a comparison between exhaled NO measurements and conventional tests must be conducted; the following findings have been observed. Exhaled NO and sputum eosinophils were compared against serial peak expiratory flow, spirometry, and airway responses to β-agonists and oral glucocorticoids in diagnosing asthma. In this study, 47 patients who were suspected of having asthma were enrolled, 36% of whom had asthma as demonstrated by β-agonist bronchodilating responses or methacholine challenge *(42)*. Exhaled NO of greater than 20 ppb showed a specificity of 79% and a sensitivity of 88%, and sputum eosinophils of more than 3% showed specificity of 88% and sensitivity of 86%. It was concluded that exhaled NO and sputum eosinophils are superior to conventional measures of making the diagnosis of asthma. Exhaled NO is most advantageous because the test is quick and easy and does not require a bronchial challenge with hypertonic saline to induce sputum. The clinical application of measurement of NNO and the use of the Aerocrine exhaled NO monitoring system and its recent approval by the Food and Drug Administration has been described *(43)*.

Exhaled NO is a marker of airway inflammation in asthma. However, in certain other inflammatory airway diseases, such as cystic fibrosis, NO is either normal or diminished. In chronic obstructive lung disease, particularly in smokers, NO may be normal or diminished.

The elevated levels of exhaled NO are associated with allergic inflammation and increased levels of the enzyme-inducible NO synthase in the airway mucosa of patients with asthma. CSs by decreasing inflammation also decreases the level of the inducible NO synthase in the airway epithelium cells.

Cytokines and T-Cells

It is now well recognized that the Th1–Th2 paradigm is an important characteristic of asthma. There is believed to be an imbalance in asthma, with a predominance of Th2 cytokines, including ILs-4, -5, and -13, in patients with asthma, with perhaps a relative deficiency of Th1 cytokines, such as interferon-γ or ILs-12 and -18.

The effect of anti-IL-5 has been studied in numerous preclinical and clinical trials and is effective in decreasing the number of eosinophils in the blood and sputum. It also decreased eosinophils in the airway mucosa, although it is recognized that a substantial number of eosinophils are still present in the mucosa. Nevertheless, although appearing promising in animal studies, in clinical studies an antibody to IL-5 failed to improve BHR or to protect against allergen challenge or significantly decrease asthma symptoms.

IL-4 was believed to be important in asthma pathogenesis because of its role as a Th2 promoter and in the production of IgE. In preclinical studies, as well as phase II studies, soluble IL-4 receptor was promising. The IL-4 receptor binds avidly to IL-4 and markedly decreases the level of IL-4 in serum and in bronchial lavage. It did not, however, show clinically significant improvement in patients with asthma.

Table 7
Role of Interleukin-13 in Asthma Pathogenesis

- Interleukin (IL)-13 is increased in the airways of patients with asthma and-could be a factor in causing airway hyperresponsiveness (AHR) in asthma.
- IL-13 markedly increased methacholine sensitivity in mice.
- IL-13 resulted in a marked decrease in the response to β-agonist relaxation.
- Still to be determined is whether the increased AHR and decreased response to β-adrenergic agonist after IL-13 are causally related.

IL-13, however, has not yet tested yet, in humans. However, in several animal models, particularly in the mouse model, it produces numerous effects relevant to asthma. IL-13 switches on IgE. IL-13 is both necessary and sufficient to cause AHR in an animal model *(44,45)*. In fact, it produced a degree of AHR similar to that induced by allergen challenge in allergen-sensitized mice. IL-13 increases airway goblet cells and mucous and is more potent than IL-4. IL-13 also increases the blood eosinophils. Therefore, it raises the question, "Is IL-13 the cause of AHR and asthma?" (*see* Table 7).

IL-13 has several significant properties, including that IL-13 is increased in the airways of patients with asthma and could be a factor in causing AHR in asthma *(46)*. The authors, as well as a number of other investigators, have demonstrated that IL-13 markedly increases sensitivity to methacholine in allergen-naïve mice. IL-13 resulted in a marked decrease in the response to β-agonist relaxation *(46)*. Still to be determined is whether the increased AHR and decrease response to β-adrenergic agonist, after IL-13, are causally related.

IL-13 is an immunoregulatory cytokine secreted by activated Th2 cells. It is also produced by eosinophils and mast cells. IL-13 is a mediator in the pathogenesis of allergic inflammation. It is important in the development of AHR and mucous production. It inhibits the production of proinflammatory mediators, such as IL-1 and TNF-α by monocytes and macrophages. It has a direct effect on eosinophil survival, activation, and recruitment, and it also has important functions in endothelial cells, smooth muscle cells, fibroblast, and epithelial cells.

IL-13 has many diverse functions on various cell types that are relevant to the pathogenesis of asthma (*see* Table 8).

IL-13 is one of the most attractive, common, novel, potential targets for therapeutic intervention in the treatment of asthma. There are now at least five different biotech or pharmaceutical companies involved in development of IL-3 blockers. The authors' laboratory has looked at the so-called decoy receptor IL-13 R-α-2 *(46)*, which is present on the surface of cells containing the IL-13 R-α-1 receptor. This decoy receptor has a high affinity for IL-13. In this sense, it "mops-up" IL-13 in the circulation and competes for the IL-13 R-α-1 receptor that is involved in the signal transduction pathway of IL-13. It has been demonstrated that IL-13 R-α-2 protects against bronchoconstriction in sensitized mice and restores the response to β-adrenergic agonist *(44–46)*. The authors have tested the hypothesis that the response to albuterol is diminished in sensitized mice and this effect is mediated by IL-13. When sensitized mice are treated with the decoy receptor IL-13 R-α-2 to inhibit the effect of IL-13, the response to albuterol is restored *(46)*. In allergen-sensitized and challenged mice, the response to albuterol is diminished, and this effect is mediated by IL-13. Indeed, it is our conclusion that the

Table 8
Functions of Interleukin-13 on Inflammatory Cells in Asthma

- **Respiratory epithelium**
  Increased chemokine expression, mucous hypersecretion, and goblet cell metaplasia.
- **Airway smooth muscle**
  Increase of smooth muscle proliferation and increased sensitivity to bronchoconstrictor agents.
- **B-lymphocyte**
  Induces immunoglobulin (Ig) E production.
  ○ Macrophage, increases low-affinity IgE expression.
  ○ Mast cells, modulates of the high-affinity IgE receptor and IgE priming. Upregulates the IgE receptor.
  ○ **Eosinophils**
  Recruitment and activation.
  Increased numbers of eosinophils.
  ○ **Vascular endothelium**
  Expression of vascular cell adhesion molecules.
  Increased chemokine expression.
  ○ **Fibroblasts**
  Increased collagen and fibrosis remodeling of the airways?

mechanism whereby IL-13 is both sufficient and necessary for inducing BHR results from inhibition of the β-adrenergic response.

IL-13 induces BHR to methacholine, and the IL-13 blocker (IL-13 R-α-2) significantly inhibits the bronchoconstriction in response to methacholine challenge. Furthermore, in vitro studies involving mouse trachea, IL-13 also inhibits the relaxation response to β-agonist, and this response is restored by the IL-13 R-α-2. The ability of IL-13 R-α-2 to restore the effect of β-agonists, such as albuterol, provides insight into the potential clinical treatment of asthma. IL-13 produced in the airway by several cells, such as T-cells, eosinophils, and mast cells, may mediate AHR through its combined actions on epithelial and smooth muscle cells. Specifically, IL-13 has several effects on airway epithelium, such as induction of calcium activation chloride channels genes and increased goblet cell mucous content and impaired mucociliary clearance, all of which are contributory to airway obstruction. IL-13 impairs NO production by airway epithelial cells, which presumably would lead to heightened smooth muscle tone as NO is a bronchodilator. Furthermore, IL-13 can induce production of anaphylatoxin and complement factor C-3, which is important in the induction of BHR. Finally, and perhaps most important, IL-13 can directly impair β-adrenergic receptor mediated relaxation of airway smooth muscle.

Asthma Pathogenesis Conclusion: Mice, Men and Cytokines

In conclusion, having extensively reviewed the tenets of the β-adrenergic blockade theory and in light of the recent developments and understanding of the role of the Th2 cytokine IL-13 *(46)*, the authors can say that the effects of IL-13 are consistent with the β-adrenergic blockade theory of asthma. In this regard, the pharmacological abnormality, that is, the increased BHR and the decreased response to β-agonist, which are two essential components of the β-blockade theory, are adequately demonstrated by the effects of

IL-13. Furthermore, the increased IgE and the increased number of eosinophils, as well as the mucous hypersecretion and edema and goblet cell metaplasia that occurs in asthma (as well as in the pertussis-sensitized mouse model) are striking features of the effect of IL-13.

Pediatric Asthma Issues

As discussed in the earlier parts of this chapter (*see* pages 4–5), pediatric asthma, especially during infancy, is difficult to diagnose because the demonstration of wheezing does not necessarily mean persistent asthma. Nevertheless, the mechanisms outlined of the β-adrenergic blockade theory and the potential role of IL-13 should equally apply to all ages of people with asthma. The future potential to measure exhaled NO even in small children may provide insight into separating those young children who have wheezing without asthma from those that are more likely to develop persistent asthma. This would have significant advantage over other parameters, such as bronchial biopsy for demonstration of inflammatory cells in asthma and bronchial lavage. Furthermore, the levels of exhaled NO is a much more sensitive indicator of the effect of therapeutic modalities. In small children, where it is not possible (or practical) to measure pulmonary function by conventional methods, it is easy to measure NO.

Although AHR is the *sine-qua-non* of asthma, it is difficult to measure in small children. Although this can be done in research programs, bronchial challenges in infancy are markedly limited in this age group. The longitudinal evaluation of lung function in wheezing infants shows that the persistent wheezer shows a gradual and significant loss of lung function from the age of birth through age 16, which is in contrast to the transient early wheezers who regain most of the pulmonary function during the same time period. NO and sputum eosinophils are the most sensitive and significant parameters for asthma and a therapeutic response to anti-inflammatory agents. Collecting sputum eosinophils or indeed collecting sputum at all in small children is difficult. When measurable, serial peak expiatory flows, spirometry, and airway responses are the standard techniques for identifying pediatric asthma.

Adult Asthma Issues

Adult asthma is characterized by bronchoconstriction, eosinophilia, BHR, and inflammation. Although adult-onset asthma is frequently nonallergic as compared to asthma in childhood and early adult years, it still has the primary characteristics of asthma. Thus, there is the same level of AHR and the same decreased response to β-agonists in light of the occurrence of severe epinephrine fast and status asthmaticus occurring in both allergic and nonallergic asthma. ILs-4 and -13 are necessary for producing an increased IgE, but there is evidence that IL-13 can produce production of features of asthma that are independent of IgE production, such as the generation of anaphylatoxin C3A and its effect on various cells involved in asthma, including its effect on decreasing response to β-agonist and increasing eosinophilia. Furthermore, because it induces release of transforming growth factor-β from epithelial cells that enhances fibroblast secretion, IL-13 consistent with its effect on airway remodeling.

Former Asthmatics

It has been observed that approximately one-third of children with asthma will cease to have symptoms typically around the time of puberty (especially in boys), another one-third will remain the same, and the rest will have perhaps even worsening of their asthma.

However, it remains to be determined which children cease to have asthma symptoms. Our group pursued this observation in studying 43 students at Creighton University who had definite history of asthma, who had asthma for an average of 7 yr, and have been free of any asthma symptoms or medication use for an average of 8.5 yr *(47)*. In these studies, the authors observed that 85% of these children who had been asthma-free anywhere from 1 to 22 yr still had measurable BHR to methacholine. The authors interpreted their findings as that although asthma may go into remission, the genetic and physiological abnormalities, particularly BHR may persist, although clinically quiescent. Indeed, it is now recognized that individuals who have had asthma and are in remission can, a number of years later, have a recurrence of asthma (*see* "Relapse Asthma" section). This particularly may occur in response to a respiratory infection or a combination of events, such as a respiratory infection and exposure to environmental allergens or to occupational sensitizers.

CONCLUSIONS

Asthma is a common but complex disease, with increasing prevalence in the United States and throughout the developed, and eventually, the developing nations. Pediatric asthma has strong familial and allergic backgrounds, whereas adult-onset asthma has less specific associations. Exaggerated BHR is central to the disease in all ages. Asthma's scope and effect require continued investigation into its causes. The authors have attempted to describe the origins and characteristics of asthma and can say that their understanding of asthma has come a long way from Osler's original description of asthma as a neurosis to modern day molecular biology and the effect of various cytokines on its receptors in relation to the clinical signs and symptoms of asthma.

ACKNOWLEDGMENT

The authors thank the secretarial contributions of Joni Bohan.

REFERENCES

1. Martinez FD, Wright AL, Taussig LM, et al. Asthma and wheezing in the first six years of life. The Group Health Medical Associates. *N Engl J Med* 1995; 332: 133–138.
2. Arif AA, Delclos GL, Lee ES, Tortolero SR, Whitehead LW. Prevalence and risk factors of asthma and wheezing among US adults: an analysis of the NHANES III data. *Eur Respir J* 2003; 21: 827–833.
3. Global burden of asthma report. Available at: http://207.159.65.33/wadsetup/materials.html. Last accessed November 23, 2004.
4. Asthma prevalence and control characteristics by race/ethnicity United States, 2002. Centers for Disease Control and Prevention CDC. *MMWR Morb Mortal Wkly Rep* 2004; 53: 145–148.
5. National Health Interview Survey (NHIS). Series 10. Available at: http://www.cdc.gov/nchs/products/pubs/pubd/series/sr10/ser10.htm. Last accessed November 23, 2004.
6. Gupta R, Sheikh A, Strachan DP, Anderson HR. Burden of allergic disease in the UK: secondary analyses of national databases. *Clin Exp Allergy* 2004; 34: 5–20.
7. Akinbami LJ, LaFleur BJ, Schoendorf KC. Racial and income disparities in childhood asthma in the United States. *Ambul Pediatr* 2002; 2: 382–387.
8. Litonjua AA, Carey VJ, Burge HA, Weiss ST, Gold DR. Parental history and the risk for childhood asthma. Does mother confer more risk than father? *Am J Respir Crit Care Med* 1998; 158: 176–181.
9. Hoffjan S, Nicolae D, Ober C. Association studies for asthma and atopic diseases: a comprehensive review of the literature. *Respir Res* 2003; 4: 142–144.

10. Cook DG, Strachan DP. Health effects of passive smoking. 3. Parental smoking and prevalence of respiratory symptoms and asthma in school age children. *Thorax* 1997; 52: 108–194.
11. Stein RT, Sherrill D, Morgan WJ, et al. Respiratory syncytial virus in early life and risk of wheeze and allergy by age 13 years. *Lancet* 1999; 354: 541–545.
12. McConnochie KM, Roghmann KJ. Wheezing at 8 and 13 years: changing importance of bronchiolitis and passive smoking. *Pediatr Pulmonol* 1989; 6: 138–146.
13. Illi S, vonMutius E, Lau S, et al. Multicenter Allergy Study Group. The natural course of atopic dermatitis from birth to age 7 years and the association with asthma. *J Allergy Clin Immunol* 2004; 113: 925–931.
14. Rodriguez MA, Winkleby MA, Ahn D, Sundquist J, Kraemer HC. Identification of population subgroups of children and adolescents with high asthma prevalence: findings from the Third National Health and Nutrition Examination Survey. *Arch Pediatr Adolesc Med* 2002; 156: 269–275.
15. Hopp RJ, Townley RG, Biven RE, Bewtra AK, Nair NM. The presence of airway reactivity before the development of asthma. *Am Rev Respir Dis* 1990; 141: 2–8.
16. Smith GCS, Wood AM, White IR, et al. Neonatal respiratory morbidity at term and the risk of childhood asthma. *Arch Dis Child* 2004; 89: 956–960.
17. The 2002 Behavioral Risk Factor Surveillance System (BFRSS). Available at: http://www.cdc.gov/asthma/brfss/default.htm. Last accessed November 23, 2004.
18. Genes for asthma? An analysis of the European Community Respiratory Health Survey. *Am J Respir Crit Care Med* 1997; 156: 177–180.
19. deMarco R, Pattaro C, Locatelli F, Svanes C. ECRHS Study Group. Influence of early life exposures on incidence and remission of asthma throughout life. *J Allergy Clin Immunol* 2004; 113: 845–852.
20. Toelle BG, Xuan W, Peat JK, Marks GB. Childhood factors that predict asthma in young adulthood. *Eur Respir J* 2004; 23: 66–70.
21. Burrows B, Lebowitz MD, Barbee RA, Cline MG. Findings before diagnoses of asthma among the elderly in a longitudinal study of a general population sample. *J Allergy Clin Immunol* 1991; 88: 870–877.
22. Postma DS, Boezen HM. Rationale for the Dutch hypothesis. Allergy and AHR as genetic factors and their interaction with environment in the development of asthma and COPD. *Chest* 2004; 126(Suppl): 96S–104S.
23. Mean Body Weight, Height, and Body Mass Index, United States 1960–2002. Available at: http://www.cdc.gov/nchs/Default.htm. Accessed November 23, 2004.
24. Segala C, Priol G, Soussan D, et al. Asthma in adults: comparison of adult onset asthma with childhood onset asthma relapsing in adulthood. *Allergy* 2000; 55: 634–640.
25. Sears MR, Greene JM, Willan AR, et al. A longitudinal, population based, cohort study of childhood asthma followed to adulthood. *N Engl J Med* 2003; 349: 1414–1422.
26. Hopp RJ. Asthma in young adults: from whence it came? *Clin Rev Allergy Immunol* 2002; 22: 45–52.
27. Cookson DU, Reed CE. Comparison of the effects of isoproterenol in the normal and asthmatic subject. *Am Rev Respir Dis* 1963; 88: 636.
28. Shelhamer JH, Metcalfe DD, Smith LJ, Kaliner M. Abnormal beta adrenergic responsiveness in allergic subjects: analysis of isoproterenol-induced cardiovascular and plasma cyclic adenosine monophosphate responses. *J Allergy Clin Immunol* 1980; 66: 52–60.
29. Hopp R, Bewtra A, Watt G, Nair N, Townley R. Genetic analysis of allergic disease in twins. *J Allergy Clin Immunol* 1984; 73: 265–270.
30. Lang D, Hopp RJ, Bewtra AK, et al. Distribution of methacholine inhalation challenge responses in a selected adult population. *J Allergy Clin Immunol* 1987; 79: 533–540.
31. Hopp RJ, Bewtra AK, Nair N, Townley RG. Specificity and sensitivity of methacholine inhalation challenge in normal and asthmatic children. *J Allergy Clin Immunol* 1984; 74: 154–158.
32. Townley RG, Bewtra A, Wilson A, et al. Segregation analysis to methacholine inhalation challenge in families with and without asthma. *J Allergy Clin Immunol* 1986; 77: 101–107
33. Townley RG, Trapani IL, Szentivanyi A. Sensitization to anaphylaxis and to some of its pharmacological mediators by blockade of the beta adrenergic receptors. *J Allergy* 1967; 39: 177–197.
34. Szentivanyi A. The beta adrenergic theory of the atopic abnormality in bronchial asthma. *J Allergy* 1968; 42: 203–233.
35. Townley RG, McGeady S, Bewtra A. The effect of beta-adrenergic blockade on bronchial sensitivity to acetyl-beta-methacholine in normal and allergic rhinitis subjects. *J Allergy* 1976; 57: 358–366.

36. Reed CE, Cohen M, Enta T. Reduced effect of epinephrine on circulating eosinophils in asthma and after beta-adrenergic blockade or Bordetella pertussis vaccine. With a note on eosinopenia after methacholine. *J Allergy* 1970; 46: 90–102.

37. Mano K, Akbarzadeh A, Townley R. Effect of hydrocortisone on beta-adrenergic receptors in lung membranes. *Life Sci* 1979; 25: 1925–1930.

38. Townley RG, Daley D, Selenke W. The effect of agents used in the treatment of bronchial asthma on carbohydrate metabolism and histamine sensitivity after beta-adrenergic blockade. *J Allergy* 1970; 45: 71–76.

39. Robinson DS. The role of the mast cell in asthma: induction of airway hyperresponsiveness by interaction with smooth muscle? *J Allergy Clin Immunol* 2004; 114: 58–65.

40. Covar RA, Szefler SJ, Martin RJ, et al. Relations between exhaled nitric oxide and measures of disease activity among children with mild-to-moderate asthma. *J Pediatr* 2003; 142: 469–475.

41. Dupont LJ, Demedts MG, Verleden GM. Prospective evaluation of the validity of exhaled nitric oxide for the diagnosis of asthma. *Chest* 2003; 123: 751–756.

42. Smith AD, Cowan JO, Filsell S, et al. Diagnosing asthma: comparisons between exhaled nitric oxide measurements and conventional tests. *Am J Respir Crit Care Med* 2004; 169: 473–478.

43. Silkoff PE, Carlson M, Bourke T, et al. The Aerocrine exhaled nitric oxide monitoring system NIOX is cleared by the US Food and Drug Administration for monitoring therapy in asthma. *J Allergy Clin Immunol* 2004; 114: 1241–1256.

44. Wills-Karp M, Luyimbazi J, Xu X, et al. Interleukin-13: central mediator of allergic asthma. *Science* 1998; 282: 2258–2261.

45. Walter DM, McIntire JJ, Berry G, et al. Critical role for IL-13 in the development of allergen-induced airway hyperreactivity. *J Immunol* 2001; 167: 4668–4675.

46. Townley R, Horiba M. Airway hyperresponsiveness: a story of mice and men and cytokines. *Clin Rev Allergy Immunol* 2003; 24: 85–110.

47. Townley RG, Ryo UY, Kolotkin BM, Kang B. Bronchial sensitivity to methacholine in current and former asthmatic and allergic rhinitis patients and control subjects. *J Allergy Clin Immunol* 1975; 56: 429–442.

II PATIENT MANAGEMENT

2 Diagnosing Allergic Asthma

Gerald L. Klein, MD

CONTENTS

KEY POINTS

- Most patients with asthma have allergic asthma, and, therefore, allergies may exacerbate their symptoms.
- The optimum treatment of allergic asthma requires identifying the offending allergens so they can be eliminated, avoided, or treated.
- The essential elements of this diagnosis require a careful allergy history, physical examination, and diagnostic allergy tests, such as skin tests, radioallergosorbent (RAST) tests, and/or challenge tests.
- The major categories of allergens affecting bronchial asthma consist of pollens, environmentals, food, and animals.

INTRODUCTION

The incidence and severity of allergy, asthma, and allergic asthma has been increasing *(1)*, and this makes diagnosing allergic asthma even more important. It is not sufficient to make the diagnosis of bronchial asthma without determining whether the patient is atopic, and if so, to what allergens. These allergens can be classified into the following broad categories:

- Pollens.
- Environmental.
- Animals.
- Foods.

When specific allergens have been identified as eliciting symptoms, they can frequently be eliminated, avoided, or decreased. Antimite avoidance measures, such as the

From: *Current Clinical Practice: Bronchial Asthma:*
A Guide for Practical Understanding and Treatment, 5th ed.
Edited by: M. E. Gershwin and T. E. Albertson © Humana Press Inc., Totowa, NJ

use of mattress encasings *(2)*, HEPA filters *(3)*, and frequent dusting and vacuuming, may significantly improve the symptoms of the patient with asthmas who is mite sensitive. Allergen-specific therapy, such as allergy immunotherapy, may be undertaken as part of the patient's overall therapeutic regimen. This may prevent the seasonal exacerbations of asthma that plague many patients who have allergic asthma.

Allergic asthma manifests itself in the form of food allergy in many infants and young children. Although it may be somewhat difficult to diagnose the offending food, the removal of the offending food from the child's diet may be critical to the child's health.

Another important group of allergens that significantly affects children, as well as adults, is animals. Exposure to pets or animal parts can either cause acute exacerbations are be an underlying cause of chronic symptoms. This exposure can occur at both work (some occupations have large exposures to animal allergens) and home, even if there are no pets in the home. Studies have shown that because of the large number of dogs and cats, more than 1 million *(4)*, present in the United States *(5)*, almost everyone has animal allergens in his or her home, regardless of whether they have pets *(6,7)*. The animal hair and dander are transferred from pet owners to non-pet owners. These allergens are then brought into the nonsuspecting person's home from their clothes, so the diagnosis and subsequent cleaning and avoidance of offending animal allergens should be part of all optimum treatment plans for patients with allergic asthma *(8)*.

The importance of identification and avoidance of culpable allergens is often critical in preventing allergic asthma symptoms, exacerbations, and hyperactive airways.

ALLERGENS

The self-reported prevalence of bronchial asthma by individuals at least 18 yr old in the United States is 11% *(9)*, reported by the Behavioral Risk Factor Surveillance System in 2001. The mean prevalence for asthma had been estimated at 7.2%, with a range of 5.3–9.5% *(10)*. The survey also found that 78% of these patients with asthma had symptoms within the last 30 d. The role of allergy in the pathology, epidemiology, prevention, and treatment of bronchial asthma has gained in significance in the last decade. It is understood now that most people who develop asthma are believed to be extrinsic or have an underlying allergic diathesis *(11)*.

Allergic asthma triggers can be divided into four categories—pollens, environmental, food, and animal—which consist of the allergens cited in Table 1.

Pollens

The symptoms of pollen-induced allergic asthma tend to exacerbate seasonally, usually in the spring (grass and trees) and fall (weeds) when the pollen counts are the highest *(12)*. This effect varies greatly depending not only on pollen counts but also on microclimate, geography, and individual sensitivities *(13)*. These patients have the following signs and symptoms associated with pollen-induced asthma:

- Genetic predisposition.
- Family members usually have allergic asthma and other allergic diseases.
- Allergic asthma that most often begins in childhood.
- Usually accompanied by allergic rhinitis.
  - May have had atopic dermatitis in childhood.

Table 1
Allergic Asthma Triggers

Pollens	Environmental	Food	Animals
Grass	Dust mite	Milk	Dogs
Weeds	Cockroach	Eggs	Cats
Trees	Miscellaneous insects	Wheat	Birds
	Mold	Peanut	Horses
		Corn	Rabbits
		Pork	Mice and rats
		Shellfish	Hamsters and gerbils
		Fish	Guinea pigs

- Asthma is frequently also exacerbated by other allergens, mite, mold, etc.
- Positive skin and radioallergosorbent (RAST) tests to pollen.
  - Positive inhalation allergen test (not frequently performed).
- Seasonal exacerbations.
- Allergy immunotherapy may improve symptoms.
- Exercise-induced asthma worse during exposure to pollen.
  - Running outside during increased pollen counts (e.g., during football practice).
- Increased bronchial reactivity to irritants.
- Methacholine.
- Smoke.
  - Noxious aerosols.

Environmental Allergens

Patients who are allergic to the indoor environmental allergens (Tables 2–4) will have a yearlong or perennial symptoms but not seasonal exacerbations *(14)*. However, many patients are allergic to both pollen and indoor environmentals. House dust mites increase during periods of high humidity *(15)*. They thrive at sea level and do not survive in high altitudes *(16)*. Mites are primarily found in bedding, carpets, rugs, and furniture *(14)*. They are not usually airborne unless the air currents are disturbed by such events as opening or closing doors *(17,18)*. House dust mites are one of the most common allergens and may cause significant morbidity. The mites most likely to cause allergic asthma and rhinitis are *Dermatophagoides pteronyssinus (19)* and *Dermatophagoides farinae (20)*. Patients who are allergic to these allergens frequently have symptoms associated with exposure to vacuuming and dusting.

Cockroaches are commonly found in the inner cities *(21)*. The German cockroach, *Blattella germanica,* is the most common roach found in the United States *(22)*. Cockroaches increase in the warm, humid periods. They are believed to be one of the reasons for the high incidence and high morbidity of asthma in the urban areas.

Mold thrives in damp *(23)* and dark locations, contaminated food, and humid climates (*see* Table 3). The effect of mold is controversial. Mold is known to cause allergic reactions. Alternaria has caused severe bouts of allergic asthma *(24)*. It is debatable regardless of whether mold releases a toxin that causes allergic or other medical complications *(25,26)*.

Table 2
Common Pollen Allergens

Grass pollen	
Common name	*Genus and species*
Johnson grass	*Sorghum halepense*
Berumda grass	*Cynodon dactylon*
Orchard grass	*Cactylis glomerata*
Meadow fescue	*Festuca elatior*
Perennial rye	*Lolium perenne*
Kentucky bluegrass	*Poa pratensis*
Redtop grass	*Agrostis alba*
Sweet vernal	*Anthoxanthum odoratum*
Timothy grass	*Phleum pratense*

Weed pollen	
Common name	*Genus and species*
Short ragweed	*Ambrosia artemisiifolia*
Giant ragweed	*Ambrosisa trifida*
Mugwort	*Artemsia vulgaris*
English plantain	*Plantago lanceolata*
Lambs quarters	*Chenopodium album*
Russinan thistle	*Salsola kali*
False ragweed	*Franseria acanthicarpa*

Tree pollen	
Common name	*Genus*
Elm	*Ulmus*
White oak	*Quercus*
Beech	*Fagus*
Birch	*Betula*
Chestnut	*Castanea*
Cypress	*Cupressus*
Cedar	*Juniperus*
Pine	*Pinus*
Pine	*Fraxinus*
Olive	*Olea*
Maple	*Acer*
Walnut	*Juglans*
Hickory	*Carya*
Cottonwood	*Populus*
Willow	*Salix*
Mesquite	*Prosopis*
Privet	*Ligustrum*

Common molds	
Penicillium	Fusarium
Cladosporium	Claviceps
Cladosporium	Rhizopus
Alternaria	Epicoccum
Aspergillus	Helminthosporium

Modified from ref. *27*.

Table 3
High Indoor Mold Concentrations

Mold	Characteristic
Total mold	Temperature in child's bedroom (5°F above the rest of the home)
	Forced air heating
	Reported water, dampness, or leaks in any room in past 12 mo
	Observed evidence of moisture or leaks in child's bedroom
	Reported cat living in home within past 6 mo
Alternaria	Reported water, dampness, or leaks in any room in past 12 mo
Aspergillus	Season (winter)
	Forced air heating
	Observed evidence of cockroaches in child's bedroom
	Reported cat living in home within past 6 mo
Cladosporium	Observed evidence of moisture or leaks in child's bedroom
Penicillium	Season (winter vs other)
	Observed musty smell in child's bedroom

Modified from ref. *27a.*

Table 4
Environmental Allergens

Allergen	Location
Cockroaches	Inner city
Mold	Dark, damp, humid locations
Miscellaneous insects	Ubiquitous
House dust mites	Lower elevations, bedding, and mattress

Animal Allergy

Allergies to pets and other animals are common and often denied by patients and family members *(28)*. Cats cause severe bouts of asthma and allergy symptoms *(29)*. The allergens from pets can come from their hair, skin, fur, saliva, urine, or feces *(4)*, so people can be exposed in a diverse manner. The most common pets causing allergy are dogs, cats, birds, mice, rabbits, gerbils, guinea pigs, and ferrets.

In the United States, it has been estimated that there are 105 million dogs and cats *(30)*. Studies have shown that almost everyone has cat hair and dander in his or her home *(31)*. This occurs even if a cat has never been in the home. The large number of these animals causes the almost ubiquitous nature of this allergen that is probably transferred from one person's clothes to another and they are into their home or office *(32,33)*.

Allergy to pets is frequently denied, making the diagnosis more difficult *(3)*. Many pet owners claim that they would rather give up their allergic spouse rather than parting with their pet. Pets can not only cause an acute exacerbation but also add to the total cumulative allergy load. This exposure has been compared with a glass of water. If some pollen is put into a glass followed by mite allergen, mold allergen, and then when you add pet allergens, the glass begins to overflow (as do patients' symptoms).

Food Allergy

Food allergy is common and has a more important role in infancy and early childhood *(34)*. Sicherer and Furlong studies have shown that approximately 4% of the US population and 6% of children under the age of 3 yr have food-induced hypersensitivity *(35)*. Allergic reactions to foods occur immediately or several hours later, making it difficult to determine the cause and effect of the child's wheezing *(36)*. This makes it is more complicated to ascertain if specific food is a factor in allergic asthma in this age group. The most common foods that cause allergy in childhood are as follows *(37)*:

Milk	Egg albumin
Casein	Yolk
β-lactaglobin	Pork
α-lactaglobin	Corn
Whey	Peanuts
Albumin	Fish
Eggs	Wheat

Food allergy should be suspected in adults who have persistent asthma or who have intermittent exacerbations with no apparent trigger. They may also have the following signs and symptoms *(38)*:

- History of atopic dermatitis in childhood.
- Family history of food allergy.
- History of colic or feeding difficulties.
- Persistent or refractory asthma.
- No known triggers to explain exacerbations.
- History of positive skin or RAST test to a food.

Food allergy can cause severe bouts of bronchial asthma *(39)*. In one study, 50% of adults with difficult-to-treat asthma had food allergy *(40)*. Allergic reactions are sometimes, but not commonly, caused by inhalation of the vapor of the food being cooked *(41)*. The inhalation of peanut dust on an airplane causing anaphylaxis is an example of this *(42)*.

Children have a higher incidence of food allergy than adults. The overall incidence is increasing, but it is difficult to detect the exact number of people who are plagued with this problem *(35)*. Table 5 lists the estimated incidence of food allergy *(34)* to common foods in both children and adults.

Food allergy in childhood has been well established to cause symptoms of allergic rhinitis *(43)*, atopic dermatitis *(44)*, asthma *(45)*, urticaria *(46)*, and pruritus *(47)*. This type of allergy also causes the following gastrointestinal symptoms *(48)*:

- Bloating.
- Nausea and vomiting.
- Gas and flatulence.
- Abdominal pain.
- Colic and cramps.
- Diarrhea.
- Bloody diarrhea.
- Heartburn.

Table 5
Prevalence of Food Allergies in the United States

Food	Young children, %	Adults, %
Milk	2.5	0.3
Egg	1.3	0.2
Peanuts	0.8	0.6
Tree nuts	0.2	0.5
Fish	0.1	0.4
Shellfish	0.1	2.0
Overall	6	3.7
Food-induced wheezing	7	
Atopic dermatitis	35	

Table 6
Commonly Used Allergy Tests

Test	Problems	Types of test	Conclusion
Skin test	Inaccurate results	Prick test	Not definitive, a guide
	May be dangerous	Intradermal	Not routinely performed
RAST	Not accurate	Cap-RAST	Good as a guide, especially if a severe reaction was suspected
DBFCT	Difficult to perform May be dangerous, expensive	Food challenge	Most accurate
Single-blind food challenge test	Difficult to perform and interpret	Food challenge	Not as accurate as DBFCT
Basic diet and challenge	Time consuming and difficult	Diet manipulation	Requires families to cooperate
Elimination diet and challenge	Diet manipulation	Diet manipulation	Easier for families to follow

RAST, radioallergosorbent test; DBFCT, double-blind food challenge test.

The diagnosis of food allergy is made by a careful history, physical examination, and diagnostic tests (49). Food allergy skin tests and RAST tests, unlike other allergy tests, such as pollen or hymenoptera, are used as more of a guide than as a definitive test (50). Food allergy testing has a higher rate of false-positive and false-negative test results (36). Table 6 lists the commonly used tests for food allergy (51,52).

There are many false-positive and false-negative food allergy tests (53). Many patients (and physicians) have difficult understanding that a "positive skin" test to a food does not equate to a food allergy. Food allergy skin testing can be dangerous and difficult to interpret (54). It is usually not advisable to perform this type of testing on patients who have a history of an anaphylactic reaction to the suspected food (55). Food allergy skin tests should always begin with a prick test (1/100) and only proceed by dilution (1/1000) intradermal testing by experienced allergists who is prepared to treat anaphylactic reactions (56). Food allergy testing is usually done both as a screening procedure during routine skin testing and for specific food allergies that were elicited during the allergy history. RAST tests can also be used instead of skin testing, but they are not as accurate as a properly applied and interpreted skin test (57). However, if a severe food allergy is suspected, a RAST test is safer than a skin test.

Once a food is suspected by history and skin or RAST test, a diagnostic challenge should occur, except for when severe food allergy reactions have occurred or are suspected by previous testing. The gold standard in this type of testing is the double-blind food challenge test (DBFCT) (58). In the DBFCT, both the suspected food allergen and a placebo are usually lyophilized and disguised in either capsules, "shakes," or other vehicles, so that it is impossible to tell them apart (59). This eliminates bias so that it is the most objective way of food challenge testing. The DBFCT has some drawbacks in that it is expensive and time consuming, no Food and Drug Administration-approved product for testing is available, and it also has the possibility of causing anaphylactic reactions in extremely sensitive patients (52). People who are experienced and prepared to treat anaphylaxis should, therefore, only conduct this test. Like any test, the DBFCT is not 100% foolproof and can have some false-positive and false-negative results, but it is the most accurate test of food allergy. Antihistamines must be discontinued at least 48 h before the challenge. The suspected food should be removed from the child's diet for at least 1 wk before the food challenge test is undertaken. The initial challenge usually begins with 125–500 mg of the suspected food and then doubled every 20–60 min, until 10 g of food have been eaten (60). If the food allergy tests are negative, the food is given to the patient in the office, in an open challenge.

Children frequently outgrow their food allergy, so that in the nonanaphylactic forms of food allergy, elimination diet and challenge testing may be performed every 6 mo.

In the single-blind placebo controlled food challenge test (SBFCT), it is not possible to blind the investigator; only the patient can be blinded. The results, therefore, have some investigator bias, and the test is not as objective as the DBFCT.

Like the SBFCT, elimination diets are not as objective as the DBFCT, but they are much easier and cheaper to undertake (49). Elimination diets consist of two types, a so-called basic diet and a regular diet that systematically eliminates and then challenges patients with the eliminated food. Basic diets consist of foods that are believed to have a low risk of causing food allergy, such as lamb, rice, potato, carrot, sweet potato, and pear. After 1 wk of eating such a diet, a new food is introduced every 3 d. If the new food causes a suspected allergic reaction, that food is removed from the diet and then subsequently reintroduced (unless a dangerous reaction may occur) or challenged into the diet. In this manner, elimination diets and challenge may detect the food allergen. Elemental basic diets are mainly used in infants and toddlers.

SKIN TESTS

Allergy skin tests are probably the most important diagnostic test in identifying allergic asthma but RAST is equally reliable (see Tables 7 and 8). Skin tests are accurate and reproducible (61). A positive, histamine, and negative saline test must always be used to compare the test allergens. If the histamine test does not elicit a classic positive test, then the testing is not valid. This usually occurs when patients have not stopped taking antihistamines within the prior allotted time period. Patients should return in 48–72 h for repeat skin tests and be instructed to stop taking all antihistamines. An abnormal positive saline test is found when a patient has dermatographism, as a result of the device or technique, or when the saline test material was contaminated by either a histamine or an allergen (62).

Table 7
Allergy Skin Testing

Pros	Cons
Easy to perform	Skin must be intact and no dermatographism
Rapid results	Experience needed in interpretation
High sensitivity	Somewhat dependent on methodology and technician
Reproducible	
Inexpensive	Medication must be withheld (antihistamines, systemic steroids, and tricyclics)
Many allergens available	Remote possibility of systemic reaction
Accurate for pollens and environmentals	Results not as exact for foods

Note. Infants as well as adults can be tested. Some patients are reluctant to undergo testing owing to fear of needles.

The two types of skin tests performed today are the prick-puncture test and the intradermal or intracutaneous test. The skin-prick test is the most accurate way to perform this type of testing (63). In this method, a small drop of allergen is placed on the skin and a needle is used to inject the material in the skin by lifting or "pricking" the skin. The allergens should be placed at least 2 cm apart so the individual tests do not run into each other and accurate results can be measured. The puncture has to be done carefully so that the skin is sufficiently punctured but that bleeding does not occur. Insufficient puncture can result in a false-negative test, and bleeding can lead to false-positive tests. The results consist of the swelling or "wheal" and the erythema or "flare." A positive test is considered if the wheal is 3 mm larger than a saline control (64). If a patient has a negative reaction to both the histamine and the saline, he or she probably has not stopped taking antihistamines. This type of patient may have to return in 48 h for repeat skin testing. In general, antihistamines should be withheld for 48 h and hydroxyzine for 72 h.

These prick tests are either measured or graded on a scale from 0 to 4. Intradermal tests are usually injected with a 25- or 26-gage needles and disposable 1-mL syringe. The allergens are more dilute than the solutions used for the prick tests (1:1000 or 1:5000). When using this methodology approx 0.02 mL of the allergen is injected in the epidermis so that a small bleb forms similar to a purified protein derivative test for tuberculosis (65). These tests are less sensitive but more specific than the prick test, and more false-positive tests result from this type of testing (66). Intradermal testing causes more systemic reactions than the prick test, so the prick test should be used initially (67). Therefore, only patients with a negative prick test should undergo an intradermal test. Intradermal tests are usually reserved for hymenoptera, pollen, mite, and, occasionally, mold. Food intradermal tests are avoided because of the difficulty in interpreting the results and the increased chance of a systemic reaction.

PREVENTING ERRORS WITH ALLERGY SKIN TESTING

General (68)

1. Instruct patient not to use any antihistamines or tricyclics for 48–72 before testing.
2. Use caution in testing an extremely allergic patient, especially during his or her susceptible "season" with too many allergens in one setting.
3. Have epinephrine readily available to treat a systemic reaction.

Table 8
Laboratory Measurement of Allergic Disease *(69)*

Allergen specific	RAST testing
Screen for allergy	Multiallergen screen (adult and pediatric forms)
Other non-RAST test	
General screen	
Marker for mast cell degranulation	Tryptase, useful in anaphylaxis
Sputum screen	Eosinophils
Complete blood count	Percentage of eosinophils

4. Perform tests on normal skin.
5. Do not allow bleeding to occur.
6. Do not place tests closer than 2 cm for proper reading of results.
7. Do not skin test a patient during an asthma exacerbation.
8. Record results in approx 15 min after the tests are applied.

Prick-Puncture

1. Penetrate the skin sufficiently to prevent false-negative results.
2. Perform prick test before intradermal testing to prevent systemic reactions.
3. Do not contaminate the needles with other allergens.
4. Avoid spreading the allergen solution during testing.
5. Use to test foods that are not suspected of causing severe allergic reactions.

Intradermal Testing

1. Starting dose with a previous negative prick test should be 1000 times weaker than the concentrated dilution used for prick-puncture (or roughly 10 AU for standardized allergy extracts).
2. In general, should not be used to test foods.
3. If no bleb occurs, then a subcutaneous injection has occurred, which may lead to false-negative test.
4. Inject 0.01–0.03 mL, otherwise irritant reaction may occur.
5. One intradermal syringe per allergen per patient should be used to prevent infectious contamination.

RAST TESTING

The Phadebas RAST test was the first important and accurate in vitro test developed for the laboratory detection of allergen-specific IgE antibody *(70)*. This type of RAST test used an allergen that was coupled to a cellulose paper disk (radioallergosorbent). Human sera would then be added, so that if there was specific IgE in the sera against the coupled allergen, they would bind together. The addition of human radiolabeled antihuman IgE antibody would then bind with the bound IgE, which are detected and quantified via calibration curves. New tests, such as the Pharmacia CAP RAST, have increased the accuracy in both specificity and sensitivity of RAST testing *(71)*.

Table 9
Pros and Cons of RAST Testing

Pro	Con
In vitro test	Expensive
No patient risk	Results not immediately available
Screening test available	Fewer allergens available than for skin tests
Not affected by medication, so patients do not have to stop them	Skin tests more accurate than RAST tests

RAST, radioallergosorbent.

Table 10
Allergy History

Seasonal affects	Pollen
Worsening of symptoms at home	Environmental
Increased symptoms with exposure to pets	Animals
Children with frequent symptoms	Food

The Multiallergen IgE E screen is a qualitative RAST test that consists of 15 indoor and outdoor allergens *(57,72)*. The specific allergens vary from company to company and are not listed. In general, they consist of allergens from grass, weeds, trees, molds, mites, dog, and cats *(66)*. They are meant to be a general screening test when a patient's history conforms to any type of aeroallergen. This is designed to detect common allergens that affect adults. A pediatric multiallergen is also available that consists of common food allergens.

Despite the improvement in this in vitro allergy testing, which is now closer to the diagnostic importance of allergy skin testing, RAST testing still suffers from what is shown in Table 9 *(30)*.

CONCLUSION

All patients who are diagnosed with bronchial asthma should be diagnosed for allergy. This should consist of a detailed history (*see* Table 10).

It is critical to make this detailed diagnosis so that the proper therapeutic interventions can be instituted, such as allergen avoidance, allergy environmental control, allergy immunotherapy, and omalizumab (Xolair®) *(73)*. Referral to an allergist can assist in this diagnosis.

REFERENCES

1. Anderson HR, Pottier AC, Strachan DP. Asthma from birth to age 23: incidence and relation to prior and concurrent atopic disease. *Thorax* 1992; 47: 537–542.
2. Bush RK, Eggleston PA. Guidelines for control of indoor allergen exposure. *J Allergy Clin Immunol* 2001; 107(suppl): 3.
3. Custovic A, Simpson A, Chapman MD, Woodcock A. Allergen avoidance in the treatment of asthma and atopic disorders. *Thorax* 1998; 53: 63–72.
4. Chapman MD, Wood RA. The role and remediation of animal allergens in allergic diseases. *J Allergy Clin Immunol* 2001; 107(Suppl): S414–S421.
5. Ingram JM, Sporik R, Rose G, et al. Quantitative assessment of exposure to dog (Can f 1) and cat (Fel d 1) allergens: relation to sensitization and asthma among children living in Los Alamos, New Mexico. *J Allergy Clin Immunol* 1995; 96: 449–456.

6. Custovic A, Fletcher A, Pickering CA, et al. Domestic allergens in public places III. House dust mite, cat, dog and cockroach allergens in British hospitals. *Clin Exp Allergy* 1998; 28: 53–59.

7. Wood RA. Animal allergens: looking beyond the tip of the iceberg. *J Allergy Clin Immunol* 1999; 103: 1002–1004.

8. Arbes SJ, Jr. Dog allergen (Can f 1) and cat allergen (Fel d 1) in US homes: results from the National Survey of Lead and Allergens in Housing. *J Allergy Clin Immunol* 2004; 114: 111–117.

9. Rhodes L, Moorman JE, Redd SC, et al. Self-reported asthma prevalence and control among adults: United States, 2001. *MMWR Morb Mortal Wkly Rep* 2003; 52: 381–384.

10. Vollmer W, Osborne M, Buist A. 20-year trends in the prevalence of asthma and chronic airflow obstruction in an HMO. *Am J Respir Crit Care Med* 1998; 157: 1079–1084.

11. Beasley R, Crane J, Lai CKW, Pearce N. Prevalence and etiology of asthma. *J Allergy Clin Immunol* 2000; 105: S466–S472.

12. Barnes C, Schreiber K, Pacheco F, et al. Comparison of outdoor allergenic particles and allergen levels. *Ann Allergy Asthma Immunol* 2000; 84: 47–54.

13. Portnoy J. Clinical relevance of spore and pollen counts. *Immunol Allergy Clin North Am* 2003; 23: 389–410.

14. Platts-Mills TAE, Vervloet D, Thomas WR. Indoor allergens and asthma: report of the Third International Workshop. *J Allergy Clin Immunol* 1997; 100: S1–S24.

15. Arlian LG, Platts-Mills TA. The biology of dust mites and the remediation of mite allergens in allergic disease. *J Allergy Clin Immunol* 2001; 107: S406–S413.

16. Arlian LG, Bernstein D, Bernstein IL. Prevalence of dust mites in the homes of people with asthma living in eight different geographic areas of the United States. *J Allergy Clin Immunol* 1992; 90: 292–300.

17. Jerrim KL. Airborne dust and allergen generation during dusting with and without spray polish. *J Allergy Clin Immunol* 2002; 109: 63–67.

18. Platt-Mills TAE, Heymann PW, Longbottom JL, Wilkins SR. Airborne allergens associated with asthma: particle sizes carrying dust mite and rat allergens measured with a cascade impactor. *J Allergy Clin Immunol* 1986; 77: 850–857.

19. Chapman MD, Heymann PW, Wilkins SR, Brown MB, Platts-Mills TAE. Monoclonal immunoassays for the major dust mite (Dermatophagoides) allergens, Der p1 and Der f1, and quantitative analysis of the allergen content of mite and house dust extracts. *J Allergy Clin Immunol* 1987; 80: 184–194.

20. Luczynska CM, Arruda LK, Platts-Mills TAE, et al. Housing characteristics, reported mold exposure, and asthma in the European Community Respiratory Health Survey allergens, Der p1 and Der f1. *J Immunol Methods* 1989; 118: 227–235.

21. Rosenstreich DL, Eggleston P, Kattan M. The role of cockroach allergy and exposure to cockroach allergen in causing morbidity among inner-city children with asthma. *N Engl J Med* 1997; 336: 1356–1363.

22. Twarog FJ, Picone FJ, Strank RS. Immediate hypersensitivity to cockroach: isolation and purification of the major antigens. *J Allergy Clin Immunol* 1977; 59: 154–160.

23. Zock JP. Housing characteristics, reported mold exposure, and asthma in the European Community Respiratory Health Survey. *J Allergy Clin Immunol* 2002; 110: 285–292.

24. O'Hollaren MT, Yuninger JW, Offord KP, et al. Exposure to an aeroallergen as a possible precipitating factor in respiratory arrest in young patients with asthma. *N Engl J Med* 1991; 324: 359–363.

25. Jarvis BB. Chemistry and toxicology of molds isolated from water-damaged buildings. *Adv Exp Med Biol* 2002; 504: 43–52.

26. Institute of Medicine (US) Committee on the Assessment of Asthma and Indoor Air. *Clearing the Air: Asthma and Indoor Air Exposures*. Washington, DC, National Academy Press; 2000.

27. Lockey RF, Bukantz SC, Bosquet J. *Allergens and Allergen Immunotherapy*. New York, Marcel Deker 2004, pp.165–232.

27a. O'Conner GC, Walter M, Mithcell H, et al. Airborne fungi in the homes of children with asthma in low-income urban communities: The Inner-City Asthma Study. *J Allergy Clin Immunol* 2004; 114: 599–606.

28. Apelberg BJ, Aoki Y, Jaakkola JJ. Systematic review: exposure to pets and risk of asthma and asthma-like symptoms. *J Allergy Clin Immunol* 2001; 107: 455–460.

29. Almqvist C, Wickman M, Perfetti L, et al. Worsening of asthma in children allergic to cats, after indirect exposure to cat at school. *Am J Respir Crit Care Med* 2001; 163: 694–698.

30. Eggleston PA, Wood RA. Management of allergies to animals. *Allergy Proc* 1992; 13: 289–292.
31. Bollinger ME, Eggleston PA, Wood RA. Cat antigen in homes with and without cats may induce allergic symptoms. *J Allergy Clin Immunol* 1996; 97: 907–914.
32. Berge M, Munir AK, Dreborg S. Concentrations of cat (Fel d1), dog (Can f1) and mite (Der f1 and Der p1) allergens in the clothing and school environment of Swedish schoolchildren with and without pets at home. *Pediatr Allergy Immunol* 1998; 9: 25–30.
33. Enberg RN, Shamie SM, McCullough J, Ownby DR. Ubiquitous presence of cat allergen in cat-free buildings: probable dispersal from human clothing. *Ann Allergy* 1993; 70: 471–474.
34. Sampson HA. Update on food allergy. *J Allergy Clin Immunol* 2004; 113: 805–819.
35. Sicherer SH. Prevalence of seafood allergy in the United States determined by a random telephone survey. *J Allergy Clin Immunol* 2004; 114: 159–165.
36. Sicherer SH. Food allergy. *Lancet* 2002; 360: 701–710.
37. Bock SA, Atkins FM. Patterns of food hypersensitivity during sixteen years of double blind, placebo-controlled food challenges. *J Pediatr* 1990; 117: 561–567.
38. Warner JO. Food intolerance and asthma. *Clin Exp Allergy* 1995; 25(Suppl): 30.
39. Roberts G, Patel N, Levi-Schaffer F. Food allergy as a risk factor for life-threatening asthma in childhood: a case-controlled study. *J Allergy Clin Immunol* 2003; 112: 168–174.
40. Fogarty A, Britton J. The role of diet in the etiology of asthma. *Clin Exp Allergy* 2000; 30: 615–627.
41. Anto JM, Sunyer J, Rodriguez-Roisin R, Suarez-Cervera M, Vazquez L. Community outbreaks of asthma associated with inhalation of soybean dust. Toxicoepidemiological Committee. *N Engl J Med* 1989; 320: 1097–1102.
42. Sicherer SH, Furlong TJ, DeSimone J, Sampson HA. Self-reported allergic reactions to peanut on commercial airliners. *J Allergy Clin Immunol* 1999; 104: 186–189.
43. James JM, Bernhisel-Broadbent J, Sampson HA. Respiratory reactions provoked by double-blind food challenges in children. *Am J Respir Crit Care Med* 1994; 149: 59–64.
44. Gustafsson D, Sjoberg O, Foucard T. Sensitization to food and airborne allergens in children with atopic dermatitis followed up to 7 years of age. *Pediatr Allergy Immunol* 2003; 14: 448–452.
45. Rhodes H, Sporik R, Thomas P. Early life risk factors for adult asthma: a birth cohort study of subjects at risk. *J Allergy Clin Immunol* 2001; 108: 720–725.
46. Hamid Q. Immunopathology of food allergy. *J Allergy Clin Immunol* 2004; 113: 1006–1008.
47. Leung DY. Advances in allergic skin diseases. *J Allergy Clin Immunol* 2003; 111(Suppl): S805–S812.
48. Sampson HA. Food allergy. *J Allergy Clin Immunol* 2003; 111(Suppl): 540–547.
49. Bock SA. Prospective appraisal of complaints of adverse reactions to foods in children during the first 3 years of life. *Pediatrics* 1987; 79: 683–688.
50. Sampson HA. Utility of food-specific IgE concentrations in predicting symptomatic food allergy. *J Allergy Clin Immunol* 2001; 107: 891–896.
51. Hill DJ, Hosking CS, Reyes-Benito LV. Reducing the need for food allergen challenges in young children: a comparison of in vitro with in vivo tests. *Clin Exp Allergy* 2001; 31: 1031–1035.
52. Sampson H, Ho D. Relationship between food-specific IgE concentration and the risk of positive food challenges in children and adolescents. *J Allergy Clin Immunol* 1997; 100: 444–451.
53. Sampson HA. Diagnosing food allergy. In: Spector SL, ed. *Provocation Testing in Clinical Practice.* New York, Marcel Dekker, Inc, 1995, pp. 623–646.
54. Vlieg-Boerstra BJ, Bijleveld MA, van der Heide S, et al. Development and validation of challenge materials for double-blind, placebo-controlled food challenges in children. *J Allergy Clin Immunol* 2004; 113: 341–346.
55. Sampson HA. Anaphylaxis and emergency treatment. *Pediatrics* 2003; 111(suppl): 1601–1608.
56. Norman PS, Peebles RS. In vivo diagnostic allergy testing methods. In: Rose NR, Hamilton RG, Detrick B, eds. *Manual of Clinical Laboratory Immunology.* 6th ed. Washington, DC, American Society for Microbiology Press, 2002, pp. 875–890.
57. Hamilton RG. Clinical laboratory assessment of IgE-dependent hypersensitivity. *J Allergy Clin Immunol* 2003; 111(Suppl): S687–S701.
58. Li JT. Allergy testing. *Am Fam Physician* 2002; 66: 621–624.
59. Bock SA, Sampson HA, Atkins FM, et al. Double-blind placebo-controlled food challenge (DBFCFC) as an office procedure: a manual. *J Allergy Clin Immunol* 1988; 82: 986.
60. Hoj L, Osterballe O, Bundgaard A, Weeke B, Weiss M. A double-blind controlled trial of elemental diet in severe, perennial asthma. *Allergy* 1981; 36: 257–262.

61. Høst A. Practical aspects of allergy testing. *Paediatr Respir Rev* 2003; 4: 312–318.
62. Bernstein IL. Proceedings of the Task Force on Guidelines for Standardizing Old and New Technologies Used for the Diagnosis and Treatment of Allergic Diseases. *J Allergy Clin Immunol* 1988; 82: 487.
63. Bernstein IL, Storms WW. Practice parameters for allergy diagnostic testing. *Ann Allergy* 1995; 75: 543–625.
64. EAACI Subcommittee on Skin Tests. Position paper: allergen standardization and skin tests. *Allergy* 1993; 48(Suppl 14): 48–82.
65. Dreborg S. Skin testing in allergen standardization and research. *Immunol Allergy Clin N Am* 2001; 21: 329–354.
66. Dolen WK. Skin testing and immunoassays for allergen-specific IgE. *Clin Rev Allergy Immunol* 2001; 21: 229–239.
67. Lockey RF, Benedict LM, Turkeltaub PC, et al. Fatalities from immunotherapy and skin testing. *J Allergy Clin Immunol* 1987; 79: 660.
68. Mansmann HC Jr, Bierman CW, Pearlmlman D, ed. *Allergic disease in infancy, childhood and adolescence.* Philadelphia, WB Saunders, 1980, p. 289.
69. Wide L, Bennich H, Johansson SGO. Diagnosis by an in vitro test for allergen specific IgE antibodies. *Lancet* 1967; 2: 1105–1109.
70. Hamilton RG. Assessment of human allergic diseases. In: RR Rich, TA Fleisher, WT Shearer, HW Schroeder, B Kotzin, eds. *Clinical Immunology: Principles and Practice.* 2nd ed. London, Mosby, 2001, pp. 124.1–124.14.
71. Hamilton R. Laboratory analyses in the diagnosis of human allergic disease. *Methods* 1997; 13: 25–32.
72. Matsson P, Hamilton RG, Adkinson NF Jr, et al. *Evaluation Methods and Analytical Performance Characteristics of Immunologic Assays for Human Immunoglobulin E (IgE) Antibodies of Defined Allergen Specificities.* Wayne PA, National Committee on Clinical Laboratory Standards (NCCLS), Approved guideline, 1997; 17: 24.
73. Buhl R. Omalizumab (Xolair®) improves quality of life in adult patients with allergic asthma: a review. *Respir Med* 2003; 97: 123–129.

3

How the Pulmonary Function Laboratory Contributes to the Management of the Patient With Asthma

Richard E. Kanner, MD, *and Theodore G. Liou,* MD

CONTENTS

KEY POINTS

- Spirometry is a dynamic test that provides the best assessment of obstructive airway disease.
- The most useful value that the spirogram provides is the maximum volume of air that can be expelled with a forced expiration after a maximal inspiratory effort, the forced expiratory volume in 1 s (FEV_1).

From: *Current Clinical Practice: Bronchial Asthma:*
A Guide for Practical Understanding and Treatment, 5th ed.
Edited by: M. E. Gershwin and T. E. Albertson © Humana Press Inc., Totowa, NJ

- Lung volume measurements are static studies and are less useful in assessing airway obstruction but can demonstrate the presence of pulmonary overinflation.
- The carbon monoxide-diffusing capacity can help distinguish between asthma and emphysema in patients who smoke.
- Arterial blood gas studies can assess the consequences of bronchospasm and provide a guide for hospitalizing patients with asthma exacerbation.
- Nonspecific bronchoprovocation challenge testing with methacholine or other agents may help diagnose asthma when the clinical picture is unclear.
- Bronchoprovocation challenge testing using specific agents can help diagnose asthma caused by workplace substances.
- Standardization of technique and rigid quality control are an absolute necessity in any pulmonary laboratory.

INTRODUCTION

The pulmonary function laboratory plays an important role in the diagnosis and management of patients with bronchospastic disorders. In this chapter, the following pulmonary function tests that should be readily available to physicians treating patients with confirmed or suspected asthma are discussed.

- Spirometry and flow-volume tracings.
- Lung volume measurements.
- Pulmonary diffusing capacity.
- Arterial blood gas measurements.
- Bronchoprovocation challenge testing.
- Exercise studies.

Although these tests are best performed in a laboratory setting, physicians will also find that an office spirometer can be useful and convenient for patient evaluation.

THE "COMPARTMENTS" OF THE LUNG

The lung is subdivided into four volumes and four capacities. By definition, a volume is a compartment that cannot be further subdivided, whereas a capacity is composed of two or more volumes. Convenient reference points are maximal inspiration and maximal expiration. In addition, there is a resting point to which the lung and thoracic cage return after a normal breath, when respiratory muscles are relaxed (*see* Fig. 1).

The Volumes of the Lung

The four volumes are illustrated in Fig. 1 and are defined as follows:

1. Tidal volume (V_T) is the amount of air or of a gas that is inhaled with a normal inspiratory effort.
2. Inspiratory reserve volume (IRV). The additional amount of gas that can be inhaled after this normal inspiratory effort is called the IRV. This is an infrequently used measurement.
3. Expiratory reserve volume (ERV). After completing a normal expiratory effort that returns the lung and thorax to the resting position, an additional amount of gas can be exhaled with a voluntary effort; this is called the ERV. Thus, the ERV is the amount of

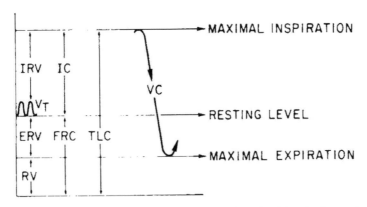

Fig. 1. Lung volumes and capacities in relation to points of maximal inspiration and expiration and the resting level. Vital capacity (VC) is an expiratory maneuver. IRV, inspiratory reserve volume; V_T, tidal volume; ERV, expiratory reserve volume; RV, residual volume; IC, inspiratory capacity; FRC, functional residual capacity; TLC, total lung capacity.

gas that can be exhaled when the expiratory effort begins at the resting position and ends at maximal expiration.

4. Residual volume (RV). At the point of maximal expiration, there is still a quantity of gas in the lung that cannot be expelled. This remaining volume is the RV.

The Capacities of the Lung

The four capacities are also shown in Fig. 1.

1. The total lung capacity (TLC) consists of all four volumes.
2. The inspiratory capacity (IC) is the maximum amount of gas that can be inhaled from the resting position. Thus, the IC is the sum of the V_T and the IRV.
3. Functional residual capacity (FRC). After a normal exhalation, the amount of gas remaining in the lung is the FRC, which consists of the ERV plus the RV.
4. The fourth capacity is the vital capacity (VC). This capacity is by definition measured as an expiratory maneuver and is the amount of gas that can be expelled from the lung when exhalation starts at the maximal inspiratory level and proceeds to the maximal expiratory level. If the VC is measured as an inspiratory maneuver going from maximal expiration to maximal inspiration, it is then called an inspiratory vital capacity (IVC). Usually the VC is measured as a forced exhalation, in which the subject is asked to inspire to the maximal inspiratory position and then empty the lungs as rapidly and completely as possible. This is termed the forced vital capacity (FVC). Because the VC measures the change in lung position from maximal inspiration to maximal expiration, it should be considered a measure of the subject's ability to change the size of the thoracic cavity. This is influenced by all the muscles of respiration and their innervation, by the elasticity of the thoracic cage and lung, and by the patency of the airways.

The FRC maintains a relatively constant level of oxygen and carbon dioxide in arterial blood. The FRC functions as a physiological equivalent of a chemical buffer. It enables the individual to maintain a relatively constant level of oxygen and carbon dioxide in arterial blood. Each breath removes carbon dioxide from the FRC and adds oxygen. If the FRC were 0, so that each breath completely filled and then emptied the lungs, the arterial oxygen and carbon dioxide partial pressures would fluctuate widely with each breath. During expiration, the entire pulmonary circulation would become a shunt resulting from the lack of gas and gas exchange in the lung; oxygen and carbon dioxide levels would remain at mixed venous (pulmonary arterial) levels. A patient with an FRC of 0 would be expected to become cyanotic at end-expiration. Inspiration would restore exchange of oxygen and carbon dioxide, and intraalveolar gases would again have essentially the same partial gas pressures as in the atmosphere. Gases in the blood rapidly equilibrate with gases in the alveoli, so marked changes would be reflected in the blood with restoration of normal arterial oxygen and carbon dioxide partial pressures and cyanosis would disappear.

The FRC physically helps keeps alveoli and airways patent. This helps prevent pulmonary arterial-to-venous shunting arising from atelectatic and thus airless portions of lung and makes the work of breathing easier, because it takes a greater effort to open and expand collapsed alveoli than to simply expand those alveoli that are already open.

In a chemical reaction, too much buffer can be bad, and this also is true for the FRC. If the FRC is too large, perhaps because of severe airway obstruction, it cannot adequately be "freshened" by each breath, leading to a decrease in arterial oxygenation and a rise in carbon dioxide tension.

DYNAMIC LUNG MEASUREMENTS: SPIROMETRY AND FLOW-VOLUME TRACINGS

- Airflow obstruction or limitation, which is usually present in patients with asthma, is best assessed by dynamic measurements, such as flow rates and the timed VC.

Spirometry is a simple procedure for obtaining flow rates and timed VC. The spirogram is a plot of volume vs time. Another technique commonly used in hospital laboratories is the flow-volume tracing. As the name indicates, this is a plot of airflow vs the expired (or inspired) lung volume.

The forced expiratory spirogram is shown in Fig. 2. In this figure, the subject is breathing normally and the V_T is recorded. The subject is asked to slowly blow all of the air out of the lungs until maximal exhalation is attained and then take a deep inspiration. This allows for measurement of the ERV, IRV, and IC, as well as the IVC. The subject is then instructed to blow all the air out of the lungs as rapidly and completely as possible. This gives a tracing of the FVC. The FVC can be subdivided into the forced expiratory volume (FEV) in 1 s, 2 s, 3 s, etc. These are volumes exhaled during each time period and are usually expressed as liters. The ratio FEV_1/FVC is a unitless number often used as an index of airflow obstruction and may be presented as a decimal fraction or as a percentage. Predicted normal (reference) values are available for the FEV_1/FVC ratio, as well as for most of the other measurements. When performed according to American Thoracic Society guidelines, these measurements are typically routinely reproducible and reliable. Less than maximal effort by the test subject leads to erroneous but easily identified results.

Another way of assessing airflow obstruction with the spirogram is to measure specific flow rates. Different FVC curve portions may be used. The most rapid flow rates occur early in expiration. The peak expiratory flow rate (PEFR) is an instantaneous rate that occurs near the beginning of a forced expiration. Average expiratory flows for specific portions of the FVC may also be measured. On the spirogram, one can measure the forced expiratory flow from 200 to 1200 mL below maximal inspiration

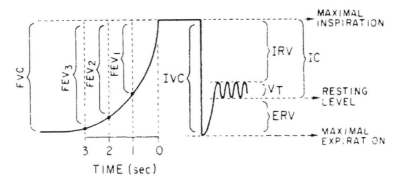

Fig. 2. Lung volumes and capacities measured by spirometry. IVC, inspiratory vital capacity; FVC, forced vital capacity; FEV_1, FEV_2, FEV_3, forced expiratory volumes in the first, second, and third seconds, respectively.

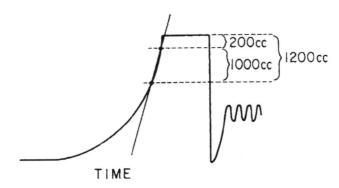

Fig. 3. Measurement of the forced expiratory flow from 200 to 1200 mL ($FEF_{200-1200}$). The expiratory flow rate is usually maximal after exhalation of the first 200 mL and before exhalation of the first 1200 mL of a forced expiration from a maximal inspiration.

($FEF_{200-1200}$) (*see* Fig. 3). Flow during the initial 200 mL of the FVC is slower than during the next liter of flow because the subject is overcoming chest wall inertia during the initial part of exhalation. The $FEF_{200-1200}$ and PEFR are useful measurements in patients with asthma who are trained to perform the forced expiratory maneuver properly. These measurements, however, are effort-dependent, and an untrained or unwilling subject may show marked variability in values on repeated efforts. Conversely, the measurements may increase with training independent of any improvement in the disease process.

The FEF from 25 to 75% of the total FVC ($FEF_{25-75\%}$) is sometimes used. It is less effort-dependent than $FEF_{200-1200}$, and thus is more reproducible. It is shown in Fig. 4. The volume of air expelled from point A in Fig. 5 (when 25% of the FVC has been expired) to point B (when 75% of the FVC has been expired) is measured, as is the time it takes to blow out the air from A to B. This gives a volume per unit time, which is a flow rate. One should be aware that comparison of separate $FEF_{25-75\%}$ measurements can only be made if the FVC on both tracings are approximately equal. This is because if one tracing has a smaller and thus incomplete FVC, the midpoint of flow is moved up to a point on the curve where flow is normally more rapid, resulting in a falsely higher $FEF_{25-75\%}$. This is shown in Fig. 5, where the solid-line tracing has a larger FVC than does the dashed-line tracing, but the initial flow rates are similar. The

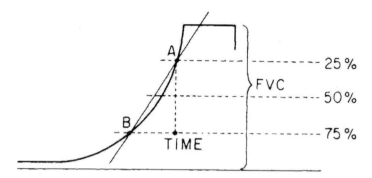

Fig. 4. Measurement of the forced expiratory flow from 25 to 75% ($FEF_{25-75\%}$) of the forced vital capacity (FVC). A and B represent the points where 25 and 75% of the FVC has been expelled. The line connecting these points forms the hypotenuse of a right triangle, of which one arm is volume and the other is time. Thus, the volume per unit time, or flow, during the middle 50% of the FVC can be measured.

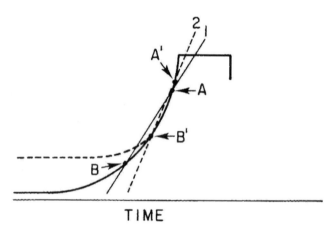

Fig. 5. Demonstration of an artificial increase in the forced expiratory flow from 25 to 75% ($FEF_{25-75\%}$) resulting from early termination of the forced vital capacity maneuver. A and B on the solid line tracing are the same as in Fig. 4. Line 1 connecting A and B is used to measure the $FEF_{25-75\%}$. The broken-line tracing is superimposed on and is identical to the solid-line tracing, except that the expiratory effort was prematurely terminated. Thus, A′ and B′ are on a steeper portion of the tracing and Line 2, which connects A′ and B′, demonstrates a more rapid $FEF_{25-75\%}$ than does Line 1. Actually, no change in flow rate has occurred. Thus, the $FEF_{25-75\%}$ cannot be used to assess bronchodilator response or patient improvement (or deterioration) unless the measured FVCs of the two studies being compared are within 5% of each other or unless the total expiratory times are similar.

major difference between the two tracings is that the dashed tracing represents an effort that was prematurely terminated. Thus, it has a steeper midportion because the slower terminal phase of a complete expiration has been eliminated. This results in a $FEF_{25-75\%}$ that is more rapid than is the value noted when exhalation has been maximal and complete. Yet when the two FVC curves are superimposed, the flow rates on both tracings are similar.

An example of what increasing degrees of airflow obstruction do to the appearance of the spirogram is shown in Fig. 6. Note that as the FRC increases (not measured by spirometry), the FEV_1 declines, and the expiratory time lengthens as the obstruction

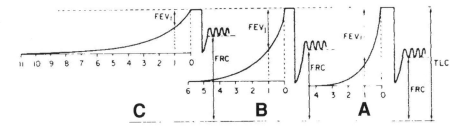

Fig. 6. Three spirometric tracings showing a normal curve (**A**), mild to moderate obstruction (**B**), and severe airflow obstruction (**C**). Although the functional residual capacity (FRC) cannot be measured by spirometry, this diagram includes this value to demonstrate the changes in this lung compartment as obstruction increases. Note that the forced expiratory volume in 1 s (FEV$_1$) decreases and the FRC increases with increasing degrees of airflow obstruction. The time it takes to complete the maneuver also increases. With severe obstruction (curve C), the FVC has decreased as well.

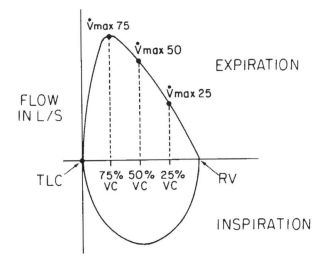

Fig. 7. Flow-vs-volume tracing. Expiration begins at the point of total lung capacity (TLC) and ends at residual volume (RV). Flow is measured at 75, 50, and 25% of the vital capacity (VC). V_{max25} = flow when 25% of the VC has been exhaled.

worsens. When severe obstruction is present, the FVC is often decreased. An increasing FRC will result in a decrease in the IRV, and thus the IRV can serve as a surrogate for the FRC.

Flow-volume tracings also allow the measurement of flow rates. Because most spirometers now have built-in electronics, the physician has the option of using either type of tracing or both simultaneously. An example of a flow-volume plot is shown in Fig. 7.

- The flow-vs-volume tracing relates flow rates to lung volumes.
- At high lung volumes, the cross-sectional area of the airways is increased, which reduces resistance and allows for higher flow rates.
- At lower lung volumes, the flow rates are more dependent on the frictional resistance in the smaller airways. When disease is present, other factors also influence the flow rates.

Using the flow-volume tracing, one can determine the flow rate at different lung volumes. At the point where 25% of the VC has been exhaled, or 75% is still in the lungs, the flow rate is termed the V_{max75}; when 50% of the vital capacity has been exhaled it is the V_{max50}, etc. However, the V_{max} values are of limited value (*see* below on this page).

The inspiratory portion of the curve is helpful in distinguishing a large airway obstruction that occurs above the level of the thoracic inlet from obstruction that occurs below this level. Large airway obstruction above the thoracic inlet results in a "plateau" of the flow rate on the inspiratory portion of the curve, whereas the expiratory portion is affected when the flow-limiting portion is within the thoracic cavity. At times, upper airway obstruction can be clinically confused with asthma (*see* page 57).

- The most useful measured flow rate taken from the spirogram is the FEV_1.
- The FEV_1 is typically reduced in patients with active asthma.

The FEV_1 is highly reproducible, and reference values derived from large normal population studies are available for patients of different ages and many ethnic and racial backgrounds. The usefulness of this measurement may be limited, however, when there is a poor start to exhalation. The FEV_1 may be artifactually altered because of uncertainty identifying the true start of exhalation. Back extrapolation may be required to determine the onset of exhalation. Nevertheless, this drawback is minor compared to the problems encountered with the other spirometric and flow-volume measurements.

The FVC is dependent on a complete exhalation, which may not occur, especially in patients with airflow obstruction. Essentially all subjects can produce a maximal effort for at least 1 s, so this is not a problem in the FEV_1 measurement. The difficulties in using the $FEF_{200-1200}$ and $FEF_{25-75\%}$ have already been discussed. The V_{max25} is believed to be sensitive when used to detect early airflow obstruction but suffers from having poor specificity; that is, it identifies too many normal subjects as being abnormal. Also, V_{max75}, V_{max50}, etc. are dependent on the actual volume of air in the lung rather than on the easily determined exhaled percentage of the VC. True lung volume is usually not known and may vary in its relation to that particular percentage of the FVC. Thus, the V_{max75}, etc. has a great deal of both intersubject and intrasubject variability.

Many pulmonologists find that the flow-volume loop is most useful in:

- Identifying upper airway obstruction where the inspiratory portion of the loop is flattened.
- Identifying poor patient performance, especially in the early phase of expiration. A poor start with a slow rise to the point of maximal flow, and an inadequate effort to produce the maximal flow can be recognized by the technician, who can then instruct the patient on how to produce a better tracing on the next effort. Many computer programs now have algorithms to assist the technician in identifying poor patient performance.
- The spirometric tracing (volume vs time) is best for evaluating the end of an FVC maneuver. A plateau should be achieved or at least set as a goal that the technician should try to get the patient to accomplish.

There are two classes of spirometers:

- Volume displacement. This type uses volume displacement of a bell or bellows to record the values. This may be in the form of a rolling seal or an inverted pail that rises and falls with inspiration and expiration.
- Integrated pneumotachometer. In this device, slight differences in pressure as exhaled air passes through a screen are measured and are electronically converted into volumes and flows.

The volume displacement type of spirometer has the advantage of maintaining its calibration from day to day without any adjustments. The disadvantages are that the equipment tends to be bulky and have moving parts that are apt to break down.

The integrated pneumotachometer has the advantage of being lightweight and without moving parts. The main disadvantage is the requirement for frequent calibration. There may be electrical drift. Also, moisture and/or particles may contaminate the screen. This can alter the pressure differences across the screen and result in falsely high values.

STATIC LUNG VOLUME MEASUREMENTS

Lung volume measurements can be useful in evaluating patients with asthma. At times, a bronchodilator response may not be evident by spirometry, but it may be demonstrated by a decrease in the RV and FRC. However, lung volume measurements are infrequently used clinically to evaluate a bronchodilator response. Because spirometry cannot measure TLC, FRC, or RV, lung volume measurements are necessary if the clinician wants to know these values. Lung volume measurements are static and, thus, will not demonstrate changes in flow rates. They do demonstrate the increases in lung volumes, especially in the RV, the FRC, and even the TLC, that may be the result of the airway obstruction. Repeat measurements performed after the use of an inhaled bronchodilator may show a decrease toward normal in these volumes.

There are two general types of lung volume measurements:

- Thoracic gas volume, which is performed in a body plethysmograph or by radiological techniques.
- Gas dilution lung volumes, which are determined by measuring the space of distribution of a tracer gas that does not cross the alveolar–capillary barrier, such as helium, neon, or methane.

Both of these two general methods are equally accurate in normal subjects. However, in the presence of airway obstruction, the gas dilution techniques may underestimate true lung volume resulting from the inhomogeneous distribution of the tracer gas in the lungs.

The radiological method of measuring thoracic gas volume can be measured in a physician's office using posterior–anterior and lateral chest radiographs (CXRs) (1). The method approximates thoracic lung volumes by estimating the volume of gas in the lobes of the lungs as a series of cylindrical ellipses and subtracting the volumes of ellipsoids that approximate the volumes of the heart and hemidiaphragms. The method requires manual measurements and estimates on physical radiographs. With the advent of filmless radiographic technology, automated measurements may be available in the near future. Because the radiographic technique measures the TLC, a VC measured (by spirometry) at the same time is necessary to determine the RV.

The body plethysmograph method is available in many hospitals in larger communities. Although the equipment is expensive, it has the value of providing measurements of airway's resistance (Raw). The reciprocal of Raw is airway conductance (Gaw). Raw and Gaw can be used to assess a response to therapy.

Gas-dilution lung volume measurements are available at most hospitals that have a pulmonary function laboratory. Usually, such a measurement is performed using a single-breath technique with a tracer gas (helium, neon, or methane) as the determination of the alveolar volume during a single-breath carbon monoxide diffusing capacity measurement (*see* "Diffusing Capacity"). There is also a commonly used rebreathing technique in which an indicator gas and its volume of distribution are measured. Washout of nitrogen from the lungs during 100% oxygen breathing is another gas-dilution technique. In this method, lung nitrogen is the indicator gas and it is collected and measured as it is displaced from the lung by 100% oxygen. Because 79% of the gas in the lung during normal breathing of room air is nitrogen, the volume of the lung can be determined using the amount of washed-out nitrogen plus corrections for the residual nitrogen in the lung and the quantity washed out of the blood.

Gas-dilution TLC measurements are less useful in measuring true lung capacity in patients with asthma than in patients without asthma because the tracer gas is not distributed throughout the lung homogeneously as a result of the airway obstruction present. This results in an underestimation of true TLC. Plethysmography is thus a better method of measurement, but with this technique, precaution must be taken to avoid overestimating true TLC. In patients with airway obstruction, pressures in the distal airways may not fully equilibrate with pressure at the mouth when the usual methodology is employed. This can lead to recording falsely large lung volumes. This can be prevented by having the subject perform the panting maneuver used in plethysmography at slow rates, e.g., less than 1/s (<1 Hz). Excessive gas volumes in the gastrointestinal tract may also contribute occasionally to a TLC overestimate.

- Raw and Gaw are sensitive, but not always specific, measures of airway obstruction.

The use of the body plethysmograph has the advantage of measuring Raw and Gaw and specific conductance (SGaw), which is Gaw divided by the thoracic gas volume at the point where Gaw is measured. These values are sensitive to changes in the larger airways and may demonstrate a bronchodilator effect not seen on routine spirometry. Thus, they may be helpful measurements in patients who are suspected of having asthma but with nondiagnostic routine spirometry. Although they are more sensitive measurements of airway obstruction and reversibility than the FEV_1, Raw, Gaw, and SGaw are, unfortunately, less specific.

DIFFUSING CAPACITY

- Single-breath carbon monoxide-diffusing capacity can help distinguish between asthma and other types of obstructive airway disease.
- The diffusing capacity may be erroneously decreased in patients who smoke because smoking elevates blood carbon monoxide tension.

The single-breath carbon monoxide diffusing capacity theoretically measures the ability of the lungs to transfer carbon monoxide from the alveoli to the hemoglobin in the circulating red blood cells. The results are reported as milliliters of carbon monoxide transferred per minute per mmHg pressure. The amount of carbon monoxide in the inspired gas is approx 0.3%. Its space of distribution and, thus, its alveolar partial pressure are determined by the addition of 10% helium (or neon or methane) to the gas mixture on the assumption that the carbon monoxide is distributed throughout the lungs in the same manner as is helium. After a 10-s breath-holding period at TLC, the exhaled gases are analyzed. Because essentially no helium crosses the alveolar capillary barrier, the ratio of $He_{expired}$ to $He_{inspired}$ is used to measure the alveolar volume, which, in people without obstructive airway disease equals the TLC. This ratio is the theoretical dilution of carbon monoxide before this gas crosses into the blood. The volume of carbon monoxide that crosses into the blood can, therefore, also be determined. Blood carbon monoxide tension is assumed to be 0, because the circulation is a "sink" for small amounts of carbon monoxide. Some care must be taken, however, because blood carbon monoxide tension can be elevated in patients who smoke. Details of the technique are available in pulmonary laboratory manuals.

ARTERIAL BLOOD GASES

Arterial blood gases are often useful in assessing the condition of a patient with asthma, especially during an acute episode. The technology for these measurements should be available in any hospital with an emergency room or where acutely ill patients are treated. Modern equipment should be able to provide accurate results within a few minutes from the time the arterial blood is collected.

QUALITY CONTROL

- Calibrated equipment, trained personnel, and adherence to published standard methods of pulmonary function testing are required to reliably diagnose and follow patients with asthma.

The value of any study is highly dependent on good quality control. Patient effort is a critical factor in most of these studies, and poor patient performance results in values that are difficult to interpret. Technicians in hospital-based pulmonary function laboratories must be trained to not only perform the various studies but also troubleshoot problems, identify poor patient performance and correct it, and accurately calibrate the equipment. Office spirometry also requires a well-trained technician and an accurate, periodically certified, calibration syringe for calibrating the spirometer if one is to be certain the values obtained are meaningful.

Recognized standards have been developed for obtaining spirometric measurements and diffusing capacity, and for calibrating the spirometer. Lung volume measurements require accurate calibration of the plethysmograph. In the gas-dilution technique, the helium meter must be linear. The diffusing capacity measurements require attention to technique and calibration of the meters. Arterial blood gas measuring instruments require frequent calibration checks for accuracy using blood or other solutions with known gas tensions.

Standardization of spirometry and diffusing capacity measurements have been developed by the American Thoracic Society and the European Respiratory Society, and have been accepted by others for use in both adult and pediatric studies (2–5). The references provided at the end of this chapter include currently used quality-control methods (6–8).

It is a good idea for each laboratory to have one or two permanent employees check their own values weekly so they can serve as the standard when questionable values are noted and thus can alert the laboratory that repairs may be indicated. These "standardmen" become indispensable should the laboratory decide to replace old equipment,

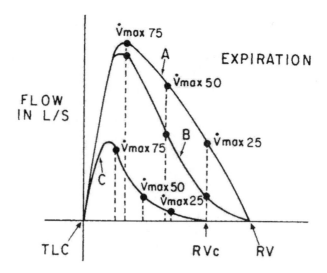

Fig. 8. A comparison of expiratory flow volume tracings in a normal subject (curve A), a subject with mild airflow obstruction (curve B), and in a subject with severe airflow obstruction (curve C). Note the decrease in the vital capacity in curve C, with the residual volume point (RVc) being shifted to the left. This indicates an increase in the RV. Also note in curve C that the points of V_{max25} and V_{max75} are shifted to the left and, thus, correspond to a different lung volume level than in curves A and B.

because they will be the determining factors in deciding if the new devices are comparable to the old equipment in providing accurate values.

PULMONARY FUNCTION MEASUREMENTS IN ASTHMA

Spirometry and Flow-Volume Studies

- The hallmark of airway obstruction is a decrease in the expiratory flow rates (*see* Figs. 6 and 8).
- The most useful single measure to follow is the FEV_1 because of its high degree of reproducibility.
- The degree of reduction of the FEV_1/FVC ratio is the standard method of categorizing the severity of airway obstruction.
- Maximal expiratory flow rates are frequently used to detect changes in asthma activity because they are easier to measure than FEV_1; however, the maximal expiratory flow rates are less reliable and can be manipulated relatively easily by patients.

In a subject with bronchospasm, a decrease in the rate of expiratory air flow is usually noted. In very mild disease, the study may be normal. The spirometric values that are most helpful are the FVC, FEV_1, and the ratio FEV_1/FVC. Using flow-volume tracings, the maximal expiratory flow rates, V_{max75}, V_{max50}, etc., are decreased. Usually in patients with asthma, some reversibility in these measurements of flow is noted after administration of a bronchodilator.

- The lack of a bronchodilator response may result from the patient taking medicine before the study and thus coming to the laboratory in a maximally bronchodilated condition.

The lack of response may also result from the refractoriness to the drug, or that the bronchospasm may be occurring in smaller airways and that lung volume measurements may be a more appropriate test. At times the measurement of Raw, Gaw, or SGaw may be more sensitive indices of bronchospasm.

- In some instances, a subject with asthma may have a decreased VC (Figs. 6 and 8).
- The degree of airway obstruction, as indicated by the FEV_1/FVC ratio, may artificially appear to be less severe in patients with a reduced VC.

Because the VC is a measure of one's ability to vary the size of the thoracic cavity, air trapping from obstructive mechanisms may limit thoracic excursions and cause a fall in VC. Airways that are physically blocked by inspissated mucous plugs or narrowed by bronchospasm may not conduct inspired air into the alveoli, resulting in a fall in VC.

- A decrease in the inspiratory flow rate suggests that the obstruction is in the central airways. Such a finding should make the clinician think of a diagnosis that may mimic asthma, such as paradoxical motion of the vocal cords or other diagnoses that can compromise the upper airways.

Lung Volume Measurements

Lung volume measurements in a patient with asthma may show an increase in the:

- RV.
- FRC.
- TLC.
- Patient with asymptomatic asthma may still have an increased RV.
- Increases in these measurements are indirect indicators of airway obstruction.

When lung volumes are measured by plethysmography, Raw, Gaw, and SGaw can also be determined; a change in these three values is a very sensitive measure of bronchodilator response. However, one should remember that changes in the FEV_1 are more specific and typically easier to measure.

Diffusing Capacity

- The single-breath carbon monoxide-diffusing capacity is sometimes increased in patients with asthma in contrast to patients with emphysema that have a reduced diffusing capacity.

The single-breath carbon monoxide-diffusing capacity is usually normal but sometimes increased in patients with asthma. Several explanations have been proposed for this supernormal value, the most plausible being an increased pulmonary capillary blood volume. This results from the more negative intrathoracic pressures generated during the 10-s breath-holding period that is part of the test performance. The more blood in the lung, the more hemoglobin is available to take up the inhaled carbon monoxide. Patients with advanced emphysema have a decrease in the single-breath diffusing capacity, so this is helpful in establishing a diagnosis in certain individuals. Anemia and an elevation in the carboxyhemoglobin can lower the measured value of the diffusing capacity. There are formulas that can correct the diffusing capacity for such abnormalities.

Arterial Blood Gas Measurements

- The arterial blood gas is not useful for diagnosing asthma.
- Arterial blood gases are a useful adjunct for identifying and following patients with respiratory failure resulting from asthma.

Table 1
Arterial Blood Gas Values in Patients With Asthma

Degree of severity	Oxygenation	PCO$_2$	Acid–base state
Mild	Relatively normal	Decreased	Compensated respiratory alkalosis
Moderate	Relatively normal to mildly decreased	Decreased	Compensated respiratory alkalosis
Severe	Marked decrease	Normal to elevated	Respiratory acidosis

- Arterial blood gas measurement is not a substitute for direct examination of a patient with potential respiratory failure.

Arterial blood gas values in subjects with asthma are shown in Table 1. In cases of mild asthma, the patient usually is able to maintain normal arterial blood oxygen tensions, although the alveolar–arterial gradient may be mildly increased. Hyperventilation is evident as the carbon dioxide tensions are decreased. The carbon dioxide tension is inversely proportional to alveolar ventilation. As airflow limitation worsens, the alveolar–arterial oxygen gradient widens and the oxygen tension falls. In severe disease, the patient can no longer maintain adequate alveolar ventilation and carbon dioxide levels start to rise. Thus, when the patient has a normal or elevated carbon dioxide level during an acute asthmatic episode, this is a sign of severe disease, because it is evidence that the body's need to eliminate carbon dioxide is not being met owing to a decrease in alveolar ventilation. It indicates that the patient should be considered for hospitalization and may be in need of ventilatory assistance.

INTERPRETATION OF RESULTS

The results obtained from the studies considered in this chapter must be compared with reference values to determine if an abnormality is present and, if so, the degree of that abnormality. Normal or reference values are available in the literature and are periodically superseded by more current studies. Ideally, every laboratory should develop its own normal standards, but this is not realistic. Recently published reference values only include subjects who are healthy lifetime nonsmokers (9,10). This is not the case in older series. Until recently, the better performed studies were done using Caucasians of European ancestry; thus, the data for other populations were either scant or less than optimal. Variations among different racial groups may exist and, thus, "normal" is less well-defined for these non-Caucasian populations. Recently, reference values for spirometry were published using the third National Health and Nutrition Examination Survey data that included 7429 asymptomatic lifelong nonsmokers of Caucasian, African-American, and Mexican-American ancestry (10). These reference values should prove helpful to many laboratories.

Normality is usually defined by convention as including 95% of a known healthy population. Thus, by definition, 1 in 20 people without any disease will have values outside this normal range. Widening the range of normal will include too many subjects with disease to make the standards useful. These problems make the term "reference values" preferable to saying "normal values." A detailed discussion and recommendations about selection of reference values and interpretative strategies have been made by the American Thoracic Society *(11)*.

There are few, if any, ideal studies of arterial blood gases in normal subjects. These results will be affected by altitude, the patient's age, and the position assumed by the subject when the sample was obtained. Reference values are available but will need revision as better studies are conducted. The reference list includes a manual with an approach for interpreting the results obtained by spirometry, lung volume measurements, diffusing capacity, and arterial blood gases *(6)*.

TESTS OF BRONCHODILATOR RESPONSE

When the presence of airflow limitation has been demonstrated, it is important to determine whether it is reversible. A therapeutic dose of a bronchodilator aerosol is given by inhalation after baseline spirometry is performed, and the measurement is repeated at an appropriate time (depending on the bronchodilator used, 5–20 min) after drug administration. Bronchodilator medications should be discontinued before testing for an appropriate time period to avoid their effects on the test results.

Choice of Bronchodilator

It is desirable to use a relatively short-acting β_2-specific bronchodilator, such as albuterol, that will act rapidly and lead to a near-peak response within 5–20 min. This will decrease the time between drug administration and the performance of the test. Some of the longer acting bronchodilators take more than 1 h to create a maximal response.

CRITERIA FOR DETERMINING A SIGNIFICANT BRONCHODILATOR RESPONSE

Table 2 provides an approach to evaluating a patient's response to an inhaled bronchodilator using spirometric values. The criteria presented are based on published studies of the responses of normal subjects to an inhaled bronchodilator and on the maximal differences noted after inhalation of a placebo. A patient should demonstrate improvement in the FEV_1 (or other measurement) that is more than 2 SDs beyond the mean improvement noted in normal subjects. The FEV_1 is, in most situations, the best measurement to use when considering the response to a bronchodilator. The FVC can be used only if the expiratory time during the postbronchodilator study is approximately equal to or is less than the prebronchodilator FVC expiratory time. Otherwise, any improvement could result from a longer period of expiration. The $FEF_{25-75\%}$ also can be used, but the range of the response in normal persons means that at least a 45% improvement must be seen before the bronchodilator response is considered significant. Also, as has been pointed out previously in this chapter on page 49 and Fig. 5, before the $FEF_{25-75\%}$ can be used to assess the response to a bronchodilator, the value for the FVC postbronchodilator must approximate the prebronchodilator value. Otherwise, the improvement noted could be the result of a shift in position of the middle 50% of the FVC to a steeper portion of the curve (Fig. 5).

Measurement of changes in Gaw before and after the inhalation of aerosolized isoetharine in 75 normal persons demonstrated a mean percentage increase (mean + SD) of 24.3 + 14.8. According to these data, normal persons may increase Gaw by as much as 53.9%, and, thus, changes exceeding this value are needed before the response is

Table 2
Spirometric Response After Bronchodilator

Category	Ratio of postbronchodilator/prebronchodilator (post/pre)		
	FVC[a]	FEV$_1$	FEF$_{25-75\%}$[b]
Markedly improved	>1.25	>1.25	>2.00
Improved	1.15–1.24	1.12–1.24	1.45–1.99
Not clearly improved	1.05–1.14	1.05–1.11	1.10–1.44
Not improved	<1.05	<1.05	<1.10

From ref. 6 with permission.

[a]Expiratory time post/pre must be less than 1.10; if not, then FVC cannot be used, because increased FVC might result solely from the increased expiratory time and not to increased flow.

[b]FEF$_{25-75\%}$ if expiratory time post/pre less than 0.90 and the FVC post/pre is not between 0.96 and 1.04, then the FEF$_{25-75\%}$ cannot be used, because reducing the expiratory time or the FVC can increase the FEF$_{25-75\%}$ in the absence of any change in flow itself.

considered significant *(12)*. Determining the therapeutic effect of a bronchodilator is more complex. Patients with low initial values may have a 15 or 20% improvement that may only be 50 or 75 mL. Such a change can result from the normal variability that can occur in repetitive studies. On the other hand, if the subject has large FVC and FEV$_1$, a 300-mL improvement may be less than a 10 or 15% change. Thus, the interpretation of prebronchodilator and postbronchodilator spirometry must always consider clinical information.

A study of the various spirometric tests and body plethysmographic measurements to evaluate the bronchodilator response of five different drug regimens concluded that the mean percentage improvement after administration of bronchodilators was greatest for the Gaw and the FEF$_{25-75\%}$. The FEV$_1$, however, statistically best differentiated among the five regimens because there is less inherent variability in measuring the FEV$_1$ than the FEF$_{25-75\%}$ or Gaw. This means that although the FEV$_1$ is a less sensitive test than the FEF$_{25-75\%}$ or Gaw, it is more specific *(13)*.

At times, a bronchodilator response may not be evident by spirometry but may be demonstrated by a decrease in the static lung volumes, such as the RV, FRC, and TLC, as shown in Fig. 9. This pattern of bronchodilator response is most apt to occur in severe disease *(14)*. When lung volume measurements are not available, watch the change in the slow VC (not FVC), because a concomitant change in a slow VC will be seen in most, if not all, of such cases.

The lack of bronchodilator response may result from the patient taking medication before the test, refractoriness to the drug used, or airflow obstruction owing to mechanisms other than bronchospasm, such as mucous plugs.

BRONCHOPROVOCATION CHALLENGE TESTING

- Bronchoprovocation challenge testing is nearly always positive in individuals with asthma; however, it is not specific and should not be the sole criterion for diagnosing asthma.
- The higher the dose of challenge agent inducing a positive response, the less specific the test.

Bronchial reactivity or responsiveness to various stimuli is a normal phenomenon in all individuals. When the degree of responsiveness exceeds that noted in normal subjects, it is

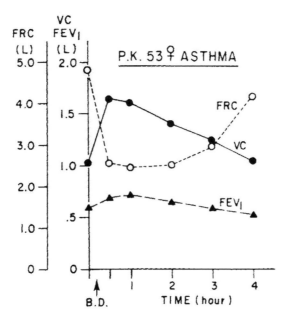

Fig. 9. A 53-yr-old female with chronic asthma. Note that after two inhalations of a short-acting bronchodilator, there is a marked reduction in functional residual capacity (FRC) as measured by body plethysmography and a concomitant increase in vital capacity (VC), with only minimal improvement in the forced expiratory volume in 1 s (FEV$_1$). She thus demonstrates a marked response to the bronchodilator despite the lack of a significant effect on the FEV$_1$.

termed *bronchial hyperresponsiveness* (BHR). BHR is noted in almost all people who have active asthma. However, this is not a specific test because increased bronchial responsiveness is noted in people with atopy, with congestive heart failure, in smokers, and in people with reduced lung function resulting from narrowed airways owing to any cause. BHR also may be seen for up to 8 wk after a viral upper respiratory infection and is more common in subjects with respiratory symptoms. In people with asthma, the degree of hyperresponsiveness is usually more marked than it is in other situations. A completely normal bronchoprovocation challenge test, with rare exceptions, excludes a diagnosis of active asthma. A positive test, especially if the patient responds to low doses of the challenge agent (a concentration of methacholine of <8 mg/mL), in the proper clinical setting, is helpful in diagnosing asthma in situations where the clinical picture is suggestive but not conclusive for making a diagnosis.

The agent used for bronchoprovocation challenge testing varies. For nonspecific challenges, the most commonly used agent in the United States is methacholine. In the United Kingdom and some other countries, histamine is preferred. Acetylcholine and other agents are sometimes used. The results obtained with histamine and methacholine are quite similar, and both are easy to use *(15)*. The test itself has only recently been standardized *(16)*, but many laboratories use their own methodology. However, this has not proved to be a great obstacle when comparing results from one laboratory to another. There are differences in the drug used, the way it is delivered, the timing of pulmonary function testing after drug delivery, the choice of pulmonary function test used, the manner of measuring the response, and the cutoff point for "normal" and "abnormal." For simplicity, use of the American Thoracic Society guidelines is recommended *(16)*.

Specific challenge testing is used to determine if a person has occupational asthma or asthma caused by specific antigens. There are no standardized methods for conducting these studies, and often it can be difficult to find the antigens in a form that is convenient and safe to use for these evaluations. The test is usually limited to situations where it is important to definitely know the cause of the patient's asthma, because this may mean a change in occupation, as well as workman's compensation considerations. It should be carried out in a negative pressure room vented to the outside to prevent sensitizing persons inside the building and to prevent exposure to those individuals who may already be sensitive to the agent. *See* Chapters 14 and 19 for a discussion of occupational asthma, disability, and legal issues for patients with asthma.

LABORATORY EVALUATION OF THE THERAPEUTIC REGIMEN

Pulmonary function testing is useful in:

- Determining the degree of the patient's impairment.
- The acute response to a bronchodilator.
- Overall evaluation of the effects of therapy.

Pharmacological agents, such as glucocorticoids, can make a patient feel much better by actions other than improving the asthmatic problem. Thus, without objective measurements (or, in selected patients, a careful physical examination of the chest), the physician may incorrectly believe that significant relief of bronchospasm has occurred, when this is not the situation. A lack of objective improvement in pulmonary function is an indication that the therapeutic regimen may need modification. With proper therapy, most people with asthma will demonstrate normal or close-to-normal pulmonary function. There are numerous individuals, however, who, despite optimum therapy, have to accept some degree of respiratory impairment. A decrease in expiratory flow rates that cannot be reversed suggests that airway remodeling has occurred as a result of chronic inflammation. If the objective tests indicate that the decrease is chronic and severe enough, the patient may be entitled to disability benefits *(17,18)*.

LABORATORY INDICATIONS FOR HOSPITALIZATION DURING AN ACUTE EPISODE OF BRONCHOSPASM

Pulmonary function testing can be an aid in determining when a patient in acute bronchospasm needs hospitalization. These are:

- Severe hypoxemia.
- Carbon dioxide retention.
- A marked decrease in FEV_1 to 1 L or less.

All the above are signs of a severe exacerbation and may be ominous signs. Unless the clinician can be certain these are chronic and not acute changes, these findings indicate that hospitalization is the safest treatment for the patient.

PROGRESSION OF DISEASE

Pulmonary function studies also can monitor the progression of obstructive lung disease. Although progressive airway obstruction is considered to be a sign of chronic obstructive pulmonary disease, including emphysema, there are patients with asthma who demonstrate this problem. In a few long-term studies of patients with chronic bronchitis and emphysema, a small number of subjects with asthma were included, and some of these had marked declines in lung function. These may represent a biased sample but at the same time serve as a warning to physicians that this phenomenon can occur. Periodic pulmonary function testing can identify these individuals, and possibly this accelerated decline can be reversed with more aggressive therapy.

REFERENCES

1. Harris TR, Pratt PC, Kilburn KH. Total lung capacity measured by roentgenograms. *Am J Med* 1971; 50: 756–763.
2. Gardner RM, Baker CD, Broennle AM, et al. ATS statement—snowbird workshop on standardization of spirometry. *Am Rev Respir Dis* 1979; 119: 831–838.
3. Crapo RO, Hankinson JL, Irvin C, et al. Standardization of spirometry. *Am J Respir Crit Care Med* 1995; 152: 1107–1136.
4. Crapo RO, Hankinson JL, Irvin C, et al. Single-breath carbon monoxide diffusing capacity (transfer factor), recommendations for a standard technique—1995 update. *Am J Respir Crit Care Med* 1995; 152: 2185–2198.
5. Miller MR, Crapo R, Hankinson J, et al. General Considerations for Lung Function Testing. *Eur Respir J* 2005; 26: 153–161.
6. Morris AH, Kanner RE, Crapo RO, et al. (eds.) *Clinical Pulmonary Function Testing: A Manual of Uniform Laboratory Procedures.* 2nd ed. Salt Lake City, UT, Intermountain Thoracic Society, 1984.
7. Conrad SA, Kinasewitz GT, George RB (eds.). *Pulmonary Function Testing. Principles and Practice.* New York, Churchill Livingstone, 1984.
8. Enright PL, Johnson LJ, Connett JE, et al. Spirometry in the lung health study: 1. Methods and quality control. *Am Rev Respir Dis* 1991; 143: 1215–1223.
9. Crapo RO, Morris AH, Gardner RM. Reference spirometric values using techniques and equipment that meet ATS recommendations. *Am Rev Respir Dis* 1981; 123: 659–664.
10. Hankinson JL, Odencrantz JR, Fedan KB. Spirometric reference values from a sample of the general US population. *Am J Respir Crit Care Med* 1999; 159: 179–187.
11. Becklake M, Crapo RO, Buist S, et al. Lung function testing: Selection of reference values and interpretative strategies. *Am Rev Respir Dis* 1991; 144: 1202–1218.
12. Watanabe S, Renzetti AD Jr, Begin R, et al. Airway responsiveness to a bronchodilator aerosol. *Am Rev Respir Dis* 1974; 109: 530–537.
13. Light RW, Conrad SA, George RB. The one best test for evaluating the effects of bronchodilator therapy. *Chest* 1977; 72: 512–516.
14. Woolcock AJ, Read J. Lung volumes in exacerbations of asthma. *Am J Med* 1966; 41: 259–273.
15. Juniper EF, Frith PA, Dunnett C, et al. Reproducibility and comparison of responses to inhaled histamine and methacholine. *Thorax* 1978; 33: 705–710.
16. Crapo RO, Casaburi R, Coates AL, et al. Guidelines for methacholine and exercise challengetesting—1999. *Am J Respir Crit Care Med* 2000; 161: 309–329.
17. Chan-Yeung M. Occupational asthma. *Chest* 1990; 98(Supplement): 148S–161S.
18. Chan-Yeung M, Harber P, Bailey W, et al. Guidelines for the evaluation of impairment/disability in patients with asthma. A statement of the American Thoracic Society. *Am Rev Respir Dis* 1993; 147: 1056–1061.

4 Treatment of Asthma in Children

Christopher Chang, MD, PhD

CONTENTS

KEY POINTS

- The incidence of asthma has increased dramatically during the past 20 yr, with the highest increases in the urban areas of developed countries.
- Asthma treatment goals in children include decreasing mortality and improving quality of life.
- Specific asthma treatment goals include decreasing inflammation, improving lung function, decreasing clinical symptoms, reducing hospitalizations and emergency department visits, reducing work or school absences resulting from asthma, and reducing rescue medication requirements.
- Nonpharmacological techniques that can help achieve asthma treatment goals include identification of asthma triggers, determination of environmental exposure to allergens and irritants, environmental control (including allergen avoidance), patient education, regular monitoring of lung function, and formulation of a complete asthma management plan.
- Achieving asthma treatment goals reduces direct and indirect costs of asthma and is economically cost-effective.

From: *Current Clinical Practice: Bronchial Asthma:*
A Guide for Practical Understanding and Treatment, 5th ed.
Edited by: M. E. Gershwin and T. E. Albertson © Humana Press Inc., Totowa, NJ

- A comprehensive asthma treatment plan should be formulated and customized for each child with asthma.
- Developing optimal technique in the use of metered-dose inhalers in children under 12 yr of age is difficult. Ongoing instruction and review may be necessary to ensure good technique. The use of spacers can help as well.
- Asthma is a chronic disease and is accompanied by the psychological burden of chronic illness. This may have an effect on the successful treatment of the child with asthma.

INTRODUCTION

The Global Initiative for Asthma (GINA), initiated in 1989 for the World Health Organization (WHO) and the US National Heart, Lung and Blood Institute (NHLBI) of the National Institutes of Health (NIH), released its 2004 Global Burden of Asthma report earlier this year (1) The prevalence of asthma is now estimated to be more than 300 million worldwide. The incidence in both children and adults has been increasing, especially in developed countries. This increase has been accompanied by an increase in atopic sensitization, as well as other clinical entities associated with atopy, including eczema and allergic rhinitis. Urbanization has been linked to the increase of asthma prevalence, but the reasons for this are still unclear, although theories abound. The prevalence of asthma for different countries is shown in Table 1.

Asthma is estimated to be responsible for 1 in every 250 deaths worldwide. Many of these deaths are preventable, and specific issues have been identified that may contribute to this high mortality rate. These issues include slow delivery of health care, poor environmental control of exposures (including allergens and environmental tobacco smoke [ETS]), dietary changes (2), genetic barriers, cultural barriers, lack of availability of medications, poor health care practitioner education, inadequacies in governmental resources, and failure to identify asthma as a public health problem. In addition to a high mortality rate, significant morbidity exists, and this is reflected by the high number of disability-adjusted life years (DALYs) lost as a result of asthma. Currently, this figure is approx 15 million per year.

The treatment of asthma in children has undergone significant progress in the past decade, with newer classes of medications and new formulations of existing medications being developed each year. However, the mortality rate of asthma has not decreased in the last two decades. On the contrary, there has been a significant increase in asthma mortality in some countries during that time period, and it is clear that pharmaceutical advances alone are not sufficient to successfully treat asthma. Therefore, the successful management of pediatric asthma involves the use of multiple therapeutic avenues, including patient education, environmental avoidance, awareness of the severity of the individual patient, proper use of medications, and immunotherapy.

GOALS OF ASTHMA THERAPY IN CHILDREN

The two primary goals in treatment of asthma in children are to decrease mortality and to improve quality of life. To achieve these primary goals requires that we meet smaller and more specific treatment goals. These goals are shown in Table 2 and are inclusive of the treatment goals of the GINA. Achieving these goals may be difficult if there is a lack of rapport between the physician and the patient. A favorable doctor–patient relationship

Table 1
Asthma Prevalence Data by Country

Country[a]	Prevalence of asthma[b]	Country[a]	Prevalence of asthma[b]
Scotland	18.5	Germany	6.9
Wales	16.8	France	6.8
England	15.3	Norway	6.8
New Zealand	15.1	Japan	6.7
Australia	14.7	Hong Kong	6.2
Republic of Ireland	14.6	United Arab Emirates	6.2
Canada	14.1	Saudi Arabia	5.6
Peru	13.0	Spain	5.7
Trinidad and Tobago	12.6	Argentina	5.5
Costa Rico	11.9	Chile	5.1
Brazil	11.4	Italy	4.5
United States	10.9	South Korea	3.9
Fiji	10.5	Mexico	3.3
Paraguay	9.7	Denmark	3.0
Uruguay	9.5	India	3.0
Israel	9.0	Cyprus	2.4
Panama	8.8	Switzerland	2.3
Kuwait	8.5	Russia	2.2
Ukraine	8.3	China	2.1
Ecuador	8.2	Greece	1.9
South Africa	8.1	Georgia	1.8
Finland	8.0	Romania	1.5
Czech Republic	8.0	Albania	1.3
Columbia	7.4	Indonesia	1.1
Turkey	7.4		

[a]Selected countries.
[b]Prevalence of asthma (% of population).
(Adapted from ref. *138*.)

Table 2
Specific Treatment Goals in Asthma

Reduction in mortality
Improvement in quality of life
    Fewer nighttime awakenings
    Ability to participate in sports
    Fewer work or school days lost
    Reduction of cough or wheeze
    Reduction in the need for rescue medications
    Easy compliance with medications with minimal disruption in daily life
    Reduction in side effects of asthma medications
    Reduction in number and severity of asthma exacerbations
    Reduction in emergency or urgent visits for asthma
    Reduction in the need for systemic steroids
    Prevention of "airway remodeling"

Table 3
Ancillary Treatment Modalities of Asthma

Asthma education
Peak flow monitoring
Pulmonary function testing
Allergy skin testing
Environmental exposure analysis
Asthma diary sheets
Asthma action plans
Allergen avoidance
Use of spacer devices
Exercise regimen
Asthma camps for children

is important to cement the patient's trust in the physician. Patient education for the child with asthma and his or her parents is imperative. It is important for the child to learn as he or she grows up that asthma is a chronic condition, and although the intensity may wax and wane, it is something that the child will have to address for a significant part of his or her lifetime. Recognition and acceptance of this is the first step toward implementing other supportive and preventive measures to improve clinical symptomatology and to reduce the frequency of asthma attacks, doctor's visits, and hospitalizations.

MANAGEMENT OF ASTHMA

The successful treatment of childhood asthma begins with identifying the child's clinical signs and symptoms and establishing the diagnosis. Once the correct diagnosis is made, triggers and exposure patterns must be identified and a plan that combines nonpharmacological and pharmacological aspects of the treatment must be provided to the patient. Nonpharmacological therapeutic modalities help to achieve the goals discussed in Table 2. Table 3 shows examples of ancillary therapeutic modalities.

MAINTENANCE THERAPY OF ASTHMA

Evaluation and Monitoring of the Disease State

CLINICAL PARAMETERS

Despite advances in medical technology, the diagnosis of asthma remains primarily a clinical diagnosis. In making the diagnosis, it is important to ask about cough (specifically nocturnal cough), wheezing, nighttime awakenings, duration and frequency of symptoms, associated allergy symptoms (such as nasal or ocular symptoms), and the need for bronchodilator and other medications. Although wheezing is the most common sign associated with asthma, other diseases in children can present with wheezing. In fact, wheezing is often confused with other breathing sounds, as in the case of stridor, transmitted upper airway sounds, snoring, and so on. A differential diagnosis of wheezing or "noisy breathing" is shown in Table 4. Other history that may help in establishing the diagnosis of asthma include family history, known triggers of symptoms, and exposure to allergens. Making the diagnosis can be facilitated by the use of chest radiograph (CXR), methacholine challenge testing, or spirometry before and after bronchodilator treatment.

Table 4
Differential Diagnosis of Cough, Wheezing, or Other
Abnormal Breathing Sounds

Asthma
Foreign body aspiration
Pneumonia
Smoke inhalation
Toxic inhalations
Bronchiolitis
Other infections
    Viral
    Bacterial
    Mycobacterial
    Fungal
Gastroesophageal reflux (cough)
Sinusitis (cough)
Hypersensitivity pneumonitis
Cystic fibrosis
Vocal cord nodules
Immunodeficiency syndromes
Subglottic stenosis (stridor)
Epiglottitis (stridor, respiratory distress)
Laryngotracheomalacia (in infants)

Once the diagnosis is established, treatment can be initiated. Both patient education and ongoing monitoring are important aspects of an asthma treatment program. The NHLBI and GINA have produced guidelines for the classification and treatment of asthma. These recommendations are shown in Table 5.

The "step" method of classifying asthma describes asthma as mild intermittent, mild persistent, moderate persistent, and severe persistent (3). All forms of the disease can involve airway inflammation and airway remodeling. The pathological features described by airway remodeling have not been defined (4), but they involve changes that can lead to irreversible damage in the airways. Features of airway remodeling have included changes in plasticity of airway smooth muscle, alterations in the mechanical properties of the airway wall, basement membrane thickening, and increase in submucosal gland area (5). Such changes can affect mortality rates, longevity, and quality of life, so it is imperative that airway inflammation be controlled. However, one cannot directly assess the extent of airway inflammation, at least not without bronchoscopy, so the identification of noninvasive surrogate markers may be an indispensable tool to monitor the success of anti-inflammatory treatment. Currently, there is no commercially available method to directly measure airway inflammation. The following two markers have been studied extensively and hold the promise for the future assessment of airway inflammation.

Nitric Oxide

Fractional exhaled nitric oxide (NO) is elevated in children with asthma (6). It has been demonstrated to be a marker of eosinophilic airway inflammation in children with asthma (7,8), and it also responds to glucocorticoid therapy (9). Measurement of fractional exhaled NO may be an effective way of monitoring airway inflammation and

Table 5
Modified National Heart, Lung, and Blood Institute Guidelines for the Diagnosis
and Treatment of Asthma

Diagnosis	Mild intermittent asthma	Mild persistent asthma	Moderate persistent asthma	Severe persistent asthma
Clinical features				
Nocturnal symptoms	<2/mo	<2/mo	>1/wk	Frequent
Use of β-agonist inhalers	Occasional	<2/wk	Daily use	Daily use
Peak expiratory flow	>80% predicted	>80% predicted	60–80% predicted	<60% predicted
Symptoms	<2/wk	>2/wk, but less than daily	Daily	Continual
Physical activity	No restrictions	May affect activity	Exacerbations affect activity	Limited
Treatment				
Anti-inflammatory agents	None	Low-dose inhaled steroids	Medium-dose inhaled steroids	High-dose inhaled steroids
		Cromolyn sodium or leukotriene pathway modifier	Cromolyn sodium or leukotriene pathway modifier	Cromolyn sodium, leukotriene pathway modifier, long-acting β-agonist (LABA)
Other control medications		None	LABA, anti-immunoglobulin (Ig) E	LABA, Anti-IgE
Quick-relief medications		Short-acting β-agonist	Short-acting β-agonist	Short-acting β-agonist

bronchial hyperresponsiveness *(10)*. However, currently, commercial use of this technique is still in the development phase.

Eosinophil Cationic Protein

Elevated eosinophil cationic protein (ECP) levels in cord blood is predictive of atopy. ECP is a marker of eosinophil activation. Serum ECP levels correlate with airway inflammation in wheezing children *(11)*. When patients with asthma are bronchial challenged with allergen, activation of eosinophils and secretion of specific eosinophilic mediators result. Evaluation and continued monitoring of eosinophil and ECP may be a way to assess efficacy of asthma therapy and airway inflammation in children with allergic asthma *(12,13)*. Both leukotriene receptor antagonists and inhaled corticosteroids (CSs) have been associated with a reduction in sputum ECP levels in patients with mild to moderate persistent asthma *(14,15)*.

Identification of Asthma Triggers

Asthma triggers are substances or conditions that can lead to a worsening of asthma. These can be inorganic, organic, or biochemicals derived from nonliving or living entities; high, low, or changes in surrounding temperature; exercise; infectious agents; postnasal drip or sinus drainage; or possibly even changes in stress level.

IRRITANTS AND ALLERGENS

Most of the chemicals that are identified as air pollutants are irritants. Irritants can be organic or inorganic compounds. The most familiar is ETS. Other gaseous irritants are NO, sulfur dioxide, formaldehyde, and other volatile organic compounds. Airborne particulates can also trigger an asthma attack. The particles may contain irritants or allergens. The smaller the particle, the greater the penetration into the airway. Particles greater than 10 μm in diameter are generally cleared in the upper airway. However, even large particles can trigger asthma by triggering early- or late-phase reactions by virtue of their contact with the upper airway. Irritants are believed to be universally injurious, whereas allergens will only affect sensitized individuals. Whether a child is sensitized to a particular allergen can be assessed by allergy testing. There are two ways to test for allergy testing. Allergy skin testing is performed by applying a small drop of allergen to the skin of the subject patient and then puncturing the skin with a short plastic hollow needle to introduce a small amount of allergen epicutaneously. Approximately 20–30 min after applying the test, the presence of a wheal-and-flare reaction is recorded. Comparison is made to a positive and negative control applied at the same time to determine sensitivity. Radioallergosorbent testing (RAST) is done by testing the patient's serum for immunoglobulin (Ig) E that is specific to various allergens. The most commonly used quantitative test is the Pharmacia-UniCAP system. The results are interpreted by comparing the raw data to specific reference values to allocate the results into various classes of reactivity, ranging from 0 to 6, with 0 being the most unlikely to be sensitized and 6 being the most likely.

Skin-Prick Testing vs RAST

Whether to select skin-prick testing or RAST as the preferred method to test for a patient's sensitivities depends on several factors. First to be considered is the sensitivity and specificity of the test. In general, skin testing is considered to be the preferred test because of its advantages in both sensitivity and specificity, by virtue of it being an in vivo test, whereas RAST is an in vitro test. Second, the age of the patient and the ability of the patient to undergo a prolonged procedure, such as skin testing, should be considered. If the child is too young to tolerate multiple skin pricks, then it may be preferable to limit the ordeal to a one-time blood draw. Sometimes, the child may tolerate skin-prick testing but may not tolerate intradermal testing. Another advantage of skin testing is that results are available immediately, because the wheal-and-flare reaction is measured from 20 to 30 min after application of the tests. Economically, skin testing costs less per test than RAST. Advantages of RAST include a less-traumatic experience, no risk of systemic reactions, and the ability to test patients who have skin conditions, such as hives or eczema, who would otherwise not be able to be skin-tested. RAST also provides the advantage that patients do not have to withhold their antihistamines before and during testing. Both skin testing and RAST can be employed in the evaluation of both environmental and food allergies. Food allergies may play a significant role in the development of atopy. Eczema is the most common presentation of atopy in infants, followed by asthma and allergies as the child gets older. Avoidance of

Table 6
Common Antigenic Determinants

Determinant	Source (common name)	Source (scientific name)
Der p 1	Dust mite	*Dermatophagoides pteronyssinus*
Der f 1	Dust mite	*Dermatophagoides farinae*
Der p 2	Dust mite	*Dermatophagoides pteronyssinus*
Der f 2	Dust mite	*Dermatophagoides farinae*
Der m 1	Dust mite	*Dermatophagoides microceras*
Blo t 1	Dust mite	*Blomis tropicalis*
Fel d 1	Cat	*Felis domesticus*
Can f 1	Dog	*Canis familiaris*
Bla g 1	Cockroach	*Blattella germanica*
Bal g 2	Cockroach	*Blattella germanica*
Rat n 1	Rat	*Rattus norvegicus*
Mus m 1	Mouse	*Mus Muscularis*
Per a 1	Cockroach	*Periplaneta Americana*
Lol p 1-5	Rye grass	*Lolium perenne*
Amb a 1-7	Ragweed	*Ambrosia artemistifolia*
Aln g 1	Alder	*Alnus glutinosa*
Bet v 1	Birch	*Betula verrucosa*
Que a 1	Oak	*Quercus alba*
Ole e 1 and Ole e 2	Olive	*Olea europea*
Cyn d 1	Bermuda grass	*Cynodon dactyilon*
Art v 1-3	Mug wort	*Artemisia vulgaris*
Dac g 1, Dac g 5	Orchard grass	*Dactylus glomerata*

certain types of foods in families where atopy is prevalent is beneficial in delaying the onset of allergic conditions. This is discussed later under "Avoidance of Allergenic Foods in the Infant."

SPECIFIC ALLERGENS

Environmental allergens can be divided into two groups: indoor and outdoor allergens. Indoor allergens include dust mites; cat, dog, and other pet danders; cockroach; and molds (16). The most prevalent of these is the dust mite. The incidence of asthma in children under the age of 5 yr correlates with exposure to high levels of dust mite (17). The primary protein determinants in dust mite have been identified and are mainly present in dust mite excrement. A list of common allergenic determinants is shown in Table 6. Cockroaches have been recently implicated as serious triggers of asthma exacerbations. Both early- and late-phase reactions have occurred in places where cockroach infestation is a problem, such as highly populated urban areas in warm climates (18). The most common of the pet allergens are dogs and cats, but small rodents, such as gerbils, hamsters, mice, rats, and guinea pigs, can also trigger an asthma attack.

Foods allergies can also trigger an asthma exacerbation. The most common allergenic foods in children are eggs, milk, soy, wheat, fish, peanuts, and citrus. Although food additives are not commonly allergenic, sulfites have been associated with severe asthma exacerbations (19).

INFECTIONS

Whether respiratory syncytial virus (RSV) infection in childhood leads to a higher incidence of asthma is debatable (20). An association has been found between prior

Table 7
An Exercise Challenge Protocol

1. Listen to patient's lungs for wheezing—chart observations.
2. Have the patient perform spirometry three times.
3. The patient then exercises for 6 min. The exercise should be enough to increase resting heart rate by 100%. Acceptable exercises include running (outdoor or indoor; treadmill is acceptable), jump rope, and swimming.
4. Immediately after exercise, listen to the patient's lungs (check for wheezing), and chart observations.
5. Have the patient perform spirometry once. If there is a decrease in forced expiratory volume in 1 s (FEV_1) of greater than 10% compared with the preexercise test, then proceed to step 9.
6. After 2 min, perform spirometry once. If there is a decrease in FEV_1 of greater than 10% compared with the preexercise test, then proceed to step 9.
7. After 5 min, perform spirometry again. If there is a decrease in FEV_1 of greater than 10% compared with the preexercise test, then proceed to step 9.
8. Listen to lungs for wheezing. If the patient is not wheezing and is not experiencing any chest tightness and if the FEV_1 did not at any time drop 10% compared with preexercise levels, this is a negative test.
9. Administer a unit-dose albuterol nebulization treatment.
10. After completion of the treatment, wait 5 min and then repeat spirometry three times.

lower respiratory tract illness with wheezing and current asthma *(21)*. Bronchiolitis in infancy may lead to decreased forced expiratory volume in 1 s (FEV_1) and $FEV_{25\%-75\%}$ in childhood, when compared with a control group of children who did not have bronchiolitis as infants *(22)*. In addition, elevated ECP and leukotriene C4 have been detected in the nasal lavage fluid of infants with RSV bronchiolitis *(23)*, suggesting perhaps a common mechanism between RSV bronchiolitis and asthma. However, it is not clear whether the development of airway inflammation in later years is triggered by the initial episode of bronchiolitis, although one prospective study of 47 children who were hospitalized for RSV bronchiolitis showed a higher incidence of airway reactivity at age 13 yr when compared with 93 matched controls *(24)*. In addition to RSV infections, other viruses that are associated with asthma exacerbations in children include rhinovirus, influenza, and parainfluenza viruses. Rhinovirus is associated with the common cold and is the major pathogen associated with hospital admissions for asthma in children *(25)*.

Children who have allergic rhinitis frequently develop acute or chronic sinusitis as a comorbid condition. If the child also has asthma, the presence of sinusitis and postnasal drip may compromise the ability to clear an asthma attack *(26–28)*. Although antibiotics should be used judiciously, children with clinical sinusitis and an asthma exacerbation should be treated appropriately.

EXERCISE

Exercise is one of the most common triggers of an asthma exacerbation in children. However, exercise itself is essential to the physical and psychological development of all children. In fact, lack of exercise causes obesity, and obesity has been linked to increased asthma severity *(29)*. The first step in the management of exercise-induced asthma (EIA) is recognition of the condition. Diagnosis of EIA can be made by an exercise challenge test. A protocol for exercise challenge testing is shown in Table 7.

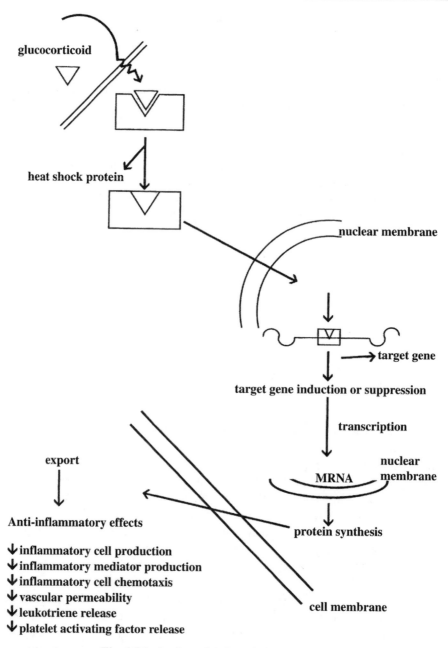

Fig. 1. Mechanism of action of glucocorticoids.

Pharmacological Options

CONTROLLER MEDICATIONS

Inhaled Corticosteroids

Inhaled CSs are the first-line medication for all forms of persistent asthma. CSs exert their action via regulation of protein synthesis. The mechanism of CS action in asthma is depicted in Fig. 1. There are five available CSs available in inhaler or nebulized form

Table 8
Daily Pediatric Doses of Inhaled Corticosteroids

Medication	Pediatric indication (age range)	Dose/ actuation (μg)	Dosing frequency	Mild persistent Number of actuations/ day	Moderate persistent Number of actuations/ day	Severe persistent Number of actuations/ day
Beclomethasone dipropionate as hydrofluoroalkanes inhaler	5–11 yr	40 80	bid bid	2	2–4 2	2
Triamcinolone acetonide	6–12 yr	100	bid to qid	4–8	8–12	8–12
Flunisolide	6–15 yr	250	bid	4	4	4
Budesonide	6 yr and older	200	bid	1	2	4
Budesonide for nebulizer	12 mo to 8 yr	Ampules of 250 or 500	bid	1 mg total daily dose	1 mg total daily dose	1 mg total daily dose
Fluticasone	12 yr and older	44 110 220	bid	2–4	4–10 2–4	4–8 2–4
Fluticasone rotadisk	4–11 yr	50 100 250	bid	2–4	1–4	2–4
Fluticasone dry powder inhaler (as component of Advair)	12 yr and older	100 250 500	bid	1–2	1–2	2–4 1–2

in the United States. These are beclomethasone dipropionate, triamcinolone acetonide, budesonide, flunisolide, and fluticasone propionate. All of the inhaled steroids can be used in the pediatric population. The dosages of inhaled steroids for mild, moderate, and severe persistent asthma are shown in Table 8. Budesonide is currently the only CS commercially available in nebulized form. Budesonide comes in two strengths of nebulizer solution, 0.25 and 0.5 mg. A multicenter study of 481 children demonstrated improvement in daytime and nighttime asthma symptoms when treated with nebulized budesonide (30).

The issue of adverse effects of inhaled steroids in children has been extensively studied. Steroids are associated with numerous side effects (see Table 9). In children with asthma, the major concerns has been the effect of inhaled CSs on growth (31–33). Studies to determine if inhaled CSs have such an effect are complicated because asthma itself is associated with growth retardation (34). Another limitation is the difficulty of correlating study data with real-life data. In the end, the bottom line is that even if there

Table 9
Adverse Effects of Asthma Medications

β-Agonists	Inhaled steroids	Systemic steroids	Anitcholinergics	Leukotriene pathway modifiers	Theophylline	Anti-immunoglobulin (Ig) E
Tremors	Dysphonia	Hyperglycemia	Dry mouth	Liver enzyme elevation	Gastritis	Anaphylaxis
Tachycardia	Oral thrush	Hypertension	Blurry vision	Churg-Strauss syndrome	Seizures	
Muscle spasms[a]	Growth retardation[a]	Osteonecrosis	Increased wheezing		Tremors[a]	
Hypokalemia	Adrenal suppression[a]	Osteoporosis			Insomnia	
Tachyphylaxis		Cushing's syndrome			Seizures	
Hyperglycemia		Adrenal suppression[a]			Nausea/vomiting	
Headache		Moon facies[a]			Tachycardia	
Hyperactivity[a]		Gastritis[a]			Hypokalemia	
		Psychological disturbances[a]			Hypoglycemia	
		Acne[a]			Central nervous system stimulation	
		Cataracts			Headache	
		Hirsutism[a]			Hyperactivity[a]	
		Decreased platelet function				
		Growth retardation[a]				

[a]Of particular importance in children.

is an effect of inhaled CSs on growth, the effect is minimal and certainly not worth compromising asthma care over a desire to be minimally taller. Adrenal suppression in children on inhaled steroids is not a significant problem, at least in those children who are on recommended dosages of inhaled steroids. In a study of 14 children on a dry-powder beclomethasone dipropionate inhaler, there was no suppression of the hypo-thalamic–pituitary–adrenal (HPA) axis. The dose of beclomethasone was 12–25 µg/kg/d *(35)*. Other studies have also failed to demonstrate adverse effects on the HPA axis *(36,37)*. On the other hand, use of high doses of fluticasone causes HPA axis suppression *(38)*. It is not known if there is any clinical significance to these observed effects.

Metered-Dose Inhalers vs Small Volume Nebulizers

Metered-dose inhalers (MDIs) are convenient and portable, have a low incidence of side effects, and, therefore, have the best therapeutic ratio. MDIs are highly dependent on bronchial microcirculation to deliver medication to the distal pulmonary airways. However, nebulizers allow for successful drug delivery to be less dependent on patient technique *(39)*. The disadvantages of nebulization treatments include lack of portability, variability between manufacturers, bacterial contamination, and the need for alternating current (AC) electricity. Medications that can be administered in nebulized form include budesonide, albuterol, levalbuterol, cromolyn sodium, and ipratropium. A comparison of different inhaler devices is shown in Table 10. Because of the damage to the ozone layer by high concentrations of chlorofluorocarbons (CFCs), most traditional inhalers will eventually be replaced by hydrofluoroalkane (HFA) inhalers or by dry-powder inhalers.

Inhaler Technique

Poor inhaler technique can negate the beneficial effects of the medications contained in the inhaler. Figure 2 illustrates options and variations in the technique of administering inhaled medications in children. There are two suggested techniques for the use of an MDI, the closed- or open-mouth technique. Either method can be used. Studies comparing the two techniques have yielded equivocal results *(40,41)*. In the closed-mouth technique, the child holds the inhaler up to the lips, creating a seal. After exhaling, the child activates the inhaler while taking a slow deep breath. The advantage to this technique is that there is no leakage of medication. The disadvantage is that coordination must be perfect. In the open-mouth technique, the child holds the spacer away from the mouth. This simulates the use of a spacer device and helps to "slow down" the spray from the inhaler, so that the delivery of the droplets into the airway is rendered more aerodynamically favorable. One point to emphasize is that the breath that is used to draw in the droplets must be slow (i.e., low inspiratory flow rate). Spacers help to improve delivery of the drug by partially obviating the need for impeccable technique *(42)*. For the very young child, spacers equipped with a mask further help to improve delivery (Fig. 2). Currently, there are two categories of spacers commercially available. One is a fixed tube, whereas the other is a collapsible plastic container, which will make a squeaky sound if the inhalation is too rapid. It is frequently difficult for the clinician to know exactly how well an MDI is working in a child. Aside from direct observation of the child's technique, the clinician has often only clinical improvement or lack thereof on which to base his or her

Table 10
Comparison of Inhaler Devices

	CFC inhalers	HFA inhalers	Autoinhalers	Dry powder inhalers	Spacer devices	Nebulizers
Availability	Widespread	Less common	Uncommon	Increasing	Common	Widespread
Portability	Easy	Easy	Easy	Easy	Some are cumbersome	Difficult
Ease of use	Difficult	Difficult	No need for coordination	Need for adequate breath actuation	Improves effectiveness of metered-dose inhaler	No coordination necessary
Age range of use	5 yr and older	5 yr and older	4 yr and older	4 yr and older	4 yr and older with spacer only, 2 yr and older with mask	Any age
Available for	SABA LABA Corticosteroids (CSs) Cromolyn Nedocromil Ipratropium bromide	SABA Corticosteroids (beclomethasone)	SABA (pirbuterol)	LABA (salmeterol, formoterol) CSs (budesonide, fluticasone)	N/A	SABA Cromolyn Nedocromil Ipratropium bromide CSs
Cost	Expensive	Expensive	Expensive	Expensive	Expensive	Expensive
Comments	80% of dose deposited in oropharynx	More will be available as chlorofluoro-carbons become unavailable owing to the destruction of the ozone layer	Cannot be used with spacer	Dose lost if child exhales through device		

HFA, hydrofluoroalkanes; SABA, short-acting β-agonist; LABA, long-acting β-agonist; N/A, not available.

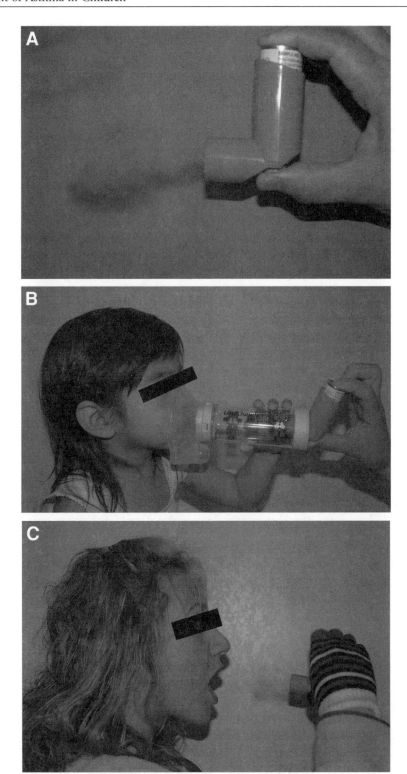

Fig. 2. Inhaler technique. (**A**) The aerosol stream from a hydrofluoroalkane inhaler. (**B**) A young child using an inhaler with spacer and mask, assisted by parent. (**C**) The "open mouth technique" without spacer. (**D**) *(opposite page)* The "closed mouth technique" without spacer.

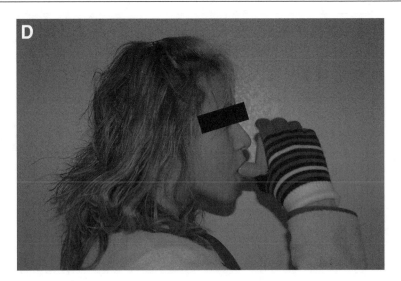

Fig. 2. *(Continued)*

assessment. Inhaler technique should therefore be continually reviewed with the patient, and the caregiver should observe and correct the patient's technique when appropriate.

Long-Acting Bronchodilators

Long-acting bronchodilators are used as combination therapy with inhaled CSs in the treatment of moderate to severe persistent asthma. The two available long-acting bronchodilators currently available are salmeterol xinafoate and formoterol fumarate.

Salmeterol xinafoate differs from short-acting β-agonists in the addition of a long hydrocarbon chain connecting the binding site and the active site of the molecule (*see* Fig. 3). Theoretically, this type of structure allows for repetitive interaction between the active site and the target receptor, while the binding site is firmly affixed to an alternate site on the cell membrane. Salmeterol is indicated down to age 4. The dose of salmeterol via MDI is two 21-µg puffs, taken twice daily. Salmeterol is also available as a dry-powder inhaler at a dose of 50 µg per puff twice daily. The terminal elimination half-life of salmeterol is 5.5 h. Previously, there was no indication for long-acting β-agonists in the treatment of acute exacerbations of asthma, but more recent studies from Europe have suggested that the use of long-acting β-agonists in mild asthma exacerbations, as well as asthma attacks, requiring hospitalization may be beneficial to the patient *(43)*. Salmeterol is available by itself in a Diskus dry-powder inhaler and also as combination therapy along with an inhaled CS in a Diskus. Formoterol is another long-acting bronchodilator with a safety profile superior to the short-acting β-agonists *(44)*.

Formoterol is available in a dry-powder inhaler form. The dry powder is contained in capsules, which must be punctured in an aerolizer device. A total of 12 µg of active drug is contained in each capsule. Formoterol is indicated for children 5 yr and older. An illustration of the differences in structure among the various β-agonists is shown in Fig. 3.

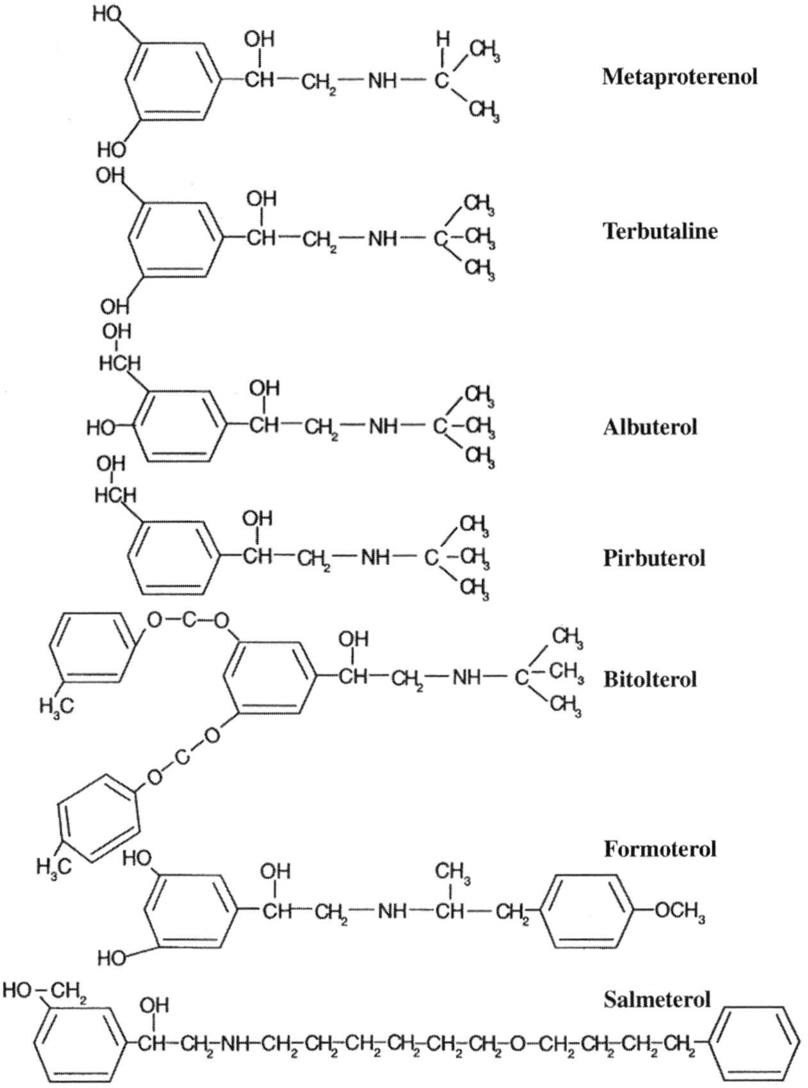

Fig. 3. Structure of the β-adrenergic agonists. Comparison of the structure of albuterol and salmeterol helps to explain the long half-life of salmeterol. The long chain connects the binding site to the active site of the molecule. The chain is theorized to swing back and forth, and allows the active portion of the drug to attach to the receptor site repeatedly, thus prolonging the action of the drug.

Leukotriene Pathway Modifiers

Leukotriene pathway modifiers originally were introduced in the early 1990s and consisted of two types, leukotriene receptor antagonists and inhibitors of leukotriene synthesis. Use of the latter group has not been widespread because of the inferior dosing frequency and high incidence of side effects. Leukotriene receptor antagonists have been particularly useful in the treatment of cough-variant asthma in children (45). Leukotrienes, prostaglandins, thromboxanes, and lipoxins are biologically active molecules belonging to the eicosanoid family. Leukotrienes LTC_4, LTD_4, and LTE_4 were previously collectively referred to as the slow-reacting substance of anaphylaxis (SRS-A).

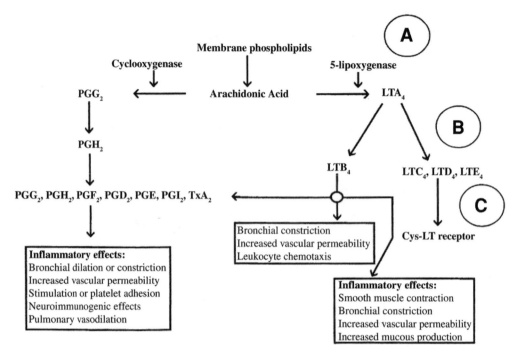

Fig. 4. Mechanism of action of leukotriene pathway modifiers.

Leukotrienes are derived from arachidonic acid, a component of membrane phospholipids, by the action of 5-lipoxygenase, via the intermediates hydroperoxyeicosatetraenoic acid and LTA_4. LTC_4, LTD_4, and LTE_4 share a common cysteinyl-leukotriene (cys-LT) receptor. LTB_4 occupies a different receptor, although it is also derived from LTA_4. The leukotriene pathway is illustrated in Fig. 4. As an inflammatory mediator in asthma, leukotrienes are 1000 times more potent than histamine *(46)*. Effects of LTC_4, LTD_4, and LTE_4 on human airways include increase in mucous production, constriction of bronchial smooth muscle, augmentation of neutrophil and eosinophil migration, increase in vascular permeability, stimulation of other inflammatory pathway mediators, and stimulation of monocyte aggregation. Figure 4 also illustrates the areas where the pathway may be regulated by pharmacological intervention.

Currently available leukotriene receptor antagonists include zafirlukast and montelukast. Newer leukotriene modifiers being investigated include pranlukast, BAY-7195 and genleuton. The latter is a 5-lipoxygenase inhibitor, whereas the others are leukotriene receptor antagonists. Side effects of leukotriene receptor antagonists are mild, with the exception of several reported cases of Churg-Strauss syndrome *(47)*. Churg-Strauss syndrome (allergic granulomatosis with angiitis) is a vasculitis associated with peripheral blood eosinophilia, an elevated serum total IgE, patchy pulmonary infiltrates, cutaneous purpuric lesions, and pleural effusions. The appearance of Churg-Strauss syndrome in patients with asthma who had been started on zileuton or zafirlukast have coincided with a concomitant decrease in steroid dosage. Whether these patients already had unrecognized Churg-Strauss syndrome that was controlled by steroid usage and that flared up when the steroid dosage was reduced is unknown. Both types of leukotriene pathway modifiers can affect the metabolism of theophylline, propranolol,

Table 11
Dosing Schedule for Omalizumab

a) Every 4-wk dosing pretreatment serum immunoglobulin (Ig) (IU/mL)	Body weight (kg)			
	30–60	>60–70	>70–90	>90–150
≥30–100	150	150	150	300
>100–200	300	300	300	
>200–300	300			
>300–400				
>400–500		See below		
>500–600				

b) Every 2-wk dosing pretreatment serum IgE (IU/mL)	Body weight (kg)			
	30–60	>60–70	>70–90	>90–150
≥30–100				
>100–200				225
>200–300		225	225	300
>300–400	225	225	300	
>400–500	300	300	375	
>500–600	300	375	Do not dose	
>600–700	375			

Adapted from Omalizumab package insert.

astemizole, calcium channel blockers, and some antiepileptics, because of their dependence on the cytochrome P450 3A4 pathway. Both zafirlukast and zileuton cause elevation of liver enzymes, although this has not been observed with montelukast. Currently, montelukast, with its safer drug profile, favorable dosing schedule, and multiple sample forms, is the only one still extensively used. Dose of montelukast is 4 mg per evening between ages 1 and 5, 5 mg per evening between ages 6 and 14, and 10 mg per evening in individuals 15 yr of age and older. Montelukast is available at various dosages in tablet, chewable tablet, and granule forms.

Monoclonal Anti-IgE

Omalizumab (Xolair®) is a recombinant DNA-derived humanized IgG1α monoclonal antibody. It binds selectively to human IgE. Binding of IgE by omalizumab inhibits both early- and late-phase reactions of asthma (48). Effects of omalizumab include a reduction in serum IgE levels and a decrease in allergen-induced bronchoconstriction (49). Omalizumab is indicated for patients 12 yr of age or older who have moderate to severe persistent asthma and whose asthma is triggered by year-round airborne allergens. Allergen-induced symptoms must be demonstrated by positive skin test or RAST allergy tests. Dosing of omalizumab is based on total serum IgE level and on body weight. A recommended dosage table is shown in Table 11. Xolair is administered subcutaneously once every 2–4 wk. Side effects observed with the use of Xolair include malignancies, anaphylactic reactions, and local injection reactions. In patients with allergic asthma, the high cost of Xolair can be potentially offset by the savings in costs of asthma exacerbations, e.g., hospital costs, outpatient emergency department visits, additional medications, and indirect costs *(50)*.

RELIEVER MEDICATIONS

Short-Acting Bronchodilators

β-AGONISTS. The mechanism of action of the β-agonists is through activation of the β_2-adrenergic receptors on airway smooth muscle cells, which leads to activation of adenylcyclase. This, in turn, leads to an increase in the intracellular concentration of cyclic adenosine monophosphate (cAMP). cAMP activates protein kinase A, causing inhibition of phosphorylation of myosin and lowering of intracellular calcium concentrations, which results in relaxation of bronchial smooth muscle. β_2-adrenergic receptors are present in all airways, from the trachea to the terminal bronchioles. Another effect of the increase in cAMP concentration is the inhibition of mediator release from mast cells. The availability of β-agonists, which exert their effect primarily on β_2-adrenergic receptors, such as albuterol, has made older, less specific β-agonists, such as metaproterenol or isoproterenol, obsolete. Adverse effects of β-agonists include paradoxical bronchospasm, cardiovascular effects, central nervous system stimulation, fever, tremors, nausea and vomiting, and unpleasant taste (*see* Table 9).

Various short acting β-agonists have been used over the years as rescue medications for asthma, including bitolterol, pirbuterol, Bronkosol, isoproterenol, and metaproterenol. But recently, the only one used on a regular basis has been albuterol. Dosing recommendations for short-acting β-agonist inhalers are shown in Table 12. Albuterol is administered at a dose of 0.083% nebulization solution. The dose of albuterol via MDI is 90 mg per puff, taken two puffs every 4 h as needed. Because β-blockers block the receptor sites for the action of β-agonists, they are contraindicated in children with asthma. β-blockers themselves are occasionally associated with worsening asthma *(51)*.

Recently, levalbuterol, a stereoisomer of albuterol, has been extensively used in nebulizers for bronchodilator therapy. Albuterol is actually a racemic mixture of the stereoisomers R-albuterol (levalbuterol) and s-albuterol. There are three available doses of levalbuterol, 0.31, 0.63, and 1.25 mg. Levalbuterol increases mean FEV_1 by 31–37% in children between the ages of 6 and 11 yr *(52)*. The elimination half-life of albuterol is 1.5 h, and that of levalbuterol is 3.3 h.

Oral β-agonists are also available for those who are unable to use an inhaler or who do not have a nebulizer. Oral albuterol is available in syrup form at a concentration of 2 mg/5mL or as a sustained-release 4-mg tablet. The dose of albuterol in children is 0.03–0.06 mg/kg/d in three divided doses (maximum dose 8 mg). Terbutaline is also available in 2.5 and 5 mg tablets. It is indicated for use in children over 12 yr of age.

ANTICHOLINERGICS. The mechanism of ipratropium bromide is through competitive inhibition of muscarinic cholinergic receptors, M2 and M3, which leads to decrease in airway vagal tone and decreased mucous gland secretion. Bronchoconstriction is also inhibited by anticholinergic agents *(53)*. Ipratropium bromide is administered by nebulization treatment (2.5 mL of a 0.02% solution = 500 µg or by MDI 18 µg/dose). Ipratropium bromide is not well absorbed from the lung or gastrointestinal tract. The elimination half-life of ipratropium bromide is 2 h when taken by MDI or administered intravenously. Ipratropium bromide is also available in combination with albuterol as an MDI. The dose of ipratropium bromide in the combination inhaler is also 18 µg per actuation.

Table 12

Characteristics of Inhaled or Nebulized Bronchodilator Preparations

Generic name	Dosage/inhalation or puff	Available delivery devices	Dosing frequency	Max puffs/day	Half-life (h)	Onset of action (min)	Time to peak effect (min)	Duration of action (h)
Albuterol	90 µg/puff or 250 µg per nebulization	MDI, D, N, C	2 puffs q4h prn	12	1.5	6	55–60	3
Levalbuterol	31, 63, or 125 µg per nebulization	N	1 tmt q8h prn	3 tmt/day	3.3	10–17	90	8
Metaproterenol	630 µg/puff or 15 mg/nebulization	MDI, N	2 puffs q4h prn	12	N/A	5–30	60–75	1–2.5
Pirbuterol	200 µg	MDI, A	2 puffs q4-6h prn	12	N/A	5	50	5
Bitolterol	370 µg	MDI, N	2 puffs q6h prn	12	N/A	3–4	30–60	5–8
Formoterol	12 µg	D	1 puff q12h	2	10	5	60	12
Salmeterol	25 µg	MDI, D	2 puffs q12h	4	5.5	10–20	45	12[a]
Ipratropium	18 µg/puff or 500 µg/treatment	MDI, C, N	2 puffs q6h prn	12	2	15	60–120	3–4

[a]Late-phase reaction may be inhibited up to 30 h.
MDI, metered-dose inhaler; A, autoinhaler; D, dry-powder inhaler; C, combination inhaler with other medication; N, solution for small volume nebulizer.

Table 13
Steroid Dose Equivalency

Scientific name	Dose equivalency (mg)	Half-life (h)	Comment
Cortisone	25	8–12	
Hydrocortisone	20	8–12	
Prednisone	5	12–36	Available in liquid or tablet form
Prednisolone	5	12–36	Available in liquid or tablet form
Methylprednisolone	4	12–36	Used in emergency departments or hospital care of asthmatics
Triamcinolone	4	12–36	
Paramethasone	2	36–72	
Dexamethasone	0.75	36–72	Generally used in croup in children
Betamethasone	0.6	36–72	

ORAL OR PARENTERAL STEROIDS.   With the development of newer, more effective medications, the need for systemic steroids in the treatment of asthma has decreased. This is particularly true for those children who previously required oral steroids as maintenance therapy. In the case of asthma exacerbations, short courses or "bursts" of oral and parenteral steroids are still used. As long as the total course of steroids is less than 7 d, no tapering of dose is necessary. A typical course of prednisone is 1–2 mg/kg/d for 5–7 d. If the course is longer than 7 d, tapering should be done gradually. Dosage equivalency for steroids is shown in Table 13. Oral steroids are available in tablet or liquid form. Liquid preparations of prednisone and prednisolone are available in concentrations of 5 mg/5 mL and 15 mg/5 mL, respectively, for children. The liquid forms of steroids are extremely unpalatable, and successful administration to children relies heavily on being able to disguise the taste.

Antihistamines and Asthma

First-generation antihistamines can cause sedation and drying of mucous membranes. Therefore, they are contraindicated in the treatment of acute asthma exacerbations.

Second-generation antihistamines, including fexofenadine, loratadine, desloratadine, and cetirizine, are distinct from older antihistamines in that the undesirable side effects of sedation and drying are significantly diminished. There is also less of an effect on cognitive performance with second-generation antihistamines. Second-generation antihistamines possess activity that may also be beneficial for patients with asthma. In addition to blocking the allergic effect of environmental allergens, cetirizine also decreases late leukocyte migration into antigen-challenge skin blister fluid chambers (54). All three inflammatory cell lines, including neutrophils, eosinophils, and basophils, were affected.

LESSER USED MEDICATIONS

Theophylline

Theophylline and aminophylline had their heyday in the 1980s, when almost every child with an asthma exacerbation that required hospital admission was started on an aminophylline drip. Similarly, most patients with asthma were placed on theophylline as maintenance therapy at that time. The use of this class of medication has decreased

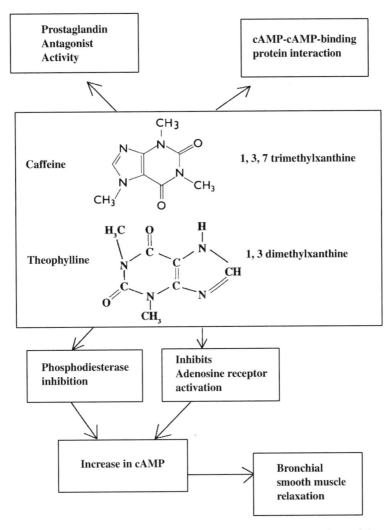

Fig. 5. Structure and bronchodilatory effects of theophylline and known actions of theophylline and caffeine. Actual mechanism for the bronchodilatory effect of methylxanthines is not completely understood. Phosphodiesterase inhibition seems to be the most obvious mechanism, but theophylline is known to have other areas of action, as shown.

significantly recently. Aminophylline is metabolized to theophylline, which is then metabolized to caffeine. Theophylline acts as a phosphodiesterase inhibitor. Its mechanism of action is illustrated in Fig. 5. As monotherapy, theophylline has had a comparable efficacy as inhaled steroids in improving symptom scores and pulmonary function test parameters *(55)*, but theophylline's side effects greatly exceed those of inhaled steroids, thus the shift away from the use of theophylline to treat asthma. Theophylline's side effects are shown in Table 9. Despite the undesirable effects of theophylline, there may still be a role for the use of theophylline as a steroid-sparing agent in patients with severe persistent asthma. Theophylline levels should be monitored regularly every 2–3 mo or more frequently if there are dosage changes or signs of any adverse effects. Theophylline is further discussed later as treatment for acute exacerbations of asthma in "Emergency Room (Outpatient) Treatment."

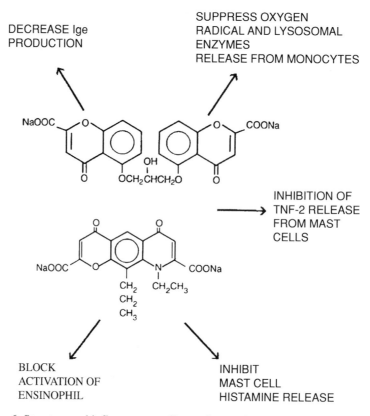

DECREASE Ige PRODUCTION

SUPPRESS OXYGEN RADICAL AND LYSOSOMAL ENZYMES RELEASE FROM MONOCYTES

INHIBITION OF TNF-2 RELEASE FROM MAST CELLS

BLOCK ACTIVATION OF ENSINOPHIL

INHIBIT MAST CELL HISTAMINE RELEASE

Fig. 6. Structure and inflammatory effects of cromolyn and nedocromil.

CROMOLYN AND NEDOCROMIL SODIUM

These two unrelated compounds have an excellent safety profile. Their chemical structures are illustrated in Fig. 6. Both are mast cell stabilizers, and both also inhibit the activation and release of inflammatory mediators from eosinophils. This appears to be mediated through blockage of chloride channels (56). Both early- and late-phase reactions to allergen challenge are affected by these two agents. Cromolyn sodium can be administered in either nebulized form or by MDI. The dose of cromolyn via MDI is 1 mg per actuation, whereas the dose of nedocromil is 2 mg per actuation delivered from the valve and 1.75 mg per actuation delivered from the mouthpiece of the inhaler. The dose of cromolyn delivered via nebulizer is 20 mg per treatment. The terminal elimination half-life of nedocromil sodium is 3.3 h. Nedocromil sodium is indicated in patients 6 yr of age and older. Cromolyn sodium is regularly used in very young children who are unable to use MDIs properly.

Because of the unfavorable dosing schedule, Cromolyn, a previously widely used medication, has given way to other inhaled or nebulized antiinflammatory medications, such as CSs. Nedocromil has an unpleasant taste and, along with Cromolyn, has fallen out of favor recently.

MUCOLYTICS

The use of mucolytics, such as *N*-acetylcysteine and *S*-carboxymethylcysteine, in childhood asthma is controversial. Mucolytics exert their action by breaking up the disulfide bonds between mucin chains and allow for easier clearance of mucous. On the other hand, they cause bronchoconstriction. Although animal studies have demonstrated that *N*-acetylcysteine can improve gas exchange after methacholine challenge *(57)*, there is currently no clinical indication for the use of mucolytics in the treatment of childhood asthma.

Pharmacological Treatment of EIA

Currently, short-acting β-agonists are widely used in the treatment of EIA, whereby the child takes two puffs of an inhaler immediately before exercise. This has the effect of shifting the stimulus response curve to the right. Inhaled albuterol or terbutaline provide relief for up to 1 h during exercise *(58)*. Other short-acting bronchodilators that have been used in EIA include fenoterol *(59)* and bitolterol *(60)*. Oral bronchodilators have provided longer relief, up to 6 h for albuterol *(61)* and 2–5 h for terbutaline *(62)*. Cromolyn and nedocromil protect against EIA for 120 and 300 min, respectively *(63,64)*. Theophylline has also been used in EIA *(65)*, but the narrow therapeutic window for this drug and the lack of benefit observed at lower doses have curtailed its use in EIA. The use of ipratropium bromide in EIA has not produced consistent results *(66)*. Controller medications that have played a role in preventing EIA include the long-acting bronchodilators salmeterol *(67,68)* and formoterol *(69,70)*, leukotriene receptor antagonists *(71–73)*, and inhaled CSs. Pediatric studies have also shown that leukotriene-receptor antagonists can offer partial protection against EIA *(74,75)*. The data on ketotifen *(76)*, calcium channel blockers *(77–79)*, and antihistamines *(80)* in the treatment of EIA is conflicting.

Nonpharmacological Modes of Therapy

ALLERGEN AVOIDANCE

It is clear from studies on allergen challenge that exposure to allergens to which a person is sensitized can bring about an asthma exacerbation *(81–83)*. When the offending allergen is removed from the patient's immediate environment, symptoms improve. Allergen avoidance has been recognized as a proven means to decrease asthma symptoms for centuries. To ensure that allergen avoidance is done in a clinically efficient and cost-effective manner, the patient's sensitivities and the environmental exposure pattern must be known. Once known, environmental control measures can be undertaken to decrease exposure. These measures are illustrated in Fig. 7.

Because of the time we spend sleeping (often one-third of our lives) and because dust mites tend to concentrate in mattresses, the bedroom should have the highest priority when outlining an allergen-avoidance program. Use of mattress and pillow encasings, high-efficiency particulate air (HEPA) filters, and reducing indoor relative humidity in the bedroom are all control measures that can be used to reduce dust mite exposure. HEPA filters are designed to filter 99% of particles down to 1 μm in diameter. HEPA filters can be standalone units or installed into existing heating, ventilation, and air-conditioning systems or may be components of vacuum cleaners. An additional defense against dust mite exposure is to wear a mask when vacuuming or cleaning the house. In addition to the generic surgical-type masks found in most hardware stores, some masks have built-in filters that protect against gaseous and particulate pollutants.

For those who are preparing to remodel or redecorate their home, replacing carpet with hardwood or linoleum (vinyl) flooring can make a significant difference in managing asthma or allergies. Blinds tend to harbor fewer dust mites than draperies; at the least, they allow for easier cleaning. Washing in temperatures above 130°F kills dust mites.

Dust mite
- Vacuum frequently
- Install allergen proof bedding and covers
- Use HEPA filter
- Buy only washable stuffed animals
- Use a damp cloth for dusting
- Keep indoor relative humidity less than 50%
- Store personal belongings in closed cabinets
- Wash bedding in water above 55°C
- Remodeling considerations
  - Remove carpets
  - Install hardwood floors
  - Remove heavy draperies
  - Install blinds

Pets
- Keep pets outdoors
- Remove pets completely
- Wash pets weekly
- Vacuum regularly
- Wash hands after contact with pet
- Keep pet off bed
- Cover the pet's bed with a washable sheet

Cockroaches
- Observe good hygienic practices
- Professional cleaning
- Insecticide bait
- Occupant education

Molds
- Circulate air
- Do not install carpeting directly onto damp floors or concrete
- Use a dehumidifier (clean and replace filters regularly)
- Remove house plants
- Select easily cleaning surfaces when remodeling kitchen
- Dry-clean carpets

Seasonal exposures (pollens)
- Plan vacations to low pollen areas or during low pollen seasons
- Stay indoors during periods of high aeroallergen seasons if possible
- Decrease early morning activity
- Wear a mask when mowing lawn
- Close car windows and use air-conditioning
- Exercise indoors during allergy season
- Do not hang linen outdoors to dry

Fig. 7. Avoidance measures for common allergens.

Avoidance of pet dander is best accomplished by getting rid of the animal. The emotional attachment that children and/or their parents and relatives have toward their pets often poses an insurmountable obstacle for the clinician attempting to achieve separation of the pet allergen and the patient. Washing the pet weekly helps to reduce exposure, but this must be done on regularly. Numerous denaturing sprays and cleaning agents are available, but their use is controversial. How often these sprays must be used and whether they sprays actually lead to an improvement on symptoms has not yet been determined.

Molds are common allergens that originate from the outdoor environment and are particularly prevalent in moist climates. If there is a high level of mold allergen indoors, when compared with outdoor levels, the more likely it is that there is a water leak or other source of indoor moisture. Keeping the humidity under 50% will reduce mold growth significantly. Substrates for mold growth include decaying living material, damp paper or books, household plants, and so on.

It is generally more difficult to avoid outdoor allergens, such as pollen grains, because these types of particles are wind-borne. It is therefore important for children and their parents to be aware of what their own sensitivities are, as well as what kind of pollens are prevalent in the environment at any given time. Common-sense measures dictate the response to this information. For example, if there is a high concentration of grass pollen and the child is known to be sensitive to grass, then the child should not increase his or her exposure by mowing the lawn. The importance of identifying environmental triggers is the reason that the National Allergy Bureau of the American Academy of Allergy, Asthma and Immunology (AAAAI) has initiated the certification of pollen-counting stations throughout the United States. Results of pollen counts from these certified locations are available on the AAAAI Web site.

AVOIDANCE OF ALLERGENIC FOODS IN THE INFANT

The question of whether avoidance of food allergens will also delay sensitization has been studied extensively. Prolonged breast-feeding decreases sensitization in high-risk children. Delayed introduction of solid foods accompanies prolonged breast-feeding. In a study of 2187 children followed from birth to 6 yr of age, non-breast-feeding increased the risk for developing allergies by 25% *(84)*. For those patients who already have a food allergy and who develop asthma symptoms when exposed to that food, avoidance is the only way to prevent an asthma exacerbation.

ASTHMA ACTION PLANS

Asthma action plans are drawn up to provide patients with instructions in the case of worsening symptoms or an asthma exacerbation. Asthma action plans contain information on a child's normal peak flow, regular medications, rescue medications that the child must have in his or her possession, and how to administer or take them. An example of an asthma action plan is shown in Fig. 8. Initially, recording symptoms and peak flow measurements on paper helps children and their parents keep better track of their disease. It may also help them to remember to take their controller medication. An example of an asthma diary is shown in Fig. 9.

PEAK FLOW METERS

Measurement of peak flow should be part of an asthma management plan. Peak flow measurements are an effective method to provide an objective assessment of the child's condition. Peak flow measurements should be done twice a day, in the morning before taking any medication and in the evening. Additional measurements should be done as necessary. Most new peak flow meters are small enough to fit in a pocket or a purse. Traditional peak flow meters come made for adult or pediatric peak flow ranges. The low range peak flow meters generally measure up to 450 L/m, whereas the high range measure up to 800 L/m. The peak flow zonal system for decision making in childhood asthma is a useful and simple method for the child or his or her parents to follow and should be a part of the asthma action plan. Data from peak expiratory flow measurements can help the child or parent decide when to give a nebulization treatment or when to seek professional help. There are electronic versions of peak flow meters as well, which can also hold data in memory. An assortment of peak flow meters and spacers is shown in Fig. 10

IMMUNOTHERAPY IN THE TREATMENT OF ASTHMA

Also referred to as hyposensitization, desensitization, or allergy shots, immunotherapy is effective in the treatment of allergic rhinitis and asthma. Studies done in children

An Asthma Action Plan developed for Name: _____ DOB: _____

Address: _____ Tel: _____ E-mail:_____

Date of diagnosis: _____ Age at diagnosis: _____

Asthma disease classification: mild intermittent   Persistent: mild   moderate   severe

Pulmonary function test done: _____ FVC: _____ FEV1: _____ PEF:_____

Personal best peak flow measurement: _____

Known triggers: Exercise   viral infections   allergies   other: _____

Allergic triggers   Action taken

Dust mite   _____

Cockroach   _____

Cat or Dog   _____

Mold   _____

Pollen   _____

❑   Measure peak flow twice daily
❑   Keep an asthma diary
❑   Take control medications as prescribed _____

Regular control medications: _____
                                      _____
                                      _____

Quick relief medications: _____
                                      _____

Asthma Exacerbation Management Plan

1. Awareness of increased exposure or condition which may lead to an asthma exacerbation
2. Evaluation of symptoms. a) Respiratory rate, b) Retractions, c) Mental status changes
3. Measure peak expiratory flow
4. Zonal system for evaluating asthma status

Green Zone – all clear No symptoms Normal daily activities Control medications effective	Peak flow above _____	Take regular control medications
Yellow Zone – action Increased symptoms Unable to perform certain tasks Increased use of β-agonist	Peak flow between _____ and _____	Increase inhaled steroid _____ to _____ puffs per day. Take b-agonist inhaler and measure peak flow. If improved, go to step 1. If not improved, repeat β-agonist, proceed to seek professional help
Red Zone – alert Symptoms > 24 hours Difficulty breathing Ineffective relief with β–agonists	Peak flow below _____	Add oral steroid _____ mg/day. Take β-agonist inhaler or nebulization treatment. If PEF remains low, proceed to seek professional help

Call 911 or proceed to hospital if danger signs occur, such as difficulty walking or talking due to respiratory distress or if lips or fingernails are blue.

Fig. 8. An asthma management plan. An asthma action plan must include information on how to assess the child. Known triggers should be listed and the PEF zonal system can be used to provide easy instructions for patients. The form also allows for entering medication dosages.

who were allergic to dust mite *(85)*, cat, dog *(86–88)*, mold *(89)*, grass *(90–92)*, ragweed *(93,94)*, olive *(95)*, and other allergens have demonstrated a beneficial effect of immunotherapy. Immunotherapy has been particularly successful in the treatment of younger patients. A study of 215 patients with dust mite allergy demonstrated that those patients with an FEV_1 greater than 90% were four times as likely to benefit from immunotherapy to house dust mite, when compared to patients with FEV_1 less than

Week 1							
Date							
	Sunday	Monday	Tuesday	Wednesday	Thursday	Friday	Saturday
Morning PEF							
Morning Sx*							
Afternoon PEF							
Afternoon Sx							
Nighttime PEF							
Nighttime Sx							
Use of β-agonists							
Regular medications							
New medications							
Exposures							
Comments							

Week 2							
Date							
	Sunday	Monday	Tuesday	Wednesday	Thursday	Friday	Saturday
Morning PEF							
Morning Sx							
Afternoon PEF							
Afternoon Sx							
Nighttime PEF							
Nighttime Sx							
Use of β-agonists							
Regular medications							
New medications							
Exposures							
Comments							

*Sx = symtoms

Fig. 9. Asthma diary sheets. A 2-wk record is a convenient period for patients to record their peak flow measurements and daily symptoms.

60%. Moreover, patients under the age of 20 yr were three times as likely to improve than those more than 51 yr of age (96). Indications for immunotherapy include clear evidence of symptom-exposure relationship, perennial symptoms, and inadequate control of symptoms with medications (3).

REFERRAL TO A SPECIALIST

It is a reality in the United States that most children with asthma receive their care from generalists and mid-level practitioners. However, despite most primary care physicians having the knowledge to treat asthma effectively, the current state of managed care medicine in the United States does not allow sufficient time for the primary care physician to formulate a comprehensive asthma treatment program, including instructions

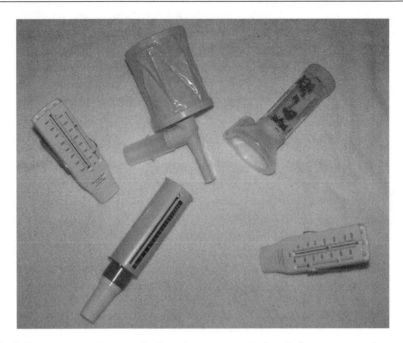

Fig. 10. Peak flow meters and spacer devises. An assortment of peak flow meters and spacer devices used in the management of asthma.

Table 14
Indications for Referral to a Specialist

- Children under 3 yr old with mild persistent, moderate persistent, or severe persistent asthma
- Patients who are receiving immunotherapy
- Patients with a history of a life-threatening asthma attack
- Patients who are not well controlled
- Patients whose symptoms are atypical or patients in whom the diagnosis has not yet been established
- Other complicating factors, such as chronic sinusitis, gastroesophageal reflux, chronic obstructive pulmonary disease, allergic rhinitis, nasal polyps, and aspergillosis
- Patients who require counseling or instructions on issues, such as compliance, environmental evaluation and control, medication usage, inhaler technique, or peak flow meter usage
- Patients who require systemic corticosteroids on a chronic basis or more than two steroid bursts in 1 yr
- Patients with exercise-induced asthma or other special circumstances
- Patients who require pulmonary function testing, rhinolaryngoscopy, skin testing, or other diagnostic procedures not routinely done by primary care providers

for asthma exacerbations, use of medicine, and overall patient education. The question frequently arises as to when a referral to a specialist is indicated. Obviously, a referral to a specialist should be made any time a primary care provider feels uncomfortable caring for the patient. Other indications may include referring for procedures that are not available to the patient under a primary care provider, such as spirometry or allergy skin testing. Table 14 provides a list of more specific indications for referral. An observed advantage of a referral to a specialist is that patients who are treated by a specialist tend to incur fewer hospitalizations, and this reduces overall economic burden of health care *(97)*.

EMERGENCY TREATMENT OF STATUS ASTHMATICUS

The management of an acute exacerbation of asthma can be divided into three separate phases, with a progressive increase in intensity of care. The first phase is management by the patient or in the case of a younger child, the parent, which usually begins in the home setting. If home management fails, the patient will present to an outpatient setting, which may be a doctor's office, an urgent care setting, or a hospital emergency department. If the patient's symptoms cannot be relieved in this setting, then further care may be indicated as an in-hospital patient. The earlier the recognition that an acute attack is occurring; the less likely the patient will require an escalation in care intensity. An algorithm outlining this procedure is shown in Fig. 11.

Home Management of an Acute Asthma Exacerbation

Home management begins well before an actual asthma exacerbation occurs. The patient must first be educated about his or her disease and must be prepared for the development of an asthma attack. Good adherence to controller medications and avoidance measures may help to prevent an attack. There is no better application of the adage, "An ounce of prevention is worth a pound of cure." Nevertheless, even with the most compliant of patients, optimal preventive care and the appropriate use of anti-inflammatory medications, asthma exacerbations will occur. Written instructions, in the form of the asthma action plans described, help the patient to remember how to recognize an imminent worsening of his or her asthma, as well as how to respond to such a scenario. Parents of younger children should supervise the asthma action plan and for school-aged children, school personnel, including school nurses, teachers, administrative staff, and coaches, should be instructed on the asthma action plan and how to adhere to it *(98)*. The patient and his or her parents or teachers should also be instructed on recognizing when to seek professional help. Having a nebulizer at home to deal with asthma episodes may help to decrease hospital visits and admissions, but there is also potential for abuse or overreliance on home nebulizers. Peak flow meters can be used to assist patients in determining the severity of their asthma exacerbation. The use of a peak flow meter in children and the zonal system is discussed under asthma action plans.

Emergency Room (Outpatient) Treatment

If home management fails, the child will present to his or her doctor's office or an urgent care setting. Frequently, the child may be experiencing an asthma episode for the first time, so the diagnosis must be made quickly and accurately, the severity of the episode assessed, and treatment initiated promptly. Clinical parameters used to evaluate an acute asthma exacerbation include heart rate, respiratory rate, use of accessory muscles, mental status changes, presence of cough or wheezing, pulsus paradoxicus, peak flow measurement, and pulse oximetry. Other causes of wheezing should be ruled out (Table 4). The diagnosis of many other conditions can be ruled out by radiographic

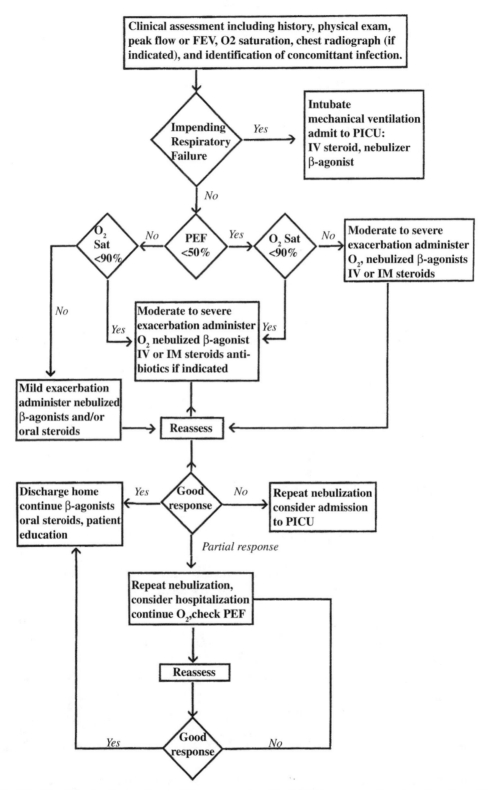

Fig. 11. Algorithm for the treatment of the acute asthmatic child. Emergency department and hospital care of the acute asthmatic child.

study. The CXR can also be useful in diagnosis other complications of asthma, including atelectasis or pneumothorax.

Once the diagnosis is made, outpatient treatment is initiated. A short-acting β-agonist, such as albuterol or levalbuterol, can be administered via small volume nebulizer. If there is time, measurement of peak flow or spirometry before and after the treatment can help to assess the effectiveness of the treatment, but one should not delay treatment if the patient's condition is serious. If the child is dyspneic, it is important to monitor vital signs and pulse oximetry. Parenteral steroids may be initiated for the moderate to severe asthma exacerbation. Methylprednisolone 1–2 mg/kg per dose can be given intravenously or intramuscularly. This can be continued every 6 h if the child requires admission. If the child's condition improves quickly and significantly, he or she may be able to be discharged home on a short course of steroids (prednisone 1–2 mg/kg/d) with close follow-up and detailed instructions. Measurement of peak expiratory flow and oxygen saturation should be done before sending the child home.

Subcutaneous epinephrine (1:1000) has been used in the treatment of the patient with acute asthma. The dose is 0.01 mL/kg to a maximum of 0.3 mL. This medication, although still important, is less commonly used because of the abundance of other medications with lesser side effects. Side effects of epinephrine include tremors, tachycardia, hypertension, neutrophil demargination, and cardiac stimulation.

The doses of emergency medications and the size of emergency equipment that is used in the pediatric population are summarized in Table 15. An intravenous line can be started in the emergency department in the case of severe respiratory distress or if the patient is dehydrated. Dehydration can result in drying up of bronchial mucous or electrolyte imbalances and should be corrected promptly. Concomitant infection, such as pneumonia or sinusitis, requires antibiotic therapy. Other medications that are used in the treatment of the patient with acute asthma include nebulized CSs, nebulized cromolyn, leukotriene-receptor antagonists, theophylline, and nebulized anticholinergic agents. Some of these are commonly viewed as maintenance medications, and some are not as widely used as before.

Currently, theophylline is much less commonly used in the treatment of an acute asthma exacerbation. However, if β-agonist nebulization is not effective in resolving respiratory distress, theophylline can be administered first as an intravenous bolus, then as a continuous drip. Once theophylline is started, the patient should be admitted. Each milligram per kilogram intravenous bolus of theophylline results in a 2 mg/dL rise in serum theophylline levels. The therapeutic window of theophylline serum levels is between 10 and 20 mg/dL. Thus, a theophylline bolus of 6 mg/kg typically results in a level well within the therapeutic window. An intravenous theophylline drip of 0.8 to 1 mg/kg per hour will usually result in a steady serum level. Theophylline levels must be monitored carefully because of the serious side effects that can occur at higher serum levels (Table 9). Another disadvantage of using theophylline is that multiple factors can affect theophylline metabolism, leading to variations in levels. These factors are shown in Table 16.

The use of leukotriene-receptor antagonists in the treatment of an acute asthma exacerbation has been reported (99). In a recent study of 201 patients, montelukast administered intravenously led to a significantly improved FEV_1 after 20 min when compared to patients who were given placebo (100). The effect lasted longer than 2 h, and patients

Table 15
Endotracheal Tube Sizes and Emergency Medication Doses in Children

		Emergency medication dosages			
Drugs		Epinephrine SQ	Epinephrine IV	Atropine	Sodium bicarbonate
Concentrations		1:1000	1:10000	0.1 mg/mL	0.5 mEq/mL (4.2%) for children under 3 mo, 1.0 mEq/mL more than 3 mo old
Age	Weight (kg)	Subcutaneous epinephrine	Intravenous epinephrine	Atropine	Sodium bicarbonate (volume in mL)
Newborn	3.0	0.03	0.3	1.0	6.0
1 mo	4.0	0.04	0.4	1.0	8.0
3 mo	5.5	0.055	0.55	1.1	11.0
6 mo	7.0	0.07	0.7	1.4	7.0
1 yr	10.0	0.1	1.0	2.0	10.0
2 yr	12.0	0.12	1.2	2.4	12.0
3 yr	14.0	0.14	1.4	2.8	14.0
4 yr	16.0	0.16	1.6	3.2	16.0
5 yr	18.0	0.18	1.8	3.6	18.0
6 yr	20.0	0.2	2.0	4.0	20.0
7 yr	22.0	0.22	2.2	4.4	22.0
8 yr	25.0	0.25	2.5	5.0	25.0
9 yr	28.0	0.28	2.8	5.6	28.0
10 yr	34.0	0.34	3.4	6.8	34.0

		Emergency equipment sizes			
Age	Weight (kg)	Self-inflating bag size	O_2 ventilation mask size	Endotracheal tube size	Laryngoscope blade size
Premature newborn	<2.5	Infant	Newborn small	<3.0	0
Newborn	2.5–4.0	Infant	Newborn	3.0–3.5	0–1
6 mo	7.0	Child	Child	3.5–4.0	1
1–2 yr	10–12	Child	Child	4.0–4.5	1–2
5 yr	16–18	Child	Child	5.0–5.5	2
8–10 yr	24–30	Child/adult	Small adult	5.5–6.5	2–3

in the treatment group received less β-agonist and had fewer treatment failures compared to the placebo group.

In-Patient Treatment

The decision regarding whether to admit the patient depends on several factors, the most important being the efficacy of outpatient therapy, the intensity of the outpatient therapy, and the duration. Clearly, the initiation of a theophylline drip, intubation, reduced oxygen saturation, and abnormal blood gas parameters are all indications for hospitalization. It is important not to wait until the child is in impending respiratory

Table 16
Factors and Drugs That Affect Theophylline Metabolism

Drugs	Effect on theophylline levels
Antibiotics	
Ketolides	Increase
Ciprofloxacin	Increase
Rifampin	Decrease
Macrolides: erythromycin, clarithromycin	Increase
Antiepileptics	
Phenobarbital	Decrease
Carbamazepine	Decrease
Phenytoin	Decrease
Other drugs	
Aminoglutethimide	Decrease
Disulfiram	Increase
Ticlopidine	Increase
Propranolol	Increase
Cimetidine	Increase
Allopurinol	Increase
Calcium channel blockers	Increase
Methotrexate	Increase
Diet	Increase/decrease
Obesity	Increase
Hypoxia	Increase
Smoking	Decrease
Viral illness	Usually increase
Pediatric and geriatric population	Usually increase

arrest before considering intubation because resuscitation is more difficult in children with respiratory failure. If intubation is necessary, blood gas measurements and chest radiography should be done to document successful intubation and proper tube placement.

When in the hospital, oxygen, nebulized or oral bronchodilators, parenteral steroids, and/or theophylline should be continued and the child's progress monitored closely. It may be necessary to monitor arterial blood gases or oxygen saturations using pulse oximetry. Dehydration sets in more easily in children than adults because of their greater body surface area to weight ratio and because of the inherently higher respiratory rate in children. Additional, concomitant infection can lead to fever, which can accelerate the onset of dehydration. Electrolyte imbalance can result from dehydration but also from the frequent use of albuterol nebulization treatments, so these must be monitored closely as well. Once the child has begun to recover, management can be focused on preparing for discharge. This would include switching the parenteral medications to oral forms, weaning of oxygen, increasing activity, reducing intravenous hydration rate, and advancing of diet.

The child will be discharged on a tapering dose of oral steroids and/or a nebulized or inhaled steroid. The child should also be discharged on a β-agonist administered via inhaler or nebulizer and any other additional and appropriate anti-inflammatory therapy. Close follow-up should be provided to monitor for relapse.

USE OF ACUPUNCTURE AND HERBAL MEDICATIONS IN THE TREATMENT OF ASTHMA

Patients in the United States spend more out-of-pocket money on alternative medicine than they do on traditional Western medicine. Acupuncture is effective in many disorders, including pain management, nausea, and vomiting. For asthma, however, studies have been inconclusive *(101–103)* The evaluation of homeopathic remedies for asthma has lead to similar results *(104)*.

PROGNOSIS OF CHILDHOOD ASTHMA

Although no one really "outgrows" his or her asthma (there is a significant genetic basis for asthma that cannot be excluded), many children will have variations in the severity of their disease during their lifetime. Indeed, there are environmental factors that may modulate the expression of the disease at various life stages. Hormonal factors may affect the clinical nature of the disease, and changes in the immune system as a result of new exposures to allergenic or nonallergenic environmental entities may lead to a change in a patient's asthma. In any case, as the child matures, he or she should be aware that asthma is an inflammatory disease and that years of chronic exposure to pollutants, irritants, and allergenic triggers may potential lead to a fixed obstructive disorder, whereupon clinical reversal of an asthma attack may become impossible.

Future Directions

NEW MEDICATIONS IN ASTHMA

Platelets

Platelet-activating factor (PAF) and prostaglandins are known mediators on airway inflammation. PAF has been associated with EIA and allergen-induced asthma. Inhibition of platelet activation diminishes the late-phase reaction of asthma *(105–107)*. Several medications currently used to treat asthma, including the glucocorticoids and ketotifen, normalize platelet survival times *(108)*. Platelets also secrete platelet factor 4 *(109)*, platelet-derived growth factor *(110,111)*, arginine-glycine-aspartic acid, thrombospondin, and transforming growth factor-α and -β *(112)*, all of which play a role in inflammation. Platelets also produce adenosine diphosphate, 5-hydroxytryptamine, thromboxane A2, 12-hydorxyeicosatetranoic acid, β-lysin, platelet-derived histamine-releasing factor, and platelet-derived histamine-releasing inhibitory factor, which may also play a role in airway inflammation. Platelets are thus themselves inflammatory and possess low-affinity receptors for IgE and IgG on their surface. Platelets also release adhesion molecules and secrete inflammatory cell chemoattractants, such as RANTES *(113)*. The anti-inflammatory agents cromolyn sodium *(114)* and nedocromil sodium *(115)* inhibit IgE-induced platelet activation. Cetirizine also has a similar effect *(116)*. Strategic manipulation of platelet-associated mediators may play a role in the future treatment of asthma in children.

CYTOKINES

Cytokines are biologically active molecules that can be secreted by or interact with inflammatory cells *(117)* and that regulate inflammatory cell recruitment, activation, and secretion of mediators. These molecules are classified as T-helper 1 (Th1) or Th2 (Th2) cytokines. Sometimes the differentiation is not clear. Primary Th2 cytokines, which favor airway inflammation, include interleukins (IL)-4, -13 *(118)*, and -5, and tumor necrosis factor-α. Th1 cytokines, whose function may inhibit airway inflammation, include IL-10 and -12, and interferon-γ. Table 17 shows the effect of cytokines on asthma. Ongoing research is being conducted involving several cytokines in the treatment of asthma *(119,120)*. Current studies have targeted modulation of the Th2-driven inflammatory process using solubilized IL receptors or antibodies to IL molecules *(117,120,121)*. Currently, there are no cytokine-related products commercially available to treat asthma.

OTHER NEW CLASSES OF MEDICATIONS

Targets for new treatment modalities in asthma include IgE, eosinophils, cytokines, chemokines, cell-signaling pathways, adhesion molecules, and inflammatory mediators *(122,123)*. Currently, phosphodiesterase-4 inhibitors *(124)*, peroxisome proliferators-activated receptor-γ agonists, nuclear factor κB, phosphoinisotide-3-kinase γ *(125)*, lipoxins, and p38 mitogen-activated protein kinase inhibitors are antiinflammatory drugs that are being investigated in the treatment of asthma *(126)*.

GENE THERAPY

There does not appear to be one single gene that controls an individual's predisposition to develop asthma or atopy. In contrast, asthma is polygenic *(127)*. Gene polymorphisms also may play a role in asthma and asthma severity *(128,129)*. Gene–gene interactions, as well as gene–environment interactions, also influence severity of asthma *(130)*.

New Advances in Immunotherapy

There are several ways to improve on the efficacy of immunotherapy. One way is to develop new techniques to administer traditional immunotherapy. Sublingual or oral immunotherapy has been studied with house dust mite extract, birch pollen, and grass pollen extracts, with some promise, and side effects were generally mild *(131)*. Potential side effects of sublingual immunotherapy include systemic reactions, angioedema, urticaria, or gastrointestinal symptoms *(132)*. In studies on children, sublingual immunotherapy has shown promise when used to treat dust mite and grass pollen allergy *(133–135)*. Nasal or inhaled routes of administering immunotherapy have shown promise in early studies *(136)*. Other developments include the use of peptide-based vaccines in immunotherapy *(137)*.

ECONOMIC IMPLICATIONS OF A COMPLETE ASTHMA MANAGEMENT PLAN

With the increase in prevalence of allergies and asthma has come an increase in healthcare costs. The average healthcare dollar spent per child with asthma is significantly higher than that of a child without asthma. Direct costs of asthma include pharmaceuticals, in-hospital costs, outpatient costs, the cost of procedures, and supplies, such as peak flow meters and spacer devices. Indirect costs of asthma include losses in productivity, school or workdays lost, cost of hiring additional care personnel, and so on. It is estimated that indirect costs from asthma are actually in the same order of magnitude as direct costs, each of which exceeds several billion dollars annually. The

Table 17
Cytokines Involved in Asthma

Cytokine	Effect	Related products under development	Results	References
Interleukin (IL)-1	Airway smooth muscle proliferation	None	N/A	
IL-2	Increases T-cell activation and expression of CD25 IL-2 receptors	None	N/A	
IL-3	Increases lifespan of eosinophils	None	N/A	
IL-4	Upregulation of immunoglobulin (Ig) E synthesis, Th2 lymphocyte differentiation, production of VCAM-1, effects low affinity CD23 IgE receptors	Soluble IL-4 receptors	Early studies promising	
IL-5	Stimulates differentiation and activation of eosinophils	Monoclonal antibody to IL-5	Blockage of eosinophils, reduces eosinophil numbers	140
IL-6	Downregulation of inflammatory cell infiltration and enhancement of airway remodeling	None	N/A	141
IL-8		None	N/A	
IL-10	Inhibits allergen-induced airway hyperresponsiveness and inflammation	None	N/A	
IL-12	Immunomodulatory cytokine, favors Th1 response	R-848	Reduces airway inflammation after allergen challenge	142,143

IL-13	Proinflammatory cytokine produced by T-cells	Anti-IL13	Antibody to IL-13 suppressed AHR, eosinophil infiltration, proinflammatory cytokine/chemokine production, serum IgE in mice	144
IL-18	Primarily Th1 cytokine, but can still be a promoter of airway inflammation	None	N/A	
IL-19	Function unknown, suggested that it may alter balance of Th1/Th2 cells in favor of Th2; Increases proportion of IL-4 producing cells	None	N/A	145
GM-CSF	Increase lifespan of eosinophils	None	N/A	
Interferon-γ	Increased production in asthmatics, though favors Th1 response	None	N/A	
Tumor necrosis factor (TNF)-α	Proinflammatory cytokine	Etanercept (decoy)	Blockade of TNF-α has shown some benefit	146
Metalloelastase	Reduction of levels of chemotactic factors and other proinflammatory cytokines	None	N/A	147
RANTES	Eosinophilic attractant	None	N/A	
CCR3	Eosinophil chemotaxis	CCR3 antagonists	Block eosinophil chemotaxis	
CXCR2	Neutrophil and monocyte chemotaxis	CXCR2 antagonists	Block neutrophil and monocyte chemotaxis	148

GM-CSF, granulocyte macrophage colony-stimulating factor.

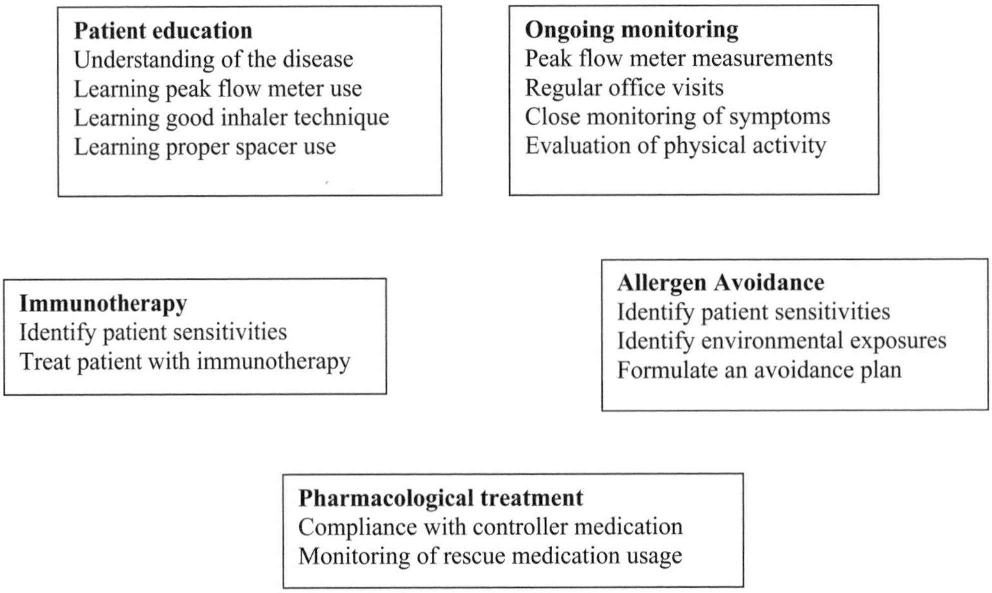

Patient education
Understanding of the disease
Learning peak flow meter use
Learning good inhaler technique
Learning proper spacer use

Ongoing monitoring
Peak flow meter measurements
Regular office visits
Close monitoring of symptoms
Evaluation of physical activity

Immunotherapy
Identify patient sensitivities
Treat patient with immunotherapy

Allergen Avoidance
Identify patient sensitivities
Identify environmental exposures
Formulate an avoidance plan

Pharmacological treatment
Compliance with controller medication
Monitoring of rescue medication usage

Fig. 12. A comprehensive asthma treatment program.

Table 18
Asthma Resources for Physicians and Patients

Asthma organizations	Internet links
American Academy of Allergy, Asthma and Immunology (AAAAI)	www.aaaai.org
American College of Allergy, Asthma and Immunology (ACAAI)	www.acaai.org
American Lung Association	www.lungusa.org
JAMA Asthma Information Center	www.ama-assn.org/special/asthma
American Thoracic Society	www.thoracic.org
Asthma and Allergy Foundation of America	www.aafa.org
National Technical Information Service	www.ntis.gov
National Asthma Education and Prevention Program	www.nhlbi.nih.gov/about/naepp/
National Heart, Lung and Blood Institute Information Center	www.nhlbi.nih.gov
National Jewish Medical and Research Center	www.njc.org
Allergy and Asthma Network/Mothers of Asthmatics	www.aanma.org

use of controller medications alone can reduce health care costs (138). Implementation of a comprehensive asthma treatment plan that includes both nonpharmacological and pharmacological remedies can further help decrease health care costs. Asthma education is an important part of a comprehensive asthma management plan. An abundance of information for both physician and patient is widely available on the internet. A sampling of these resources is shown in Table 18.

CONCLUSIONS

Our understanding of the pathogenesis of asthma as a primarily inflammatory disease has generated a gamut of improved medications to control and treat asthma in the past two decades. However, in developed countries, asthma mortality in children has not decreased during this time *(139)*. Ultimately, the primary goals of treatment should be to decrease mortality and to improve quality of life. To achieve this, therapy must focus on decreasing airway inflammation, improving asthma symptoms scores, reducing nighttime cough or nighttime awakenings, normalizing peak flows, decreasing missed school or work days, reducing the effect of asthma on daily activity (such as sports or school), reducing the need for emergency outpatient visits and hospital admissions, and reducing the need for rescue medications. These goals are achieved through integration of pharmacological and nonpharmacological modes of therapy. The components of such a comprehensive asthma treatment program are shown in Fig. 12. Nonpharmacological modes of therapy include identification of asthma triggers, identification of allergen exposures, patient education, monitoring of peak flows and symptoms, and an asthma action plan. Inhaled CSs are still the mainstay of controller therapy in all forms of persistent asthma. Other controller medications that can be added to inhaled CSs include long-acting bronchodilators, leukotriene-receptor antagonists, and monoclonal anti-IgE. In children, leukotriene-receptor antagonists are also beneficial in treating cough-variant asthma and EIA. The availability of nebulized CSs has improved outcomes in treating infants and toddlers with asthma. Everything possible should be done to ensure that the child can lead as normal a lifestyle as possible, including getting adequate exercise and being able to participate fully in sports.

REFERENCES

1. Masoli M, Fabian D, Holt S, Beasley R. The global burden of asthma: executive summary of the GINA Dissemination Committee report. *Allergy* 2004; 59(5): 469–478.
2. Chang CC, Phinney SD, Halpern GM, Gershwin ME. Asthma mortality: another opinion—is it a matter of life and bread? *J Asthma* 1993; 30(2): 93–103.
3. NHLBI. *Guidelines for the Diagnosis and Management of Asthma. Expert Panel Report 2*. National Institutes of Health, National Heart, Lung and Blood Institute. NBIH Publication 1997; 97: 4051.
4. James A. Airway remodeling in asthma. *Curr Opin Pulm Med* 2005; 11(1): 1–6.
5. Chen FH, Samson KT, Miura K, et al. Airway remodeling: a comparison between fatal and nonfatal asthma. *J Asthma* 2004; 41(6): 631–638.
6. Byrnes CA, Dinarevic S, Shinebourne EA, Barnes PJ, Bush A. Exhaled nitric oxide measurements in normal and asthmatic children. *Pediatr Pulmonol* 1997; 24(5): 312–318.
7. Mattes J, Storm van's Gravesande K, Reining U, et al. NO in exhaled air is correlated with markers of eosinophilic airway inflammation in corticosteroid-dependent childhood asthma. *Eur Respir J* 1999; 13(6): 1391–1395.
8. Warke TJ, Fitch PS, Brown V, et al. Exhaled nitric oxide correlates with airway eosinophils in childhood asthma. *Thorax* 2002; 57(5): 383–387.
9. Baraldi E, Azzolin NM, Zanconato S, Dario C, Zacchello F. Corticosteroids decrease exhaled nitric oxide in children with acute asthma. *J Pediatr* 1997; 131(3): 381–385.
10. del Giudice MM, Brunese FP, Piacentini GL, et al. Fractional exhaled nitric oxide (FENO), lung function and airway hyperresponsiveness in naive atopic asthmatic children. *J Asthma* 2004; 41(7): 759–765.
11. Shields MD, Brown V, Stevenson EC, et al. Serum eosinophilic cationic protein and blood eosinophil counts for the prediction of the presence of airways inflammation in children with wheezing. *Clin Exp Allergy* 1999; 29(10): 1382–1389.
12. Ahlstedt S. Clinical application of eosinophilic cationic protein in asthma. *Allergy Proc* 1995; 16(2): 59–62.
13. Bousquet J, Chanez P, Lacoste JY, et al. Eosinophilic inflammation in asthma. *N Engl J Med* 1990; 323(15): 1033–1039.
14. Perng DW, Huang HY, Lee YC, Perng RP. Leukotriene modifier vs inhaled corticosteroid in mild-to-moderate asthma: clinical and anti-inflammatory effects. *Chest* 2004; 125(5): 1693–1699.
15. Basyigit I, Yildiz F, Kacar Ozkara S, Boyaci H, Ilgazli A, Ozkarakas O. Effects of different anti-asthmatic agents on induced sputum and eosinophil cationic protein in mild asthmatics. *Respirology* 2004; 9(4): 514–520.

16. Chang CC, Halpern GM, Tam AY, Lau YL, Yeung CY. Evaluation of serum total IgE in Chinese allergic children using different assays. *Allergol Immunopathol (Madr)* 1992; 20(2): 51–56.

17. Polk S, Sunyer J, Munoz-Ortiz L, et al. A prospective study of Fel d1 and Der p1 exposure in infancy and childhood wheezing. *Am J Respir Crit Care Med* 2004; 170(3): 273–278.

18. Koh YY, Choi JW, Lee MH, et al. A preceding airway reaction to one allergen may lead to priming of the airway responses to another allergen. *Allergy* 1997; 52(3): 284–292.

19. Picado C. Classification of severe asthma exacerbations: a proposal. *Eur Respir J* 1996; 9(9): 1775–1778.

20. Kalina WV, Gershwin LJ. Progress in defining the role of RSV in allergy and asthma: from clinical observations to animal models. *Clin Dev Immunol* 2004; 11(2): 113–119.

21. Oddy WH, de Klerk NH, Sly PD, Holt PG. The effects of respiratory infections, atopy, and breast-feeding on childhood asthma. *Eur Respir J* 2002; 19(5): 899–905.

22. McBride JT. Pulmonary function changes in children after respiratory syncytial virus infection in infancy. *J Pediatr* 1999; 135(2 Pt 2): 28–32.

23. Dimova-Yaneva D, Russell D, Main M, Brooker RJ, Helms PJ. Eosinophil activation and cysteinyl leukotriene production in infants with respiratory syncytial virus bronchiolitis. *Clin Exp Allergy* 2004; 34(4): 555–558.

24. Sigurs N, Gustafsson PM, Bjarnason R, et al. Severe respiratory syncytial virus bronchiolitis in infancy and asthma and allergy at age 13. *Am J Respir Crit Care Med* 2004.

25. Johnston SL, Pattemore PK, Sanderson G, et al. The relationship between upper respiratory infections and hospital admissions for asthma: a time-trend analysis. *Am J Respir Crit Care Med* 1996; 154(3 Pt 1): 654–660.

26. Downey P, Cox R. Update on the management of status asthmaticus. *Curr Opin Pediatr* 1996; 8(3): 226–233.

27. Kraft M. The role of bacterial infections in asthma. *Clin Chest Med* 2000; 21(2): 301–313.

28. Nelson HS. Allergen and irritant control: importance and implementation. *Clin Cornerstone* 1998; 1(2): 57–68.

29. Akerman MJ, Calacanis CM, Madsen MK. Relationship between asthma severity and obesity. *J Asthma* 2004; 41(5): 521–526.

30. Mellon M, Leflein J, Walton-Bowen K, Cruz-Rivera M, Fitzpatrick S, Smith JA. Comparable efficacy of administration with face mask or mouthpiece of nebulized budesonide inhalation suspension for infants and young children with persistent asthma. *Am J Respir Crit Care Med* 2000; 162(2 Pt 1): 593–598.

31. Allen DB, Mullen M, Mullen B. A meta-analysis of the effect of oral and inhaled corticosteroids on growth. *J Allergy Clin Immunol* 1994; 93(6): 967–976.

32. Balfour-Lynn L. Growth and childhood asthma. *Arch Dis Child* 1986; 61(11): 1049–1055.

33. Balfour-Lynn L. Effect of asthma on growth and puberty. *Pediatrician* 1987; 14(4): 237–241.

34. Russell G. Childhood asthma and growth—a review of the literature. *Respir Med* 1994; 88 (Suppl A): 31–36; discussion 6–7.

35. Chang CC, Tam AY. Suppression of adrenal function in children on inhaled steroids. *J Paediatr Child Health* 1991; 27(4): 232–234.

36. Doull IJ, Freezer NJ, Holgate ST. Growth of prepubertal children with mild asthma treated with inhaled beclomethasone dipropionate. *Am J Respir Crit Care Med* 1995; 151(6): 1715–1719.

37. Goldstein DE, Konig P. Effect of inhaled beclomethasone dipropionate on hypothalamic-pituitary-adrenal axis function in children with asthma. *Pediatrics* 1983; 72(1): 60–64.

38. Boorsma M, Andersson N, Larsson P, Ullman A. Assessment of the relative systemic potency of inhaled fluticasone and budesonide. *Eur Respir J* 1996; 9(7): 1427–1432.

39. O'Connell E J. Optimizing inhaled corticosteroid therapy in children with chronic asthma. *Pediatr Pulmonol* 2005; 39(1): 74–83.

40. Chhabra SK. A comparison of "closed" and "open" mouth techniques of inhalation of a salbutamol metered-dose inhaler. *J Asthma* 1994; 31(2): 123–125.

41. Thomas P, Williams T, Reilly PA, Bradley D. Modifying delivery technique of fenoterol from a metered dose inhaler. *Ann Allergy* 1984; 52(4): 279–281.

42. Dubus JC, Anhoj J. Inhaled steroid delivery from small-volume holding chambers depends on age, holding chamber, and interface in children. *J Aerosol Med* 2004; 17(3): 225–230.

43. Hospenthal MA, Peters JI. Long-acting beta2-agonists in the management of asthma exacerbations. *Curr Opin Pulm Med* 2005; 11(1): 69–73.

44. Kaae R, Agertoft L, Pedersen S, et al. Cumulative high doses of inhaled formoterol have less systemic effects in asthmatic children 6–11 years-old than cumulative high doses of inhaled terbutaline. *Br J Clin Pharmacol* 2004; 58(4): 411–418.

45. Kopriva F, Sobolova L, Szotkowska J, Zapalka M. Treatment of chronic cough in children with montelukast, a leukotriene receptor antagonist. *J Asthma* 2004; 41(7): 715–720.

46. Taylor IK, O'Shaughnessy KM, Fuller RW, Dollery CT. Effect of cysteinyl-leukotriene receptor antagonist ICI 204.219 on allergen-induced bronchoconstriction and airway hyperreactivity in atopic subjects. *Lancet* 1991; 337(8743): 690–694.

47. Martin RM, Wilton LV, Mann RD. Prevalence of Churg-Strauss syndrome, vasculitis, eosinophilia and associated conditions: retrospective analysis of 58 prescription-event monitoring cohort studies. *Pharmacoepidemiol Drug Saf* 1999; 8(3): 179–189.

48. Buhl R. Anti-IgE antibodies for the treatment of asthma. *Curr Opin Pulm Med* 2005; 11(1): 27–34.

49. D'Amato G, Liccardi G, Noschese P, Salzillo A, D'Amato M, Cazzola M. Anti-IgE monoclonal antibody (omalizumab) in the treatment of atopic asthma and allergic respiratory diseases. *Curr Drug Targets Inflamm Allergy* 2004; 3(3): 227–229.

50. Gendo K, Lodewick MJ. Asthma economics: focusing on therapies that improve costly outcomes. *Curr Opin Pulm Med* 2005; 11(1): 43–50.

51. Lewis RV, Lofthouse C. Adverse reactions with beta-adrenoceptor blocking drugs. An update. *Drug Saf* 1993; 9(4): 272–279.

52. Gawchik SM, Saccar CL, Noonan M, Reasner DS, DeGraw SS. The safety and efficacy of nebulized levalbuterol compared with racemic albuterol and placebo in the treatment of asthma in pediatric patients. *J Allergy Clin Immunol* 1999; 103(4): 615–621.

53. Ihre E, Larsson K. Airways responses to ipratropium bromide do not vary with time in asthmatic subjects. Studies of interindividual and intraindividual variation of bronchodilatation and protection against histamine-induced bronchoconstriction. *Chest* 1990; 97(1): 46–51.

54. Charlesworth EN, Massey WA, Kagey-Sobotka A, Norman PS, Lichtenstein LM. Effect of H1 receptor blockade on the early and late response to cutaneous allergen challenge. *J Pharmacol Exp Ther* 1992; 262(3): 964–970.

55. Tinkelman DG, Reed CE, Nelson HS, Offord KP. Aerosol beclomethasone dipropionate compared with theophylline as primary treatment of chronic, mild to moderately severe asthma in children. *Pediatrics* 1993; 92(1): 64–77.

56. Alton EW, Norris AA. Chloride transport and the actions of nedocromil sodium and cromolyn sodium in asthma. *J Allergy Clin Immunol* 1996; 98(5 Pt 2): S102–S105; discussion S5–S6.

57. Ueno O, Lee LN, Wagner PD. Effect of N-acetylcysteine on gas exchange after methacholine challenge and isoprenaline inhalation in the dog. *Eur Respir J* 1989; 2(3): 238–246.

58. Campbell LM. From adrenaline to formoterol: advances in beta-agonist therapy in the treatment of asthma. *Int J Clin Pract* 2002; 56(10): 783–790.

59. Konig P, Hordvik NL, Serby CW. Fenoterol in exercise-induced asthma. Effect of dose on efficacy and duration of action. *Chest* 1984; 85(4): 462–464.

60. Walker SB, Bierman CW, Pierson WE, Shapiro GG, Furukawa CT, Mingo TS. Bitolterol mesylate in exercise-induced asthma. *J Allergy Clin Immunol* 1986; 77(1 Pt 1): 32–36.

61. Francis PW, Krastins IR, Levison H. Oral and inhaled salbutamol in the prevention of exercise-induced bronchospasm. *Pediatrics* 1980; 66(1): 103–108.

62. Sly RM, O'Brien SR. Effect of oral terbutaline on exercise-induced asthma. *Ann Allergy* 1982; 48(3): 151–155.

63. Debelic M, Stechert R. [Exercise-induced asthma—protection with disodium cromoglycate alone and in combination with fenoterol]. *Monatsschr Kinderheilkd* 1988; 136(8): 448–452.

64. Patel KR, Wall RT. Dose-duration effect of sodium cromoglycate aerosol in exercise-induced asthma. *Eur J Respir Dis* 1986; 69(4): 256–260.

65. Merland N, Cartier A, L'Archeveque J, Ghezzo H, Malo JL. Theophylline minimally inhibits bronchoconstriction induced by dry cold air inhalation in asthmatic subjects. *Am Rev Respir Dis* 1988; 137(6): 1304–1308.

66. Thomson NC, Patel KR, Kerr JW. Sodium cromoglycate and ipratropium bromide in exercise-induced asthma. *Thorax* 1978; 33(6): 694–649.

67. Green CP, Price JF. Prevention of exercise induced asthma by inhaled salmeterol xinafoate. *Arch Dis Child* 1992; 67(8): 1014–1017.

68. Newnham DM, Ingram CG, Earnshaw J, Palmer JB, Dhillon DP. Salmeterol provides prolonged protection against exercise-induced bronchoconstriction in a majority of subjects with mild, stable asthma. *Respir Med* 1993; 87(6): 439–444.

69. Boner AL, Spezia E, Piovesan P, Chiocca E, Maiocchi G. Inhaled formoterol in the prevention of exercise-induced bronchoconstriction in asthmatic children. *Am J Respir Crit Care Med* 1994; 149 (4 Pt 1): 935–939.

70. Daugbjerg P, Nielsen KG, Skov M, Bisgaard H. Duration of action of formoterol and salbutamol dry-powder inhalation in prevention of exercise-induced asthma in children. Acta *Paediatr* 1996; 85(6): 684–687.

71. Finnerty JP, Wood-Baker R, Thomson H, Holgate ST. Role of leukotrienes in exercise-induced asthma. Inhibitory effect of ICI 204219, a potent leukotriene D4 receptor antagonist. *Am Rev Respir Dis* 1992; 145(4 Pt 1): 746–749.

72. Makker HK, Lau LC, Thomson HW, Binks SM, Holgate ST. The protective effect of inhaled leukotriene D4 receptor antagonist ICI 204,219 against exercise-induced asthma. *Am Rev Respir Dis* 1993; 147(6 Pt 1): 1413–1418.

73. Robuschi M, Riva E, Fuccella LM, et al. Prevention of exercise-induced bronchoconstriction by a new leukotriene antagonist (SK&F 104353). A double-blind study versus disodium cromoglycate and placebo. *Am Rev Respir Dis* 1992; 145(6): 1285–1288.

74. Moraes TJ, Selvadurai H. Management of exercise-induced bronchospasm in children: the role of leukotriene antagonists. *Treat Respir Med* 2004; 3(1): 9–15.

75. Peroni DG, Piacentini GL, Ress M, et al. Time efficacy of a single dose of montelukast on exercise-induced asthma in children. *Pediatr Allergy Immunol* 2002; 13(6): 434–437.

76. Tanser AR, Elmes J. A controlled trial of ketotifen in exercise-induced asthma. *Br J Dis Chest* 1980; 74(4): 398–402.

77. Barnes PJ, Wilson NM, Brown MJ. A calcium antagonist, nifedipine, modifies exercise-induced asthma. *Thorax* 1981; 36(10): 726–730.

78. Foresi A, Corbo GM, Ciappi G, Valente S, Polidori G. Effect of two doses of inhaled diltiazem on exercise-induced asthma. *Respiration* 1987; 51(4): 241–247.

79. Patel KR. Calcium antagonists in exercise-induced asthma. *Br Med J (Clin Res Ed)* 1981; 282(6268): 932–933.

80. Zielinski J, Chodosowska E. Exercise-induced bronchoconstriction in patients with bronchial asthma. Its prevention with an antihistaminic agent. *Respiration* 1977; 34(1): 31–35.

81. Naclerio RM, Meier HL, Kagey-Sobotka A, et al. Mediator release after nasal airway challenge with allergen. *Am Rev Respir Dis* 1983; 128(4): 597–602.

82. Gelfand EW, Cui ZH, Takeda K, Kanehiro A, Joetham A. Fexofenadine modulates T-cell function, preventing allergen-induced airway inflammation and hyperresponsiveness. *J Allergy Clin Immunol* 2002; 110(1): 85–95.

83. Gelfand EW, Cui ZH, Takeda K, Kanehiro A, Joetham A. Effects of fexofenadine on T-cell function in a murine model of allergen-induced airway inflammation and hyperresponsiveness. *J Allergy Clin Immunol* 2003; 112(4 Suppl): S89–S95.

84. Oddy WH, Holt PG, Sly PD, et al. Association between breast feeding and asthma in 6 year old children: findings of a prospective birth cohort study. *BMJ* 1999; 319(7213): 815–819.

85. Turner MW, Yalcin I, Soothill JF, et al. In vitro investigations in asthmatic children undergoing hyposensitization with tyrosine-adsorbed *Dermatophagoides pteronyssinus* antigen. *Clin Allergy* 1984; 14(3): 221–231.

86. Hedlin G, Graff-Lonnevig V, Heilborn H, et al. Immunotherapy with cat- and dog-dander extracts. V. Effects of 3 years of treatment. *J Allergy Clin Immunol* 1991; 87(5): 955–964.

87. Hedlin G, Graff-Lonnevig V, Heilborn H, et al. Immunotherapy with cat- and dog-dander extracts. II. In vivo and in vitro immunologic effects observed in a 1-year double-blind placebo study. *J Allergy Clin Immunol* 1986; 77(3): 488–496.

88. Hedlin G, Heilborn H, Lilja G, et al. Long-term follow-up of patients treated with a three-year course of cat or dog immunotherapy. *J Allergy Clin Immunol* 1995; 96(6 Pt 1): 879–885.

89. Horst M, Hejjaoui A, Horst V, Michel FB, Bousquet J. Double-blind, placebo-controlled rush immunotherapy with a standardized Alternaria extract. *J Allergy Clin Immunol* 1990; 85(2): 460–472.

90. Frankland AW, Augustin R. Prophylaxis of summer hay-fever and asthma: a controlled trial comparing crude grass-pollen extracts with the isolated main protein component. *Lancet* 1954; 266(6821): 1055–1057.

91. Frankland AW, Augustin R. Grass pollen antigens effective in treatment. *Clin Sci* 1962; 23: 95–102.

92. Leynadier F, Banoun L, Dollois B, et al. Immunotherapy with a calcium phosphate-adsorbed five-grass-pollen extract in seasonal rhinoconjunctivitis: a double-blind, placebo-controlled study. *Clin Exp Allergy* 2001; 31(7): 988–996.

93. Johnstone DE. Study of the role of antigen dosage in the treatment of pollenosis and pollen asthma. *AMA J Dis Child* 1957; 94(1): 1–5.

94. Mirone C, Albert F, Tosi A, et al. Efficacy and safety of subcutaneous immunotherapy with a biologically standardized extract of Ambrosia artemisiifolia pollen: a double-blind, placebo-controlled study. *Clin Exp Allergy* 2004; 34(9): 1408–1014.

95. Gonzalez P, Florido F, Saenz de San Pedro B, de la Torre F, Rico P, Martin S. Immunotherapy with an extract of *Olea europaea* quantified in mass units. Evaluation of the safety and efficacy after one year of treatment. *J Investig Allergol Clin Immunol* 2002; 12(4): 263–271.

96. Bousquet J, Hejjaoui A, Clauzel AM, et al. Specific immunotherapy with a standardized *Dermatophagoides pteronyssinus* extract. II. Prediction of efficacy of immunotherapy. *J Allergy Clin Immunol* 1988; 82(6): 971–977.

97. Vollmer WM, Swain MC. Role of the specialist in the treatment of asthma. *Curr Opin Allergy Clin Immunol* 2002; 2(3): 189–194.

98. Sapien RE, Fullerton-Gleason L, Allen N. Teaching school teachers to recognize respiratory distress in asthmatic children. *J Asthma* 2004; 41(7): 739–743.

99. Ferreira MB, Santos AS, Pregal AL, et al. Leukotriene receptor antagonists (Montelukast) in the treatment of asthma crisis: preliminary results of a double-blind placebo controlled randomized study. *Allerg Immunol (Paris)* 2001; 33(8): 315–318.

100. Camargo CA Jr, Smithline HA, Malice MP, Green SA, Reiss TF. A randomized controlled trial of intravenous montelukast in acute asthma. *Am J Respir Crit Care Med* 2003; 167(4): 528–533.

101. Bielory L, Russin J, Zuckerman GB. Clinical efficacy, mechanisms of action, and adverse effects of complementary and alternative medicine therapies for asthma. *Allergy Asthma Proc* 2004; 25(5): 283–291.

102. Birch S, Hesselink JK, Jonkman FA, Hekker TA, Bos A. Clinical research on acupuncture. Part 1. What have reviews of the efficacy and safety of acupuncture told us so far? *J Altern Complement Med* 2004; 10(3): 468–480.

103. Davis PA, Chang C, Hackman RM, Stern JS, Gershwin ME. Acupuncture in the treatment of asthma: a critical review. *Allergol Immunopathol (Madr)* 1998; 26(6): 263–271.

104. Gyorik SA, Brutsche MH. Complementary and alternative medicine for bronchial asthma: is there new evidence? *Curr Opin Pulm Med* 2004; 10(1): 37–43.

105. Coyle AJ, Page CP, Atkinson L, Sjoersdma K, Touvay C, Metzger WJ. Modification of allergen-induced airway obstruction and airway hyperresponsiveness in an allergic rabbit model by the selective platelet-activating factor antagonist, BN 52021. *J Allergy Clin Immunol* 1989; 84(6 Pt 1): 960–967.

106. Knauer KA, Lichtenstein LM, Adkinson NF Jr, Fish JE. Platelet activation during antigen-induced airway reactions in asthmatic subjects. *N Engl J Med* 1981; 304(23): 1404–1407.

107. Lupinetti MD, Sheller JR, Catella F, Fitzgerald GA. Thromboxane biosynthesis in allergen-induced bronchospasm. Evidence for platelet activation. *Am Rev Respir Dis* 1989; 140(4): 932–935.

108. Szczeklik A, Schmitz-Schumann M, Krzanowski M, Virchow C, Sr. Delayed generation of thrombin in clotting blood of atopic patients with hayfever and asthma. *Clin Exp Allergy* 1991; 21(4): 411–415.

109. Hayashi N, Chihara J, Kobayashi Y, et al. Effect of platelet-activating factor and platelet factor 4 on eosinophil adhesion. *Int Arch Allergy Immunol* 1994; 104(Suppl 1): 57–59.

110. Deuel TF, Huang JS. Platelet-derived growth factor. Structure, function, and roles in normal and transformed cells. *J Clin Invest* 1984; 74(3): 669–676.

111. Ross R, Raines EW, Bowen-Pope DF. The biology of platelet-derived growth factor. *Cell* 1986; 46(2): 155–169.

112. Roberts AB, Sporn MB, Assoian RK, et al. Transforming growth factor type beta: rapid induction of fibrosis and angiogenesis in vivo and stimulation of collagen formation in vitro. *Proc Natl Acad Sci USA* 1986; 83(12): 4167–4171.

113. Kameyoshi Y, Dorschner A, Mallet AI, Christophers E, Schroder JM. Cytokine RANTES released by thrombin-stimulated platelets is a potent attractant for human eosinophils. *J Exp Med* 1992; 176(2): 587–592.

114. Tsicopoulos A, Lassalle P, Joseph M, et al. Effect of disodium cromoglycate on inflammatory cells bearing the Fc epsilon receptor type II (Fc epsilon RII). *Int J Immunopharmacol* 1988; 10(3): 227–236.

115. Thorel T, Joseph M, Tsicopoulos A, Tonnel AB, Capron A. Inhibition by nedocromil sodium of IgE-mediated activation of human mononuclear phagocytes and platelets in allergy. *Int Arch Allergy Appl Immunol* 1988; 85(2): 232–237.

116. De Vos C, Joseph M, Leprevost C, et al. Inhibition of human eosinophil chemotaxis and of the IgE-dependent stimulation of human blood platelets by cetirizine. *Int Arch Allergy Appl Immunol* 1989; 88(1–2): 212–215.

117. Palma-Carlos AG, Palma-Carlos ML, Santos MC, Melo A. Cytokines and adhesion molecules in respiratory allergy. *Allerg Immunol (Paris)* 1995; 27(6): 178–181.

118. Kioi M, Kawakami K, Puri RK. Mechanism of action of interleukin-13 antagonist (IL-13E13K) in cells expressing various types of IL-4R. *Cell Immunol* 2004; 229(1): 41–51.

119. Ricci M, Matucci A, Rossi O. New advances in the pathogenesis and therapy of bronchial asthma. *Ann Ital Med Int* 1998; 13(2): 93–110.

120. Barnes PJ. Cytokine modulators as novel therapies for airway disease. *Eur Respir J Suppl* 2001; 34: 67s–77s.

121. Kumar RK, Herbert C, Webb DC, Li L, Foster PS. Effects of anticytokine therapy in a mouse model of chronic asthma. *Am J Respir Crit Care Med* 2004; 170(10): 1043–1048.

122. Hansel TT, Barnes PJ. Novel drugs for treating asthma. *Curr Allergy Asthma Rep* 2001; 1(2): 164–173.

123. Donnelly LE, Barnes PJ. Acidic mammalian chitinase—a potential target for asthma therapy. *Trends Pharmacol Sci* 2004; 25(10): 509–511.

124. Spina D. The potential of PDE4 inhibitors in respiratory disease. *Curr Drug Targets Inflamm Allergy* 2004; 3(3): 231–236.

125. Barnes PJ, Hansel TT. Prospects for new drugs for chronic obstructive pulmonary disease. *Lancet* 2004; 364(9438): 985–996.

126. Belvisi MG, Hele DJ, Birrell MA. New advances and potential therapies for the treatment of asthma. *BioDrugs* 2004; 18(4): 211–223.

127. Immervoll T, Loesgen S, Dutsch G, et al. Fine mapping and single nucleotide polymorphism association results of candidate genes for asthma and related phenotypes. *Hum Mutat* 2001; 18(4): 327–336.

128. Kabesch M, Tzotcheva I, Carr D, et al. A complete screening of the IL4 gene: novel polymorphisms and their association with asthma and IgE in childhood. *J Allergy Clin Immunol* 2003; 112(5): 893–898.

129. Sandford AJ, Chagani T, Zhu S, et al. Polymorphisms in the IL4, IL4RA, and FCERIB genes and asthma severity. *J Allergy Clin Immunol* 2000; 106(1 Pt 1): 135–140.

130. Howard TD, Koppelman GH, Xu J, et al. Gene–gene interaction in asthma: IL4RA and IL13 in a Dutch population with asthma. *Am J Hum Genet* 2002; 70(1): 230–236.

131. Passalacqua G, Fumagalli F, Guerra L, Canonica GW. Safety of allergen-specific sublingual immunotherapy and nasal immunotherapy. *Chem Immunol Allergy* 2003; 82: 109–118.

132. Lombardi C, Gargioni S, Melchiorre A, et al. Safety of sublingual immunotherapy with monomeric allergoid in adults: multicenter post-marketing surveillance study. *Allergy* 2001; 56(10): 989–992.

133. Novembre E, Galli E, Landi F, et al. Coseasonal sublingual immunotherapy reduces the development of asthma in children with allergic rhinoconjunctivitis. *J Allergy Clin Immunol* 2004; 114(4): 851–857.

134. Bufe A, Ziegler-Kirbach E, Stoeckmann E, et al. Efficacy of sublingual swallow immunotherapy in children with severe grass pollen allergic symptoms: a double-blind placebo-controlled study. *Allergy* 2004; 59(5): 498–504.

135. TePas EC, Hoyte EG, McIntire JJ, Umetsu DT. Clinical efficacy of microencapsulated timothy grass pollen extract in grass-allergic individuals. *Ann Allergy Asthma Immunol* 2004; 92(1): 25–31.

136. Andri L, Falagiani P. Symptomatic relief after grass nasal immunotherapy: lasting efficacy after 4–5 years. *J Investig Allergol Clin Immunol* 2003; 13(4): 228–231.

137. Alexander C, Kay AB, Larche M. Peptide-based vaccines in the treatment of specific allergy. *Curr Drug Targets Inflamm Allergy* 2002; 1(4): 353–361.

138. Jonsson B, Berggren F, Svensson K, O'Byrne PM. An economic evaluation of combination treatment with budesonide and formoterol in patients with mild-to-moderate persistent asthma. *Respir Med* 2004; 98(11): 1146–1154.

139. Baena-Cagnani CE. The global burden of asthma and allergic diseases: the challenge for the new century. *Curr Allergy Asthma Rep* 2001; 1(4): 297–298.

140. Holgate ST. Cytokine and anti-cytokine therapy for the treatment of asthma and allergic disease. *Cytokine* 2004; 28(4–5): 152–157.

141. Qiu Z, Fujimura M, Kurashima K, Nakao S, Mukaida N. Enhanced airway inflammation and decreased subepithelial fibrosis in interleukin 6-deficient mice following chronic exposure to aerosolized antigen. *Clin Exp Allergy* 2004; 34(8): 1321–1328.

142. Quarcoo D, Weixler S, Joachim RA, et al. Resiquimod, a new immune response modifier from the family of imidazoquinolinamines, inhibits allergen-induced Th2 responses, airway inflammation and airway hyper-reactivity in mice. *Clin Exp Allergy* 2004; 34(8): 1314–1320.

143. Randolph AG, Lange C, Silverman EK, et al. The IL12B gene is associated with asthma. *Am J Hum Genet* 2004; 75(4): 709–715.

144. Yang G, Volk A, Petley T, et al. Anti-IL-13 monoclonal antibody inhibits airway hyperresponsiveness, inflammation and airway remodeling. *Cytokine* 2004; 28(6): 224–232.

145. Gallagher G, Eskdale J, Jordan W, et al. Human interleukin-19 and its receptor: a potential role in the induction of Th2 responses. *Int Immunopharmacol* 2004; 4(5): 615–626.

146. Babu KS, Davies DE, Holgate ST. Role of tumor necrosis factor alpha in asthma. *Immunol Allergy Clin North Am* 2004; 24(4): 583–597, v–vi.

147. Warner RL, Lukacs NW, Shapiro SD, et al. Role of metalloelastase in a model of allergic lung responses induced by cockroach allergen. *Am J Pathol* 2004; 165(6): 1921–1930.

148. Forssmann U, Hartung I, Balder R, et al. n-Nonanoyl-CC chemokine ligand 14, a potent CC chemokine ligand 14 analogue that prevents the recruitment of eosinophils in allergic airway inflammation. *J Immunol* 2004; 173(5): 3456–3466.

5

Adult-Onset Asthma

Samuel Louie, MD, *Nicholas J. Kenyon,* MD,
Kimberly A. Hardin, MD, *and Ken Y. Yoneda,* MD

*It is better to keep your mouth shut and appear
stupid than to open it and remove all doubt.*
—Mark Twain

KEY POINTS

- Asthma in adults is composed of a complex group of reversible airway disorders in contrast to childhood asthma that is largely allergic in nature.
- Adult-onset asthma may be recently acquired in adulthood or represent various stages of long-standing disease. Atopic adults may carry the genotype of childhood asthma symptomatically into adulthood only to have the phenotype finally expressed because of a powerful trigger, e.g., specific aeroallergen(s) or infection.
- Approximately 31 million Americans suffer from asthma. The majority of patients (71%) are adults, whereas fewer than 29% (8.9 million) are children less than 18 yr of age. More women than men are affected with severe adult-onset asthma. Estrogen replacement therapy, respiratory infection with *Chlamydia* or *Mycoplasma*, certain occupations, tobacco smoking, gastroesophageal reflux, obesity, and sleep disorders are important risk factors and comorbid conditions.

From: *Current Clinical Practice: Bronchial Asthma:
A Guide for Practical Understanding and Treatment, 5th ed.*
Edited by: M. E. Gershwin and T. E. Albertson © Humana Press Inc., Totowa, NJ

- Asthma and active cigarette smoking interact to cause more severe symptoms, accelerated decline in lung function, and impaired short-term therapeutic response to corticosteroids (CSs).
- Simple spirometry, e.g., forced expiratory volume in 1 s (FEV_1) and forced vital capacity (FVC), detect expiratory flow limitations and lung volumes. Demonstration of reversible obstructive airways disease with spirometry after using albuterol or ipratropium in an adult older than 18 yr old does not alone diagnose adult-onset asthma. Methacholine challenge testing to exclude abnormal airway hyperresponsiveness is safe in adult-onset asthma patients with FEV_1 greater than 70% predicted.
- High doses of inhaled CSs should be avoided in adult-onset asthma, particularly in the elderly or those with late-onset asthma. The addition of long-acting β2-agonists or antileukotriene drugs is preferable to using high doses of inhaled CSs. All patients using β2-agonists should be monitored for adverse effects, including paradoxical bronchoconstriction.
- Given their demonstrated benefit in conditions such as heart failure, coronary artery disease, and hypertension, cardioselective β1-blockers should not be withheld from adults with mild–moderate reversible airway disease.
- Patient adherence with prescribed asthma therapy is poor, and it is clearly the overwhelming explanation for poor control of asthma in adults, leading to exacerbations and hospitalizations. Compared with younger hospitalized adults, older hospitalized adults had clear deficiencies, including lower use of peak flow meters and worse asthma self-management knowledge.
- Factors independently associated with hospitalization included being female, nonwhite, less educated, and less physically healthy and more frequent asthma symptoms. Chronological age was not an independent risk for hospitalization. Appropriate care for older adults with asthma should address asthma symptoms as in children and younger adults.

INTRODUCTION

Asthma in adults is composed of a complex group of reversible airway disorders that, in contrast to childhood asthma, is largely allergic in nature. The National Institute of Health National Asthma Education and Prevention Program (NIH-NAEPP) Guidelines (http://www.nhlbi.nih.gov/guidelines/asthma/asthgdln.htm), which rely heavily on identifying asthma phenotypes presenting with episodic dyspnea, wheezing or cough with partially reversible airways obstruction, and increased airway hyperresponsiveness (AHR), may not adequately address this issue.

Adult-onset asthma is underdiagnosed and undertreated in the United States, particularly in those ≥65 yr old, despite an ongoing campaign by the NIH-NAEPP to increase asthma awareness, diagnosis, and treatment. Atopic, adult-onset asthma (AOA) represents the most prevalent asthma phenotype in clinical practice. These patients typically respond well to anti-inflammatory drugs and bronchodilators as recommended by the NIH-NAEPP; however, many other phenotypes do not. For example, in the authors' practice, they have often encountered women with particularly debilitating AOA that is incompletely controlled with systemic corticosteroids (CSs). The NIH-NAEPP guidelines for managing typical asthma do not address the means to achieve complete control of disease in these patients, nor do they adequately address the pathophysiology of their disease. Cigarette smoking, exposure to second-hand tobacco smoke, and air pollution may contribute to asthma and confound the distinction between asthma and chronic obstructive pulmonary disease (COPD) in adults. There is significant overlap between these two reversible obstructive airway disorders. In addition, some nonatopic patients with asthma have concomitant gastroesophageal reflux disease (GERD), obesity, or atypical respiratory infections, presenting further diagnostic and therapeutic challenges not fully addressed by the NIH-NAEPP. These comorbidities may contribute to poor control of asthma symptoms, frequent acute exacerbations, and a decidedly poor quality of life.

DEFINITIONS

AOA implies the development of asthma in adulthood and is defined as asthma in an adult (18 yr or older) at the time of diagnosis. *Late-onset asthma* (LOA) is defined as asthma in a person who is 65 yr of age or older at the time of diagnosis *(1)*. However, the time of onset in a patient's life is one of many risk factors associated with AOA. In reality, onset of asthma more often reflects when asthma symptoms are first recognized in the medical record. Clinicians diagnose asthma by its phenotype or clinical appearance. Not all asthma is allergic or "extrinsic" nor is it nonallergic or "intrinsic" in nature. Whether the patient objectively has asthma as defined becomes a clinical and diagnostic laboratory challenge and even then there may be lingering doubts regarding the precise diagnosis. Asthma should be viewed more as a general set of symptoms or syndrome representing distinct diseases that express a common appearing phenotype.

Much of what we currently understand about asthma comes from the scientific study of selected animal models and patients with asthma beginning in early childhood. But there is also a large group of patients that inexplicably develop the symptoms of asthma for the first time in adulthood, even after age 65. Hence, AOA may be recently acquired in adulthood or represent various stages of long-standing disease. Atopic adults may carry the genotype of childhood asthma symptomatically into adulthood, only to have the phenotype finally expressed because of a powerful trigger, e.g., specific aeroallergen(s) or infection. The majority of patients with AOA may have had mild childhood asthma that was never appropriately diagnosed or was clinically silent.

Alternatively, long-standing AOA beginning in young adulthood may lead to chronic persistent airway obstruction and be easily mistaken for COPD caused by cigarette smoking. The majority of cases of AOA, even if first recognized in adulthood, represent chronic persistent asthma that began early in childhood. The majority of mild childhood asthma cases enter clinical remission but persistence of severe disease from childhood into adulthood is responsible for the majority of asthma in adults. In this latter group of patients, chronic asthma is linked to persistence of atopy, although in later years some older adults lose their positive skin tests to specific allergens *(2)*. However, it is important to recognize that many adults who are diagnosed with AOA do not have atopic disease. They still present with the same asthma phenotype as their atopic counterparts but probably through different mechanisms of disease.

The age of onset of asthma extends over a range of ages in both genders. Nearly 50% of all patients with asthma experience onset before age 10 yr, but 25% of all patients with asthma experience onset after age 40 yr *(3)*. The NIH-NAEPP divides patients with asthma arbitrarily into age groups: the very young (<5 yr), everyone older (adults and children 5 yr and older), and the elderly, typically over age 65. Using age to discriminate asthma, however convenient, conceals the clinical and genetic diversity of asthma in adults. Although allergic asthma remains a chronic eosinophilic bronchitis associated with bronchial smooth muscle mast cell infiltration, clinicians today must face variable presentations in adults with asthma who exhibit highly variable response to treatments, including antileukotriene drugs, bronchodilators, anti-immunoglobulin (Ig) E, and even inhaled CSs.

Physiological changes with aging cause airways to narrow through various mechanisms and alter pulmonary function tests (PFTs). Incomplete reversibility becomes more often the rule than the exception in AOA. Intermittent bronchoconstriction, loss of elastic recoil, and mucous plugging in adult airways can lead to physiological changes in lung function and symptoms of dyspnea, wheezing, cough, and poor exercise capacity. However, there are other modulating factors, including specific genetic polymorphisms and environmental determinants, that may underlie phenotype severity, observed variable response to therapy, and prognosis. Psychosocial changes from reaching adulthood and elder age ($\geq$65 yr) can delay or prevent recognition of asthma by the physician and patient. Comorbid illnesses complicate the clinical picture of asthma in adults, e.g., tobacco smoking, second-hand or environmental tobacco smoke (ETS), air pollution, obesity, and GERD. Common air pollutants can cause a decline in lung function, increased bronchial hyperresponsiveness, and acute exacerbations; however, with the exception of ETS, they have not been shown conclusively to cause asthma in adults (4).

EPIDEMIOLOGY

Approximately 31 million Americans suffer from asthma (CDC, 2002; http://www.cdc.gov/nchs/fastats/asthmahtm), 71% of whom are adults. The majority of asthma-related deaths also occurs in adults with an incidence if 1.9 per more than 100,000, compared with 0.3 deaths per 100,000 in children (CDC, 2002). High-risk groups for death today include women age 55 yr and older, blacks, and Puerto Rican-Americans. A longitudinal, population-based cohort study of children with asthma in New Zealand found that 15% of children experienced remission of their disease during adolescence but another 12% had remission followed by a subsequent relapse as adults (5).

The prevalence of asthma in the elderly ranges from 3 to 17% (see Tables 1, 2) (6). The incidence of asthma in the elderly has been reported to be 3% in individuals over age 60 yr and less than 1% in those over 70 yr of age (7). However, these studies may underestimate the true prevalence and incidence of asthma. The DIDASCO Study used screening spirometry to detect COPD and doubled the number of patients with COPD in their patient population (8). Similar results may be realized in the patient populations with undiagnosed asthma in primary care settings. The number of patients identified with significant airway obstruction was doubled. Significant overlap between asthma and COPD can exist (see Fig. 1). The degree of overlap among asthma, chronic bronchitis, and emphysema can vary considerably with the community, region, country, and the prevalence of cigarette smoking and air pollution. For example, in Melbourne and Victoria, Australia, 50% of adults with asthma had chronic bronchitis and 73% of adults with chronic bronchitis had asthma in a 2002 survey (9).

The number of deaths from asthma in the United States declined in 2002 from between 5000 and 6000 annually to 4261 or 1.5 per 100,000 (CDC, 2002). Public awareness of asthma has increased; however, it is unclear if this awareness alone or in part is responsible for the mortality reduction. Physician and patient adherence to best practice guidelines remain decidedly poor (10).

Table 1

Estimated Annual Number of Persons With Self-Reported Asthma (1980–1996) or an Episode of Asthma or Asthma Attack (1997–1999) During the Preceding 12 mo by Race, Sex, and Age Group

	1980	1985	1990	1995	1996	1997	1998	1999
	Self-reported asthma prevalence during the preceding 12 mo					Episode of asthma or asthma attack during the preceding 12 mo		
Race								
White	5,975,000	7,425,000	8,544,000	12,161,000	11,764,000	8,924,000	8,352,000	8,226,000
Black	899,000	1,119,000	1,413,000	2,217,000	2,310,000	1,629,000	1,680,000	1,535,000
Other	102,000[a]	68,000[a]	353,000	461,000	522,000	559,000	581,000	727,000
Sex								
Male	3,438,000	3,863,000	4,741,000	6,673,000	5,751,000	4,592,000	4,550,000	4,310,000
Female	3,538,000	4,748,000	5,570,000	8,166,000	8,845,000	6,522,000	6,063,000	6,178,000
Age group (yr)								
0–4	369,000	661,000	840,000	1,227,000	805,000	812,000	915,000	825,000
5–14	1,530,000	1,720,000	2,270,000	3,215,000	2,771,000	2,391,000	2,321,000	2,288,000
15–34	2,251,000	2,855,000	2,898,000	4,443,000	5,139,000	3,380,000	2,853,000	3,208,000
35–64	2,056,000	2,339,000	3,220,000	4,715,000	4,441,000	3,655,000	3,599,000	3,451,000
≥65	769,000	1,036,000	1,082,000	1,238,000	1,445,000	875,000	925,000	717,000
Total[b]	6,975,000	8,611,000	10,310,000	14,838,000	14,601,000	11,113,000	10,613,000	10,488,000

Relative standard error of the estimate is 30–50%, the estimate is unreliable.

[a]National Health Interview Survey—United States, (1980–1999). All relative standard errors are <30%, unless otherwise indicated.

[b]Numbers for each variable might not add up to total because of rounding error.

Table 2

Estimated Annual Prevalence[a] of Self-Reported Asthma (1980–1996) or an Episode of Asthma or Asthma Attack (1997–1999) During the Preceding 12 mo by Race, Sex, and Age Group

	1980	1985	1990	1995	1996	1997	1998	1999
	Self-reported asthma prevalence during the preceding 12 mo					Episode of asthma or asthma attack during the preceding 12 mo		
Race								
White	31.4	37.0	41.5	54.5	53.6	40.5	37.5	37.6
Black	33.1	38.6	45.8	64.8	65.5	45.4	46.7	42.7
Other	19.9[b]	12.8[b]	40.2	44.4	43.2	34.7	33.7	38.9
Sex								
Male	30.5	33.8	39.1	48.6	43.0	33.0	31.7	31.6
Female	31.9	38.9	44.2	61.1	65.5	47.9	44.4	44.5
Age group (yr)								
0–4	23.0	36.7	44.0	60.5	40.1	41.2	46.4	42.1
5–14	45.1	50.9	63.7	82.0	69.8	60.0	57.8	56.4
15–34	30.0	36.1	37.3	57.8	67.2	44.2	37.5	42.2
35–64	29.9	30.8	38.4	50.1	46.2	37.0	35.7	33.4
≥65	31.9	38.6	36.3	39.4	45.5	27.3	28.7	22.1
Total[c]	31.4	36.6	41.9	55.2	54.6	40.7	39.2	38.4

All relative standard errors are <30%, unless otherwise indicated.

[a]National Health Interview Survey—United States, 1980–1999, per 1000 population.

[b]Age-adjusted to 2000 US population.

[c]Relative standard error of the estimate is 30–50%: the estimate is unreliable.

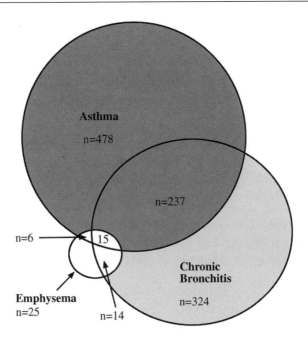

Fig. 1. Number of patients reporting asthma, chronic bronchitis, and/or emphysema. Adapted with permission from ref. *9.*

RISK FACTORS AND SPECIFIC SYNDROMES

Atopy

Chronic asthma in adults and children is most often related to underlying atopy (*see* Fig. 2 and Table 3). Atopic children generally remain atopic to varying degrees when they enter adulthood. AOA may persist clinically with exacerbations despite changes in skin test reactivity *(2,11)*. Little known about the prevalence of atopy in elderly patients with asthma. Bochenska-Marciniak and colleagues investigated the prevalence of atopy using skin-prick tests in 274 patients with AOA age 60 yr and older *(12)*. They found the prevalence of atopy ranged between 40% in those with late-onset asthma (defined in the study as asthma developed before age 40) and 57% in all others groups that experienced asthma at an earlier age. Eight percent of patients with early-onset asthma (defined by the investigators as asthma developed before age 30) and 4% of patients with LOA had negative skin-prick tests. Dust mite, feathers, grass, and tree pollen were the most common allergens that caused a positive skin-prick tests in the study.

Gender

Gender is linked inseparably to reproductive hormones. More women experience AOA than men. Postmenopausal women who take estrogen hormone replacement for 10 yr or more are more likely to develop asthma than women who never used estrogen. Women with asthma are more likely to have a severe attack immediately before or during their menstrual period, perhaps related to levels of estradiol. The Formoterol and Corticosteroid Establishing Therapy (FACET) study found that women are at higher risk and experience more severe asthma exacerbations than men *(13)*.

Siroux and colleagues found a relationship between eosinophils, IgE, and atopy with asthma according to gender and age of onset and hormone-related events. Using data from the Epidemiological Study on the Genetics and Environment of Asthma, Bronchial Hyperresponsiveness and Atopy, adults and children with asthma were recruited in chest clinics ($n = 313$) and first-degree relatives of patients with asthma ($n = 214$) were compared with controls without asthma ($n = 334$) and first-degree relatives without asthma ($n = 595$). Among women with asthma, eosinophilia was significantly associated with perimenstrual asthma independently from age, smoking, and asthma severity (eosinophils/mm^3, 330 vs 194; $p = 0.01$). In women without asthma, IgE level was significantly decreased (by 50%) and atopy decreased with menopause, and IgE increased with oral contraceptive use, independently from age and smoking. Comparing both genders, the increase of eosinophil counts with asthma was significantly greater in women with childhood-onset asthma than in women with AOA or in men in general. No interaction between gender and asthma was observed for eosinophils in children and for IgE level and atopy in children and adults *(14)*.

Estrogen Replacement

It is important to mention that published clinical studies that link the use of a particular drug(s) with asthma do not explain conclusively whether the drug caused asthma in the patients or population studied or whether the drug therapy exacerbated the airway inflammation in clinically silent asthma to cause the phenotype to be overtly recognized. There is an impulse to assign guilt by association, but convincing evidence is lacking in most circumstances.

Estrogen or hormone replacement therapy (HRT) increases the risk of AOA in women but not COPD. Previous randomized, clinical studies have suggested that HRT may modulate the development of asthma and COPD. The longitudinal Nurses Health Study initiated in 1976 was a prospective cohort study of more than 121,000 female registered nurses age 30–55 yr who became menopausal *(15)*. Barr and colleagues evaluated whether postmenopausal hormone use was associated with an increased rate of newly diagnosed AOA and, separately, newly diagnosed COPD *(15)*. A link was found between HRT use and the development of new asthma. From 1984 to 1996, Barr et al. found 756 women acquiring new diagnoses of asthma, 409 had new diagnoses of COPD, and 345 had both. During 546,259 person-years of follow-up, current use of estrogen alone was associated with an increased rate of asthma (multivariate rate ratio, 2.29; 95% confidence interval [CI], 1.59–3.29) compared with those who never used hormones. Current users of estrogen plus progestin had a similarly increased rate of newly diagnosed asthma. Rate ratios increased with certainty of diagnosis of asthma. In contrast, rates of newly diagnosed COPD were the same among hormone users and nonusers (multivariate rate ratio, 1.05; 95% CI, 0.80–1.37). HRT users had an 80% higher risk of asthma than did those women who never used HRT. The effect was similar among women who took conjugated estrogen only and among those who received the combination of estrogen plus progestin. Asthma risk increased in magnitude with higher does of estrogen and with longer duration of estrogen use. There was no association between HRT use and the new diagnosis of COPD. It is not clear what the underlying mechanisms for this finding. HRT may worsen inflammation or bronchospasm by increasing systemic activation of mast cells releasing histamines, leukotrienes, and interleukins (ILs). Cyclical release of proinflammatory mediators may be responsible for causing airway inflammation and chronic asthma in adult women.

Concern regarding HRT and asthma should not discourage clinicians from prescribing estrogen replacement therapy, if indicated, to reduce the risk of osteoporosis and heart disease in postmenopausal women. The incidence of asthma in the elderly has been reported to be 3% in individuals over age 60 yr and less than 1% in age over 70 yr. Increasing the risk of developing asthma by 80% is obviously significant to women who develop asthma on HRT. However, it should also be recognized that asthma severity has been linked perimenstrually to the reproductive hormones and to the use of oral contraceptives, the state of pregnancy, and the onset of menopause regardless of whether HRT is used *(14)*.

Drug-Induced Conditions

Certain drugs can trigger asthma symptoms in adults, particularly aspirin, nonsteroidal anti-inflammatory drugs (NSAIDs), nonselective β-blockers, and angiotensin-converting enzyme inhibitors. The mechanisms involved in drug-induced AOA often result from the direct nontherapeutic effects. The most practical approach is to avoid or cautiously use such drugs in AOA if possible. Adenosine, β-blockers, antibiotics (e.g., penicillins and cephalosporins), cholinergic drugs, NSAIDs (including aspirin, indomethacin and cyclooxygenase [COX]-1 and COX-2 inhibitors), pentzocaine, and tartrazine dye are among the more commonly recognized causes of drug-induced asthma in AOA.

Aspirin-Induced Asthma

Aspirin-induced asthma is a distinct form of AOA that is potentially life threatening. It is often part of the triad of asthma, nasal polyposis, and aspirin sensitivity in adults known as Samter's syndrome or Samter's asthma. The published prevalence before 2004 was 4–10%. However, aspirin-induced asthma is more prevalent than previously recognized. Jenkins et al. reviewed the literature retrospectively and determined that diagnosis was highest when determined by oral aspirin provocation testing. The new prevalence of aspirin-induced asthma in adults is 21% and 16% in children *(16)*. Cross-sensitivity to doses of over-the-counter NSAIDs was present in most patients with aspirin-induced asthma: ibuprofen, 98%; naproxen, 100%; and diclofenac, 93%. Interestingly, cross-sensitivity to acetaminophen was 7%.

Two theories exist to explain aspirin-induced asthma. Inhibition of COX-1 shunts arachidonic acid metabolism away from production of prostanoids and toward cysteinyl leukotrienes (cys-LT) production, leading to bronchoconstriction and bronchospasm. Alternatively, aspirin may cause a structural change in COX-2 that once again leads to a dramatic increase in the production of cys-LT. Indeed, these patients typically have elevated levels of cys-LT in urine, sputum, and blood even before exposure to aspirin and NSAIDs. Recently, a genetic polymorphism of the *LTC4S* gene has been identified consisting of an A to C transversion of 444 nucleotides upstream of the first codon. This is associated with a relative risk of aspirin-induced asthma of 3.89. Carriers of the C444 allele instead of the A444 allele show a dramatic increase in urine LTE4 after aspirin administration, and these patients respond better to leukotriene receptor antagonists and 5-lipoxygenase inhibitors *(17)*.

When there is a clinical necessity to use aspirin or an NSAID and there is uncertainty about safety, oral provocation testing should be performed under strict physician monitoring in the clinic or hospital. CSs typically do not control aspirin-induced asthma well. Antileukotriene drugs have helped patients considerably in controlling bronchospasm in this group of patients presumably by preventing the production of leukotrienes or blocking receptors for leukotrienes. Patients with aspirin-induced asthma can still develop anaphylaxis or an anaphylactoid reaction with aspirin, despite being on controller therapy.

Tobacco Smoking

Tobacco smoking has been linked to both asthma and COPD. Although the two obstructive airway disorders are different, the clinical similarities between the definition of asthma and the definition COPD (GOLD, 2003 http://www.goldcopd.com) are apparent, e.g., airway obstruction reversibility (albeit incomplete and occasionally absent), after bronchodilator treatment, and presence of airway inflammation. The early diagnosis and proper treatment of different reversible obstructive airway disorders is therefore a challenge in adults.

Smokers with asthma experience an excessive and rapid decline in PFTs compared with nonsmokers (18). In most developed countries, approx 25% of adults with asthma are active cigarette smokers. Asthma and active cigarette smoking interact to cause more severe symptoms, accelerated decline in lung function, and impaired short-term therapeutic response to CSs. Cigarette smoking may modify inflammation that is associated with asthma, although there is limited published data on airway pathology in smokers with asthma. The mechanisms of CS resistance in smokers with asthma are unexplained but could be a result of alterations in airway inflammatory cell phenotypes (e.g., increased neutrophils or reduced eosinophils), changes in the glucocorticoid receptor-α to -β ratio, e.g., overexpression of glucocorticoid receptor β, and increased activation of proinflammatory transcription factors, e.g., nuclear factor-κB or reduced histone deacetylase activity. Every effort should be made to encourage patients with asthma to stop smoking even in light of the low, sustained abstinence rates (19).

Pregnancy

Asthma is estimated to affect approx 3.7–8.4% of pregnant women in the United States. One out of every 500 expectant mothers experiences serious consequences from uncontrolled asthma during pregnancy, including preeclampsia and maternal and/or perinatal death. Approximately one-third of pregnant women experience worsening of their asthma during gestation, one-third remain the same, and one-third improve. The explanation of these clinical observations remains unclear. Uncontrolled asthma is a much greater risk to the mother and unborn baby than any known risk from asthma medications. However, it is important to evaluate the risk–benefit of any medication before prescribing it to the pregnant woman based on the safety of the medication in prior studies. Smoking by the mother, particularly smoking during pregnancy, is linked with development of asthma in the child in later life. The most common errors by health care providers and pregnant women are: (1) to underestimate the severity of asthma during pregnancy, (2) to not implement appropriate environmental control measures, (3) to undertreat chronic persistent asthma, and (4) to delay treatment of acute severe exacerbations, including the use of oral CSs, which can be life-saving to both mother and fetus (20).

Gastroesophageal Reflux Disease

GERD is an asthma trigger that is clinically silent in 50% of patients who have asthma who also have GERD. GERD is not an epidemiological risk factor of AOA but may explain why patients are diagnosed as adults. In addition, patients with AOA have a higher prevalence of hiatal hernias *(21)*, and asthma medications, such as β2-agonists and theophylline, can aggravate GERD by reducing lower esophageal sphincter pressure.

A 1- to 3-mo empiric trial with a proton pump inhibitor in a poorly controlled patient with AOA is recommended to ascertain if GERD hinders asthma control *(22)*. There is no other way to quickly determine which patients with AOA would benefit from proton pump inhibitors. The authors only recommend esophageal pH testing after the empiric trial with proton pump inhibitors fails and the clinical symptoms of GERD persist.

Control of GERD can independently improve asthma outcomes, but medical treatment for GERD does not consistently improve asthma control. The Cochrane Library analyzed clinical trials conducted in children and adults and found seven of nine studies associating antireflux therapy with at least one significantly improved asthma outcome *(23)*. In patients with asthma who also have GERD, there was no overall improvement in asthma after treatment for GERD. Subgroups of patients may gain benefit, but it appears difficult to predict responders. Adults over age 19 yr with AOA and GERD may be at higher risk factor for hospitalization for poorly controlled asthma *(24)*.

Infection

Asthma is a prevalent disease with marked effects on quality of life and economic societal burden. However, the cause of asthma and its pathophysiology are not completely defined. Recently, the possibility that chronic infection may play a role has been suggested. Martin and colleagues sought to define the association between *Mycoplasma* and *Chlamydia* species and chronic asthma. They performed a comparison study of patients with asthma and normal control subjects *(25)*. Fifty-five patients with chronic stable asthma were compared with 11 normal control subjects by using polymerase chain reaction (PCR), culture, and serology for *Mycoplasma* species, *Chlamydia* species, and viruses from the nasopharynx, lungs, and blood. Bronchoalveolar lavage cell count and differential, as well as tissue morphometry, were also evaluated. Computer-generated scoring for the degree of chronic sinusitis in patients with asthma was additionally evaluated. Thirty-one of 55 patients with asthma had positive PCR results for *Mycoplasma* ($n = 25$) or *Chlamydia* species ($n = 6$), which were mainly found on lung biopsy specimens or in lavage fluid. Only 1 of 11 normal control subjects had positive PCR results for *Mycoplasma* species. The distinguishing phenotype between patients with asthma with positive and negative PCR results was the significantly greater number of tissue mast cells in the group with positive results. A significant number of patients with chronic stable asthma demonstrate the presence of *Mycoplasma* species, *Chlamydia* species, or both in their airways, with the distinguishing feature of increased mast cell number. These findings need further delineation but may help us to understand the pathophysiology of asthma and new treatment options *(25)*.

Obesity

Current estimates are that 25% of Americans are obese and half of the country is overweight. The obesity epidemic has shadowed the asthma epidemic since the 1970s. In the

Nurses' Health Study, after controlling for diet and physical exercise, body mass index (BMI) greater than 30 (BMI = weight/ht^2) was directly correlated to an increased incidence of asthma in these adult nurses. Obesity may be viewed as an inflammatory state with increased levels of cytokines IL-6 and IL-8. In women who are obese, obesity increases estrogen levels that can cause inflammatory events through mast cell activation. There is currently great interest to determine whether obesity and asthma are linked to the same candidate genes, which would explain the parallel appearance of both epidemics *(26)*.

Several studies have identified obesity as a risk factor for asthma in both children and adults. An increased prevalence of asthma in subjects with GERD and obstructive sleep apnea syndrome has also been reported. In a 5- to 10-yr follow-up study of the European Community Respiratory Health Survey in Iceland, Norway, Denmark, Sweden, and Estonia, a postal questionnaire was sent to previous respondents. A total of 16,191 participants responded to the questionnaire. Reported onset of asthma, wheeze, and nocturnal symptoms, as well as nocturnal GERD and habitual snoring, increased in prevalence along with the increase in BMI. After adjusting for nocturnal GERD, habitual snoring, and other confounders, obesity (BMI >30) remained significantly related to the onset of asthma, wheeze, and nighttime symptoms. This study adds evidence to an independent relationship among obesity, nocturnal GERD, and habitual snoring and the onset of asthma and respiratory symptoms in adults *(27)*.

Sleep Disorders and Chronobiology

The relationship among asthma, GERD, obesity, and sleep disorders is complex and is the subject of excellent recent reviews *(28)*. However, it is important to know all of the above diseases and disorders disturb sleep. All are important in the chronobiology of asthma, as expounded by Kraft and colleagues *(29)*. This relatively new area, termed chronobiology, describes how time-related events shape our daily biological responses and apply to any aspect of medicine regarding altering pathophysiology and treatment response. For example, normally occurring circadian (daily cycles, approx 24 h) events, such as nadirs in epinephrine and cortisol levels that occur in the body around 10 PM to 4 AM and elevated histamine and other mediator levels that occur between midnight and 4 AM, play a major role in the worsening of asthma during the night. In fact, this nocturnal exacerbation occurs in the majority of patients with asthma. Because all biological functions, including those of cells, organs, and the entire body, have circadian rhythms, understanding the pathophysiology and treatment of disease must be viewed with these changes in mind. Biological rhythms are ingrained, and although changing the wake–sleep cycle can change them over time, these alterations occur over days. However, sleep itself can adversely affect the pathophysiology of asthma and other diseases. During the afternoon, patients who sleep the night before generally achieve their best lung function. Hence, many patients with asthma are more healthy and functional, bringing clinicians to suspect anything but asthma.

Normal circadian rhythm changes in lung function, e.g., forced expiratory volume in 1 s (FEV$_1$) decline in an exaggerated manner in AOA who experience nocturnal awakening. An abnormal decrease in FEV$_1$ and increase in airway inflammation can be detected during the sleep cycle. Monitoring for nocturnal symptoms is an important key to asthma control *(30)*. Nocturnal death from asthma is high, with 53% of asthma-related deaths occurring between 6 PM and 4 AM *(31)*.

Occupation

Occupational asthma is an important cause of AOA, particularly in men. Isocyanates remain the most important single cause of occupational asthma worldwide. Other industrial chemicals, biological enzymes, animal secretions, and dusts at work (e.g., toluene diisocyanate, metals salts, laundry detergents, flour dust causing Baker's Asthma, and cockroach allergens in buildings) are all reported to cause occupational asthma but are often overlooked in the management of AOA. The key is a clinical history focused to reveal the link between occupational exposures and clinical exacerbations *(32)* Absence from work during weekends or medical leave nearly always brings about clinical remission, only to have the symptoms of asthma recur with return to work and to the offending workplace environment. However, 20–30% of patients have persistent symptoms that do not resolve, despite prolonged absence from the work environment. In addition, one must not forget men or women who work at home who may develop AOA as a consequence of a domestic or household trigger *(33)*. School teachers, professors, and health care professionals may have unusual forms of occupational asthma caused by contact with students, patients, and poor building conditions, e.g., molds and cockroaches in the inner cities.

GENETIC AND IMMUNOLOGICAL INSIGHTS

Genetic Insights

Several asthma susceptibility genes have been identified, and the topic has been expertly reviewed. A functional polymorphism in the regulated on activation, normal T-cell expressed and secreted (RANTES) gene promotor is associated with the development of late-onset asthma *(34)*. RANTES is an important CC chemokine involved in asthma inflammation that is a potent chemoattractant for T-cell lymphocytes, eosinophils, basophils, monocytes that become macrophages, and mast cells. Both atopic asthma and nonatopic asthma are associated with increased levels of RANTES in bronchoalveolar lavage fluid, and RANTES contributes to the influx of activated eosinophils into the asthmatic airways. Furthermore, all of the aforementioned cells, as well as epithelial cells, fibroblasts, and endothelial cells, can generate and secrete RANTES. Hizawa and colleagues noted the −403A and −28G alleles of the RANTES promoter region exhibit significantly enhanced promoter activity in reporter constructs in vitro. They investigated the genetic influence of these alleles on the development of asthma using case–control analysis in 298 Japanese patients with asthma and 311 control subjects. Given the evidence for heterogeneity of asthma according to age at onset, they divided patients with asthma into three subgroups: 117 patients with LOA (defined by investigators as onset at >40 yr of age), 83 patients with middle-onset asthma (onset at 20–40 yr of age), and 98 patients with early-onset asthma (onset at <20 yr of age). The −28G allele was significantly associated with LOA (odds ratio = 2.033; 95% CI, 1.379–2.998; corrected $p < 0.0025$) but was not associated with the other two asthma subgroups. The −403A allele was not associated with any of the asthma subgroups. Further evidence of the importance of the −28G allele was a significant increase in the production of RANTES in vitro in individuals who carried this allele. Their findings suggest that among Japanese, the −28G allele of the RANTES promoter region confers susceptibility to LOA *(42)*. However, what actually triggers the immunological events leading to AOA in this population is unknown.

Childhood asthma → Adolescent asthma → Persistent Adult asthma
                                            Adult-onset asthma
                                            Late-onset asthma
                                            Samter's asthma
                                            Drug-induced asthma
                                            Occupational asthma
                                                    ↑
                                            Contributing Morbidities
                                            Occupation
                                            GERD
                                            Gender
                                            Obesity
                                            Sleep disorder
                                            Lack of exercise
                                            Tobacco smoking
                                            Air pollution
                                            Pregnancy

Fig. 2. Development of syndromes of adult-onset asthma.

Genotype-specific responses are clinically relevant. Polymorphism at the 16th amino acid residue of the β2 receptor is associated with adverse effects of β2-agonist use in patients with asthma. Patients with the Arg/Arg genotype improved when β2-agonist therapy was withdrawn and replaced with the anticholinergic ipratropium bromide. Patients with the Gly/Gly genotype had better control of their asthma with regular albuterol use. It is estimated that one-sixth of the population with asthma in the United states have the Arg/Arg genotype, and the prevalence is present in approx 20% of Americans of African descent and 15% of whites. In the β-Adrenergic Response by Genotype (BARGE) Study, Israel and colleagues *(35)* suggest that patients with Arg/Arg genotype may benefit from discontinuing the use of albuterol as a rescue inhaler, using ipratropium bromide in its place for regular and rescue use.

Recent studies by McGraw and colleagues in transgenic mice support the hypothesis that the decline in lung function after regular or as-needed use of albuterol may trigger cellular mechanisms different from those normally associated with smooth-muscle bronchodilation. Paradoxically, frequent triggering of the β2 receptors may cause bronchoconstriction instead of bronchodilation. Altering the expression of bronchial smooth muscle β2 receptors in transgenic mice affects the function of other airway receptors, such as muscarinic receptors, that are also important in controlling airway contractility. These effects may be mediated through a phospholipase C-β pathway *(36)*.

Immunological Insights

Lung parenchyma in asthma remains largely normal unlike in COPD, where the lung parenchyma is slowly destroyed by oxidative stress and proteolytic processes. Small airways inflammation are prominently involved in both asthma and COPD, but the cellular populations and clinical response to drug therapy differ markedly. Eosinophils, mast cells, CD4+ T-lymphocytes, and macrophages characterize the cellular inflammation in asthma *(see* Fig. 3). In contrast, cellular inflammation in COPD consists of neutrophils, macrophages, CD8+ T-lymphocytes, and, during clinical exacerbations, eosinophils. This topic of airway inflammation has been reviewed exhaustively *(37,38)*.

Cellular populations and their mediators appear changed with disease progression in AOA. The bronchial eosinophilic inflammation is orchestrated by mast cells and CD4+

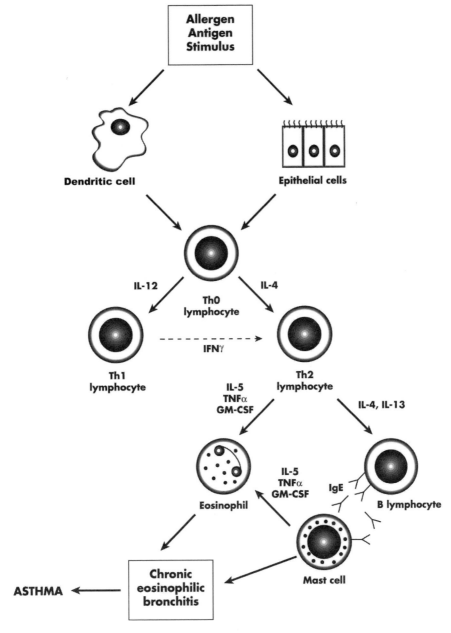

Fig. 3. Role of cytokines in airway inflammation in asthma. Reproduced with permission from ref. *39.*

T-lymphocytes in childhood asthma and asthma that extends into adulthood. However, eosinophils and neutrophils become increasingly more important with AOA and in severe cases of persistent asthma in adults. The relationship was explored by Wenzel and colleagues to determine whether phenotypic differences exist between early-onset severe asthma as compared with late-onset disease and whether the presence or absence of eosinophilia influences the phenotypes. Differentiating severe asthma by age at onset and presence or absence of eosinophils identifies phenotypes of asthma, which could benefit subsequent genetic and therapeutic studies. Eighty participants were divided into those with asthma onset before age 12 yr ($n = 50$) vs after age 12 yr ($n = 30$) and by the presence or absence of lung eosinophils. Subjects with early-onset severe asthma had significantly more allergen sensitivity (skin test positivity, 98 vs 76%, $p < 0.007$) and more allergic symptoms than subjects with LOA. In contrast, subjects with LOA had lower lung function than subjects with early-onset asthma, despite a shorter illness duration. Both groups had a high degree of general asthma symptoms, but those with persistent eosinophils from either age at onset group had significantly worse symptoms. Similarly, the presence of eosinophils in either age at onset group was associated with the lowest lung function. Although LOA was associated with the highest numbers of lung eosinophils, only early-onset severe asthma was associated with a lymphocytic/mast cell inflammatory process. Finally, subjects with LOA without eosinophils had no subepithelial basement membrane thickening, suggesting a different pathological process (38).

For many years it has been supposed that the production of an excess of nitric oxide (NO) by inducible NO synthase (iNOS) plays a major role in inflammatory diseases, including asthma. However, recent studies indicate that a deficiency of beneficial, bronchodilating constitutive NOS-derived NO is important in allergen-induced AHR. Although several mechanisms are proposed to explain the reduction of constitutive NOS activity, reduced substrate availability, caused by a combination of increased arginase activity and decreased cellular uptake of L-arginine, plays a key role (40). Recent evidence also indicates that iNOS-induced pathophysiological effects involve substrate deficiency. At low concentrations of L-arginine iNOS produces both NO and superoxide anions, which results in the increased synthesis of the highly reactive, detrimental oxidant peroxynitrite. Based on these observations, a relative deficiency of NO caused by increased arginase activity and altered L-arginine homeostasis may be a major factor in the pathogenesis of allergic asthma. Morris and colleagues found that patients with asthma (median age 14, range 2–52 yr) exhibited a significant reduction in plasma arginine levels during acute exacerbations compared with normal control subjects without asthma (41). High arginase activity in patients with asthma may contribute to low circulating arginine levels, thereby limiting arginine bioavailability and creating a NO deficiency that induces hyperreactive airways. Addressing the alterations in arginine metabolism may result in new strategies for treatment of asthma.

DIAGNOSIS

Until genetic screening becomes available, clinicians must rely on clinical curiosity, a carefully acquired clinical history (e.g., family history, cigarette smoking, or exposure to ETS, or urban air pollution), and deliberate use of PFTs, including spirometry before and after bronchodilator challenge with albuterol or albuterol and ipratropium bromide, methacholine bronchoprovocation tests (i.e., PC_{20}), and carbon monoxide-diffusing capacity (see Table 4).

A longitudinal, population-based cohort study of 613 children followed from age 3 yr to age 26 yr and found that clinicians should not rely on finding wheezing to help diagnose asthma. Only 27% of the subjects at age 26 yr never reported wheezing, 21% reported wheezing only once, and 10% had intermittent wheezing. Interestingly, 15% had remission of their asthma during adolescence, but another 12% experienced remission followed by a subsequent relapse (5).

Aging definitely affects pulmonary physiology and the results of pulmonary function testing (Table 4). The normal decline in FEV_1 is approx 25–35 mL/yr. From age

Table 3
Risk Factors for Adult-Onset Asthma

Risk factors	Specific syndromes
Atopy	Samter's asthma
Gender	Exercise-induced asthma
Drugs, estrogens, aspirin, and nonsteroidal	
anti-inflammatory drugs	Refractory asthma
Tobacco smoking	Occupational asthma
Environmental tobacco smoke	
Air pollution	
Obesity	
Pregnancy	
Respiratory infections, particularly *Chlamydia* spp.	
Gastroesophageal reflux disease	

Table 4
Clinical Differences Between Adult-Onset Asthma and Chronic Obstructive Pulmonary Disease

Adult-onset asthma	Chronic obstructive pulmonary disease
• Prevalence in women is greater than in men	• Prevalence men = women
• Airflow limitation reversible after albuterol	• Airflow limitation not fully reversible after albuterol
• Airway hyperresponsiveness (PC_{20}) very marked to methacholine and adenosine monophosphate	• Airway hyperresponsiveness variable
• DLco normal	• DLco normal with chronic bronchitis; low in emphysema
• FEV_1 improvement $\geq 12\%$ β2-agonists greater than anticholinergics	• FEV_1 improvement $\geq 12\%$ • β2 agonists = anticholinergics
• Improvement with steroids but variability in response exists	• Steroids reduce exacerbations but do not improve lung function
• Improvement with LTRA	• No improvement with LTRA unless asthma overlaps

LTRA, leukotriene receptor antagonist; DLco, carbon monoxide-diffusing capacity.

25–39 yr, the decline is approx 20 mL/yr; age older than 45 yr, 35 mL/yr. Hence, loss of spirometric function increases with age. This becomes important when trying to separate asthma from COPD using the global obstructive lung disease (GOLD) guidelines updated October 2003 at http://www.goldcopd.com (*see* Table 5).

Gas exchange, i.e., PaO_2 and $PaCO_2$, is near normal in elderly patients with asthma. One cannot rely solely on the presence of reduced expiratory flow rates on pulmonary function tests to identify AOA. PFTs detect expiratory flow limitations and lung volumes, nothing more. Demonstration of reversible obstructive airways disease with spirometry after using albuterol or ipratropium in an adult over 18 yr old does not alone AOA.

One of the hallmarks of asthma is reversibility in spirometric measurements on receiving a bronchodilator, such as inhaled albuterol (Table 2). A significant bronchodilator response is commonly seen in children with asthma after administration of

Table 5
Normal Physiological Changes in the Lungs Associated With Aging

- Increased air trapping leading to hyperinflation
- Decreased lung elastic recoil
- Decreased chest wall compliance → ↑FRC, ↑RV
- Increased restriction from kyphosis, e.g., secondary to osteoporosis and vertebral compression fractures
- Loss of height → ↓FEV_1, ↓FEV_1%, ↓VC, ↑FRC, ↑RV. No change in TLC.
- Decreased respiratory muscle strength
- Impaired respiratory reflexes
- Impaired perception of respiratory workload reduces mental cognition or awareness

FRC, functional residual capacity; RV, residual volume; VC, vital capacity; TLC, total lung capacity.

albuterol, with FEV_1 improving by at least 12% and 200 mL. The same criteria have been applied to adults, but many older patients have evidence of reduced expiratory flow rates and chest wall restriction if they develop changes in posture, e.g., osteoporosis and obesity. Lung volumes may also improve but often are not measured after bronchodilator challenge. Total lung capacity and residual volume may decrease and inspiratory capacity may increase significantly after bronchodilator administration in patients with asthma and in patients with COPD. This "volume shifting" may occur in the absence of any significant improvement in expiratory flow rates. Examination of flow-volume loops before and after bronchodilator treatment may readily disclose this phenomenon *(42)*.

Bronchoprovocation challenge tests detect the presence of nonspecific hyperresponsive airways in patients with normal spirometry and normal chest X-ray in AOA, even in the elderly (*see* Fig. 4). AHR is defined as the degree to which expiratory flow rates decline after response to a nonspecific trigger, e.g., methacholine, histamine, cold air, exercise, or adenosine-5′-monophosphate. Although these bronchoconstrictive triggers can cause expiratory flow rates to decline in everyone, adults with asthma require much less methacholine (<8 mg/mL) than normal controls. The methacholine PC_{20} is the dose of methacholine causing a 20% decrease in a patient's baseline FEV_1 measured after inhaling normal saline. A negative test, i.e., FEV_1, remains greater than 80% of baseline excludes asthma in adults with 95% certainty. A positive test confirms the presence of bronchial hyperresponsiveness but is not specific for asthma (*see* Fig. 5). Methacholine bronchial challenge is used primarily to rule out AHR in the clinical setting of normal PFTs. However, it can be used to detect AHR in AOA, particularly in the elderly. When a normal methacholine challenge is found, a diagnosis of AOA can be excluded, and the clinician should then pursue other diagnoses, including congestive heart failure, GERD, chronic pulmonary aspiration, vocal cord dysfunction, and lung cancer.

Enright has recommended an excellent algorithm employing clinical history and the aforementioned PFTs to ascertain the diagnosis of asthma or COPD in the older adult and the elderly patient suffering from asthma-like symptoms (Fig. 4) *(43)*. In his scheme, a methacholine PC_{20} less than 4 mg/mL is considered diagnostic of AHR in the older population in contrast to a PC_{20} of less than 8 mg/mL in younger adults and adolescents.

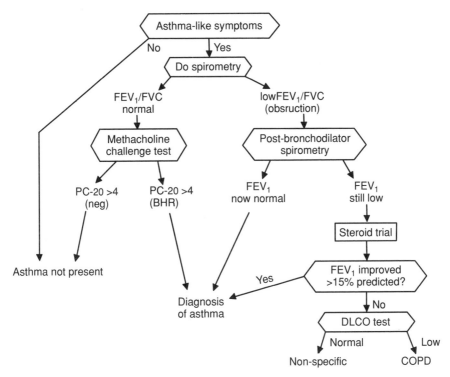

Fig. 4. Suggested algorithm to evaluate elderly patients with asthma symptoms. (Adapted with permission from ref. *42*.)

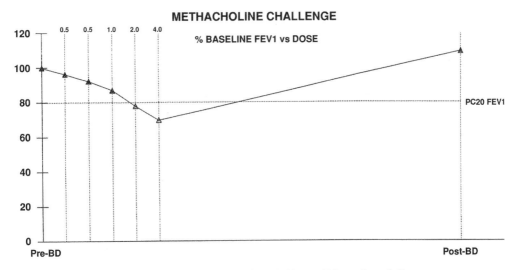

Fig. 5. A positive methacholine challenge. $PC_{20} = 2$ mg/mL.

GENETIC PROFILING

Given the heterogeneity of AOA, genetic profiling will help separate and group patients and their phenotype, e.g., clearly separate asthma from COPD. But it is uncertain whether it will improve care and long-term outcomes and, in some patients, tell clinicians which gene profile is more important than the other, e.g., the profile for asthma or the profile for

COPD. The problem becomes apparent in the patient with both asthma and COPD. Genetic profiling of asthma may eventually predict which patients will benefit from certain specific anti-inflammatory drugs, bronchodilators, and anti-IgE antibody therapy and which will not benefit, but it will not obviate the need in individual patients with asthma to do a "clinical trial of one" as the great Eugene Robin used to harangue.

In addition to aiding clinical diagnosis, genetic profiling may be best employed as a tool to keep patients away from certain treatments and adverse reactions. However, the authors suspect that patients' responses to pharmacotherapy will remain highly variable, despite knowledge of genetic profiles. Ideally, a genetic test or group of tests to predict response to therapy would be cost-effective by reducing the need to treat empirically. Genetic profiling could help patients and their physicians make better choices regarding how to treat asthma and simplify the clinical trials that each new patient must undergo with a drug. In the interim, reliance on the asthma phenotype and its response to therapy will remain the most practical approach.

TREATMENT AND MANAGEMENT

Treatment

The NIH-NAEPP guidelines basically recommend treatment by identifying a specific asthma phenotype, i.e., mild, moderate, or severe persistent, and rely on response to stepwise therapy and patient education to achieve control. Comorbid conditions should be suspected and treated when AOA becomes difficult to control in adults, e.g., GERD and rhinosinusitis. Given recent concerns about drug safety, it is vital to avoid a nonchalant approach to treatment and to carefully monitor clinical trial(s) with each drug therapy in each patient to determine safety and effectiveness.

Inhaled CSs remain the single most effective therapy for adult patients with asthma. However, for those who are unable or unwilling to take inhaled CSs, the use of leukotriene modifiers/receptor agonists is reasonable, with the caveat that clinical asthma control is achieved. Long-acting β2-agonists may be added to inhaled CSs for those who remain symptomatic despite low-dose inhaled CSs therapy and is preferred by the NIH-NAEPP. However, the long-term effects of these agents on acute exacerbations are unclear.

Sin and colleagues systematically reviewed and quantitatively synthesized the long-term effects of inhaled CSs, long-acting β2-agonists, leukotriene pathway modifiers/receptor antagonists, and anti-IgE therapies on clinical outcomes and particular clinically relevant exacerbations in adult patients with chronic asthma (44). MEDLINE, EMBASE, and Cochrane databases were searched to identify relevant randomized controlled trials and systematic reviews published from January 1, 1980 to April 30, 2004. They identified additional studies by searching bibliographies of retrieved articles and contacting experts in the field. Included trials were double-blind, had follow-up periods of at least 3 mo, and contained data on exacerbations and/or FEV_1. The effects of interventions were compared with placebo, short-acting β2-agonists, or each other.

Not surprisingly, inhaled CSs were most effective, reducing exacerbations by nearly 55% compared with placebo or short-acting β2-agonists. Compared with placebo, the use of long-acting β2-agonists was associated with 25% fewer exacerbations; when added to inhaled CSs, there was a 26% reduction above that achieved by steroid monotherapy. Combination therapy was associated with fewer exacerbations than was increasing the dose of inhaled CSs. Compared with placebo, leukotriene modifiers/receptor antagonists reduced exacerbations by 41% but were less effective than inhaled CSs. Use of monoclonal anti-IgE antibodies with concomitant inhaled CS therapy was associated with 45% fewer exacerbations. Anti-IgE therapy may be considered as adjunctive therapy for young adults with asthma who have clear evidence of allergies and elevated serum IgE levels.

Older patients may benefit from a trial of antileukotriene drugs, as Enright and others recommend (43,44). The dose of inhaled CSs can often be reduced to lower levels without compromising the response of patients to bronchodilators if needed. Antileukotriene drugs can be used as alternatives to long-acting β2-agonists in adult-onset asthma who have exercise-induced bronchospasm (45). Regular use of β2-agonist can cause tolerance and a reduction in the magnitude of bronchodilator rescue.

A double-blind, placebo-controlled study was performed at 16 centers in the United States. Patients with asthma ($n = 122$, ages 15–58 yr) whose symptoms were uncontrolled on low-dose inhaled fluticasone and who had a history of exercise-induced worsening of asthma were randomized to receive montelukast (10 mg once daily), salmeterol (50 μg twice daily), or placebo for 4 wk. The magnitude and rate of rescue bronchodilation were significantly greater with montelukast compared with salmeterol ($p < 0.001$). Five minutes after rescue β2-agonist, 92% of patients taking montelukast and 68% of those taking placebo had recovered to preexercise levels, whereas only 50% of those taking salmeterol recovered to preexercise levels. Storms and colleagues concluded that in patients whose asthma symptoms remain uncontrolled using inhaled CSs, addition of montelukast permits a greater and more rapid rescue bronchodilation with a short-acting β2-agonist than addition of salmeterol and provides consistent and clinically meaningful protection against exercise-induced bronchoconstriction.

Sims and colleagues evaluated whether montelukast or formoterol provides additive effects to patients with asthma who are not controlled by inhaled CSs by studying patients who were homozygous for the Gly/Gly-16 genotype and considered to be genetically susceptible to β2-receptor downregulation (46). Fifteen CS-treated patients with mild to moderate persistent asthma received montelukast 10 mg once daily or formoterol 9 μg twice daily for 2 wk, separated by a 2-wk placebo run-in and washout, in a double-blind, double-dummy, randomized, cross-over design. Bronchoprotection against adenosine monophosphate challenge (primary end point), spirometry, and blood eosinophils were measured at trough after placebo and first and last doses. Neither treatment significantly improved FEV_1, forced expiratory flow in 25–75 s, or peak expiratory flow rate after 2 wk. In genetically susceptible patients with the homozygous Gly/Gly-16 genotype, montelukast, but not formoterol, conferred sustained antiinflammatory properties in addition to inhaled CSs, which were dissociated from changes in lung function after 2 wk. Assessing lung function alone may deprive potentially beneficial anti-inflammatory effects of montelukast when used as add-on therapy (47).

Allergen injection immunotherapy is the only treatment currently in use with the potential for modifying the course of allergic disease. To better target mucosal allergies, new approaches of administering allergen via the sublingual or intranasal route are being developed. The use of modified allergens, allergen peptides, DNA immunization, and novel adjuvants represent alternatives to conventional immunotherapy with potential for improved efficacy with fewer side effects. For atopic asthma, novel treatment strategies aim at locally targeting inflamed airways. Nebulized monoclonal blocking antibodies and soluble IL receptors against T-helper cell type 2 cytokines have been designed. An alternative approach has been the administration of T-helper cell type 1 cytokines. Although immunomodulatory strategies provide a promising outlook for the treatment of allergic patients, more studies are needed in the future to address issues of efficacy, safety, and long-term effects of altered immune responses.

Barnes reviewed new drug therapies in asthma, including novel CSs, cytokine and chemokine inhibitors, mediator antagonists, bronchodilators (i.e., anticholinergics), and β2-agonists inhibitors of phosphodiesterase-4, p38 mitogen-activated protein kinase and nuclear factor κB *(48)*. However, their future benefit to patients with AOA may be better served with study populations that are defined by genotype and phenotype.

Management

Is it far more important to know the patient than the disease as Sir William Osler once asserted? Becoming familiar with patients with AOA is important for therapeutic and safety reasons, if anything, to try and help change behavior and lifestyle. Understanding patients' personal characteristics is generally believed to be essential for better asthma management *(49)*.

Abdulwadud and colleagues assessed the relationships between patients' related variables in asthma and identified key associations relevant to asthma management *(50)*. A total of 169 subjects participated in the study; 57% had one or more previous hospital admissions, 94% had either moderate or severe asthma, and 51% reported nocturnal symptoms in the last 6 wk. Patients who spoke only English, had been admitted to an intensive care unit, had a peak flow meter, and had an asthma action plan had significantly better asthma knowledge than those who did not. The effect of asthma was greatest in patients who had a peak flow meter, used oral steroids, had exercise limitation, and developed asthma between the ages of 31–45 yr. Female patients had better self-management skills than males. Patients with asthma-related distress were more likely to use oral steroids or theophylline and have a history of previous hospital admissions. Patient self-confidence was negatively correlated with age.

Treatment and management of asthma according to the NIH-NAEPP guidelines relies on clinical evaluation of symptoms and simple measures of lung function. A single spirometry measurement alone, even if normal, fails to predict any future asthma and correlates poorly with airway inflammation. It is the pattern or trend of expiratory flow rates combined with the clinical features of a patient with AOA, e.g., presence or absence of nocturnal awakening that is most important in evaluating control as defined by the NIH-NAEPP (http://www.nhlbi.nih.gov/guidelines/asthma/asthgdln.htm). Nocturnal awakening and/or an increased requirement for a short-acting β2-agonist are harbingers of an acute exacerbation coming. The patient with AOA who sleeps well is a controlled patient with AOA. Other investigators, notably the NIH in their Asthma Clinical Research Network (ACRN) Centers, have employed sputum eosinophils and exhaled NO in addition to traditional symptoms and spirometry in their management strategies.

Use of sputum eosinophil counts alone can be effective alternative strategy in reducing asthma exacerbations. Green and colleagues recruited 74 patients with moderate to severe asthma from hospital clinics and randomly allocated them to management either by standard British Thoracic Society (BTS) asthma guidelines (BTS group) or by normalization of the induced sputum eosinophil count and reduction of symptoms (sputum management group) *(49)*. They assessed patients nine times during 12 mo. The results were used to manage those in the sputum management group but were not disclosed in the BTS group. The primary outcomes were the number of severe exacerbations and control of eosinophilic inflammation, measured by induced sputum eosinophil count. The sputum eosinophil count was 63% (95% CI 24–100) lower for those 12 mo in the sputum management group than in the BTS management group (*p* = 0.002). Remarkably, patients in the sputum management group had significantly fewer severe asthma exacerbations than did patients in the BTS management group (35 vs 109; *p* = 0.01), and significantly fewer patients were admitted to hospital with asthma (one vs six, *p* = 0.047). The average daily dose of inhaled or oral CSs did not differ between the two groups studied. Treatment strategy directed at normalization of the induced sputum eosinophil count reduces asthma exacerbations and admissions without the need for additional anti-inflammatory treatment and should be evaluated for more widespread use in primary and subspecialty clinics *(51)*.

SAFETY ISSUES

The Patient

Patient safety is paramount during the treatment of AOA. Patient adherence with prescribed asthma therapy in the United States is poor and, in the authors' opinion, it is clearly the overwhelming explanation for poor control of asthma in AOA. In a study evaluating the adherence of 48,571 adult patients with asthma, less than 30% took inhaled CSs twice daily, less than 30% took inhaled long-acting β2-agonists twice daily, and less than 50% took a leukotriene receptor antagonist once a day at 6 and 9 mo. There was a statistically significant difference between groups with *p* < 0.004 for leukotriene receptor antagonist vs inhaled CS and long-acting β2-agonists based on medication refills *(52)*.

Inhalation of CSs permits effective delivery of the drug in high concentration to target sites within the lung while minimizing systemic exposure. Consequently, the safety profile of inhaled CSs is markedly better than that of oral CS therapy. Although it was first believed that direct delivery might eliminate systemic adverse effects, this has not been confirmed by clinical trials and experience. Inhaled CSs are absorbed from the lungs into the systemic circulation and can acutely decrease growth velocity in children, an effect that fortunately appears to be temporary and likely has no effect on final adult height. In sufficient dosages, they also produce bone mineral loss leading to osteoporosis and may increase the risk of cataracts, glaucoma, skin atrophy, and vascular changes that increase the risk of ecchymoses. High doses of inhaled CSs should be avoided in adult-onset asthma for these reasons, particularly in the elderly or those with late-onset asthma. Addition of long-acting β2-agonists, e.g., salmeterol or formoterol, or antileukotriene drugs, e.g., montelukast or zafirlukast or theophylline, is preferable (NIH-NAEPP, 2002). All patients using β2-agonists should be monitored for adverse effects, including paradoxical bronchoconstriction.

β2-Agonists

Tolerance to β2-agonist treatment after regular use in AOA has been reported in a meta-analysis of 22 studies in patients who take either a β2-agonist or placebo regularly for at least 1 wk *(53)*. Patients who took a β2-agonist regularly for at least 1 wk were less responsive to the effects of subsequent doses of β2-agonists than were patients who took placebo. Regular users developed tolerance to the effects of the β2-agonist on both bronchodilation and inflammation. Regular users demonstrated more airway inflammation than those who took placebo. It is unclear whether taking β2-agonist as needed is worse than not taking any β2-agonist at all. It is unclear whether a similar phenomenon occurs with long-acting β2-agonists because previous NIH Asthma Clinical Research Network (ACRN) studies had suggested that the return of airway inflammation was the result of, in large part, the withdrawal of inhaled CSs (54).

Recent concerns regarding the clinical significance of β2-receptor polymorphisms and lung function have been raised with the BARGE study (35). The implications of the BARGE Study led by Israel and colleagues in the NIH ACRN is that even as-needed use of albuterol may not be safe in patients with Arg/Arg genotype. Previous retrospective studies suggested that regular albuterol use produces adverse effects in Arg/Arg patients. In their prospective BARGE Study, Israel et al. suggest carefully evaluating the bronchodilator response of patients with asthma to β2-agonists before prescribing long-term therapy and rescue treatments (35). Anticholinergics may be safer in the long-term for use, at least in asthma. Only albuterol was studied in the BARGE study. Whether the effects are observed with other short-acting β2-agonist or long-acting β2-agonist is not known nor are the consequences of having Arg/Arg genotype with more severe asthma or the interaction and effect of combing β2-agonists with inhaled CSs.

Inhaled Corticosteroids

There is also evidence that marked and variable response to inhaled CSs should be expected in AOA and particularly in LOA. Szefler and colleagues in the NIH ACRN compared the relative beneficial and systemic effects in a dose–response relationship for two inhaled CSs, beclomethasone, and fluticasone (55). A 24-wk, parallel, open-label, multicenter trial examined the benefit–risk ratio of two inhaled CSs in persistent asthma. Benefit was assessed by improvements in FEV_1 and PC_{20}; risk of side effects was assessed by overnight plasma cortisol suppression. Thirty subjects were randomized to either beclomethasone (BDP) 168, 672, and 1344 µg/d ($n = 15$) or fluticasone (FP) 88, 352, and 704 µg/d ($n = 15$), both administered by means of a metered-dose inhaler (MDI) with chlorofluorocarbon propellant via a spacer, in three consecutive 6-wk intervals. This was followed by 3 wk of FP dry-powder inhaler (DPI) 2000 µg/d. The results were surprising. Maximum FEV_1 response occurred with the low dose for FP-MDI and the medium dose for BDP-MDI and was not further increased by treatment with FP-DPI. Near-maximum methacholine PC_{20} improvement occurred with the low dose for FP-MDI and the medium dose for BDP-MDI. Both BDP-MDI and FP-MDI caused dose-dependent cortisol suppression. Responsiveness to inhaled CS treatment varied markedly among subjects. Good (>15%) FEV_1 response, in contrast to poor (<5%) response, was associated with high exhaled NO, high bronchodilator reversibility (25.2 vs 8.8%), and a low FEV_1/forced volume capacity ratio (0.63 vs 0.73) before treatment. Excellent (>3 doubling dilutions) improvement in PC1o, in contrast to poor (<1 doubling dilution) improvement, was associated with high sputum eosinophil levels (3.4 vs 0.1%) and older age at onset of asthma (age, 20–29 yr vs <10 yr). Near-maximal FEV_1 and PC_{20} effects occurred with low-medium dose for both inhaled CSs in the subjects studied. High-dose inhaled CS therapy did not significantly increase the efficacy measures that were evaluated, but it did increase the systemic effect measure, overnight cortisol secretion. Significant intersubject variability in response occurred with both inhaled CSs. It is possible that higher doses of inhaled CSs are necessary to manage patients with more severe asthma or to achieve goals of therapy not evaluated in this study, such as prevention of asthma exacerbations.

Inactivation of histone deacetylase (HDAC) 2 may be responsible for CS resistance in both asthma and COPD *(56)*. Unlike patients with asthma, those with COPD are poorly responsive to CSs, providing little clinical benefit except during acute COPD exacerbations. In both diseases, multiple inflammatory genes are activated, which results from acetylation of core histones around which DNA is wound. This acetylation opens up the chromatin structure, allowing gene transcription and synthesis of inflammatory proteins to proceed. CSs recruit HDAC2 to the actively transcribing gene, which reverses this process and switches off inflammatory gene transcription. Cigarette smoking and oxidative stress, leading to a pronounced reduction in responsiveness to CSs, may impair HDAC2 function. High doses of inhaled CSs, as defined by the NIH-NAEPP, combined with one or two other long-term controllers or systemic corticosteroids (20 mg every other day) are the only viable alternative in very severe AOA or patients with refractory asthma, but evidence-based studies of their efficacy are lacking.

β1-Blockers

Numerous randomized clinical trials of β1-blockers have shown significant reduction of total mortality in patients with myocardial infarction and chronic heart failure. The life-saving therapy of myocardial infarction or chronic heart failure with β1-blockers, however, is often withheld from patients with asthma and COPD because of the fear of triggering acute bronchospasm. Recent meta-analyses in the Cochrane Library show that cardioselective β1-blockers in normally prescribed dose ranges are well tolerated by these patients without causing acute exacerbations. However, both cardioselective and noncardioselective β1-blockers can cause bronchospasm at higher dosages, and clinical suspicion should be raised the setting of glaucoma where a β1-blockers is prescribed to treat the ocular condition.

β1-blockers were previously contraindicated in congestive heart failure because of their intrinsic negative inotropic effects, but they have now been shown to be beneficial, partly as a result of their ability to enhance sensitivity to sympathetic stimulation. Similarly, new evidence has shown that cardioselective β1-blockers, such as atenolol, metoprolol, and betaxolol, are safer in patients with asthma and COPD and may actually be beneficial by enhancing sensitivity to endogenous or exogenous β-adrenergic stimulation manifest as an increased FEV_1 bronchodilator response after albuterol treatment.

Relative contraindications for β1-blockers include acute COPD exacerbations and severe to very severe stages of COPD (GOLD stage III and stage IV), as well as severe persistent asthma. β1-blockers therapy should be given with low initial doses, preferably using cardioselective drugs. Given their demonstrated benefit in conditions, such as heart failure, coronary artery disease, and hypertension, cardioselective β1-blockers should not be withheld from adults with mild–moderate reversible airway disease *(57)*.

Gaps in Asthma Care

Despite this available knowledge and collective clinical experience, gaps in asthma care in adults continue to exist. Impaired perception of dyspnea in older patients increases the risk of hospitalization and near-fatal and fatal asthma *(43,58)*. There are many opportunities to improve both the pharmacological and the nonpharmacological care of older adults with asthma. Overuse of and potentially toxic combinations of inhaled and oral sympathomimetics should be avoided. Older patients with asthma may also benefit from increased specialty referral, peak flow meter (PFM) use, allergy testing, and asthma teaching. Wolfenden and colleagues performed a prospective cohort study to arrive at these conclusions. They assessed the adequacy of asthma care reported by a group of older adults who were subsequently hospitalized for their asthma in 15 managed care organizations in the United States. Surveys of patient demographics, asthma symptoms, health status, comorbid conditions, asthma treatment, asthma knowledge, and asthma self-management at baseline and 1 yr later were conducted. Of 254 older adults, 38 (15%) reported being hospitalized for asthma at 1-yr follow-up. Of these, 22.9% owned a PFM. Of those with allergies, only about half (56%) had been told how to avoid allergens and had been referred for formal allergy testing. Adrenergic drug use was high in some patients. Nearly all (94.6%) used β2-agonist MDIs; 60% reported theophylline; 17.1% reported β2-agonist MDI overuse (>8 puffs/d); 10.5% reported β-agonist MDI overuse and theophylline; and 13.2% reported both β-agonist MDI overuse and oral β2-agonist use. Only 18.4% of respondents rated their overall asthma attack knowledge as excellent. Compared with nonhospitalized older adults, the hospitalized group reported care that was more consistent with guidelines but also higher rates of potentially toxic combinations of adrenergic drugs. Compared with younger hospitalized adults, older hospitalized adults had clear deficiencies, including lower use of PFMs (55.3 vs 22.9%) and worse asthma self-management knowledge.

Diette and colleagues tried to determine whether patterns of care were less favorable for older than younger adults with asthma and to assess whether patient characteristics, such as symptom severity and comorbid illnesses, explain the higher rate of hospitalization *(24)*. A prospective cohort study of 6590 adults with asthma in 15 managed care organizations in the United States was studied. Among 6590 adults with asthma, 554 (8%) were 65 yr or older and 1942 (29%) were aged 18–34 yr. Older patients were more likely than younger patients to be men, white, non-Hispanic, and less educated. At baseline, older patients reported a greater frequency of asthma-related symptoms, such as daily cough (36 vs 22%, $p < 0.001$) and wheezing (27 vs 22%, $p < 0.002$). They were also more likely to report comorbid conditions, such as sinusitis (50 vs 38%), heartburn (35 vs 23%), chronic bronchitis (43 vs 16%), emphysema (19 vs 1%), congestive heart failure (8 vs 1%), and history of smoking (54 vs 34%) (all $p < 0.001$). Care was better for the older patients compared with the younger, including more frequent use of inhaled CSs, greater self-management knowledge, and fewer reported barriers to care.

In the follow-up year, older patients were approximately twice as likely to be hospitalized (14%) than were younger patients (7%) ($p < 0.001$). In multivariate analysis, however, older age was not predictive of future hospitalization (odds ratio, 1.05; 95% CI, 0.68–1.61) after adjustment for sex, ethnicity, education, baseline asthma symptoms, health status, comorbid illnesses, and tobacco use. Factors independently associated with hospitalization included being female, nonwhite, less educated, and less physically healthy and more frequent asthma symptoms. Chronological age was not an independent risk for hospitalization. Appropriate care for older adults with asthma should address asthma symptoms as in children and younger adults.

CONCLUSIONS

The authors' goal was to highlight the heterogeneity of AOA and review the difficulties identifying and managing the various types of asthma presenting in adults. In the near future, genetic profiling of all types of asthma may obviate the need to emphasize the onset of disease. More importantly, genetic profiling will aid diagnosis in difficult cases and may help identify which therapies and interventions will be most effective in prevention and treatment. More effective and safer therapeutic interventions to control symptoms and disease mechanisms underlying AOA are greatly needed. Further clinical investigations are imperative to achieve the goals of chronic disease management in AOA to better long-term health care outcomes. Early diagnoses and medical interventions form only part of the greater solution. Better living conditions and psychosocial resources are desperately needed in the United States and require urban mandates and social readiness to begin reform.

REFERENCES

1. *Diagnosis and Management of Asthma in the Elderly*. Bethesda, MD, National Institute of Health, 1996. NIH Publication No. 96-3662.
2. Burrows B, Lebowitz MD, Barbee RA, et al. Findings before diagnoses of asthma among the elderly in a longitudinal study of a general population sample. *J Allergy Clin Immunol* 1991; 88: 870–877.
3. Broder I, Higgins MW, Mathews KP, Keller JB. Epidemiology of asthma and allergic rhinitis in a total community. Tecumseh, Michigan: 3. Second survey of the community. *J Allergy Clin Immunol* 1974; 53: 127–138.
4. Koenig JQ. Air pollution and asthma. *J Allergy Clin Immunol* 1999; 104: 717–722.
5. Sears MR, Greene JM, Willan AR, et al. A longitudinal, population-based cohort study of childhood asthma followed to adulthood. *N Engl J Med* 2003; 349: 1414–1422.
6. Braman SS, Kaemmerlen JR, Davis SM. Asthma in the elderly. A comparison between patients with recently acquired and long-standing disease. *Am Rev Respir Dis* 1991; 13: 336–340.
7. Derrick EH. The significance of age of onset of asthma. *Med J Aust* 1971; 1: 1317–1319.
8. Buffels J, Degryse J, Heyrman J, Decramer M. Office spirometry significantly improves early detection of COPD in general practice. The DIDASCO Study. *Chest* 2004; 125: 1394–1399.
9. Abramson M, Matheson M, Wharton C, et al. Prevalence of respiratory symptoms related to chronic obstructive pulmonary disease and asthma among middle aged and older adults. *Respirology* 2002; 7: 325–331.
10. Cabana MD, Rand CS, Powe NR, et al. Why don't physicians follow clinical practice guidelines? *JAMA* 1999; 282: 1458–1465.
11. Kjellman B, Gustafsson PM. Asthma from childhood to adulthood: asthma severity, allergies, sensitization, living conditions, gender influences and social consequences. *Respir Med* 2000; 94: 454–465.
12. Bochenska-Marciniak M, Kolomecka M, Gorski P, Kuna P. Prevalence of atopy and the diagnostic value of skin prick tests in asthmatics over the age of 60. *J Allergy Clin Immunol* 2001; 107: A862.
13. Tattersfield AE, Postma DS, Barnes PJ, et al. Exacerbations of asthma: a descriptive study of 425 severe exacerbations. The FACET International Study Group. *Am J Respir Crit Care Med* 1999; 160: 594–599.
14. Siroux V, Curt F, Oryszczyn MP, et al. Role of gender and hormone-related events on IgE, atopy, and eosinophils in the Epidemiological Study on the Genetics and Environment of Asthma, bronchial hyperresponsiveness and atopy. *J Allergy Clin Immunol* 2004; 114: 491–498.
15. Barr RG, Wentowski CC, Grodstein F, et al. Prospective study of postmenopausal hormone use and newly diagnosed asthma and chronic obstructive pulmonary disease. *Arch Intern Med* 2004;164: 379–386.
16. Jenkins C, Costello J, Hodge L. Systematic review of prevalence of aspirin-induced asthma and its implications for clinical practice. *Br Med J* 2004; 328: 434–440.
17. Hamad AM, Sutcliffe AM, Knox AJ. Aspirin-induced asthma: clinical aspects, pathogenesis and management. *Drugs* 2004; 64: 2417–2432.
18. Lang DM, Polansky M. Patterns of asthma mortality in Philadelphia form 1969 to 1991. *N Engl J Med* 1994; 331: 1542–1546.
19. Thomson NC, Chaudhuri R, Livingston E. Asthma and cigarette smoking. *Eur Respir J* 2004; 24: 822–833.
20. *Management of Asthma During Pregnancy. Report of the Working Group on Asthma and Pregnancy*. Bethesda, MD, National Institute of Health, 1993. NIH Publication No. 93-3279.
21. Harding SM. Gastroesophageal reflux and asthma: insight into the association. *J Allergy Clin Immunol* 1999; 104: 251–259.

22. Kiljander TO, Laitinen JO. The prevalence of gastroesophageal reflux disease in adult asthmatics. *Chest* 2004;126:1490–1494.
23. Gibson PG, Henry RL, Coughlan JL. The effect of treatment for gastro-esophageal reflux on asthma in adults and children. *Cochrane Database Syst Rev* 2003; 2: CD001496.
24. Diette GB, Krishman JA, Dominici F, et al. Asthma in older patients: factors associated with hospitalization. *Arch Intern Med* 2002; 121: 8–10.
25. Martin RJ, Kraft M, Chu HW, et al. A link between chronic asthma and chronic infection. *J Allergy Clin Immunol* 2001;107:595–601.
26. Camargo CA Jr, Weiss ST, Zhang S et al. Prospective study of body mass index, weight change, and risk of adult-onset asthma in women. *Arch Intern Med* 1999; 159: 2582–2588.
27. Gunnbjornsdottir MI, Omenaas E, Gislason T, et al. Obesity and nocturnal gastro-oesophageal reflux are related to onset of asthma and respiratory symptoms. *Eur Respir J* 2004; 24: 116–121.
28. Bonekat HW, Hardin KA. Severe upper airway obstruction during sleep. *Clin Rev Allergy Immunol* 2003; 25: 191–210.
29. Kraft M, Martin RJ. Chronobiology and chronotherapy in medicine. *Dis Mon* 1995; 41: 501–575.
30. Turner-Warwick M. The epidemiology of nocturnal asthma. *Am J Med* 1988; 85: 6–8.
31. Robertson CF, Rubinfeld, AR, Bowes G. Deaths from asthma in Victoria: a 12-month survey. *Med J Austr* 1990; 152: 511–517.
32. Sama SR, Hunt PR, Cirillo CI, et al. A longitudinal study of adult-onset asthma incidence among HMO members. *Environ Health* 2003; 2: 10.
33. Frew AJ. Advances in environmental and occupational diseases 2003. *J Allergy Clin Immunol* 2004; 113: 1161–1166.
34. Hizawa N, Yamaguchi E, Konno S, et al. A functional polymorphism in the RANTES gene promotor is associated with the development of late-onset asthma. *Am J Respir Crit Care Med* 2002; 166: 686–690.
35. Israel E, Chinchilli VM, Ford JG, et al. Use of regularly scheduled albuterol treatment in asthma: genotype-stratified, randomized, placebo-controlled cross-over trial. *Lancet* 2004; 364: 1505–1512.
36. McGraw DW, Almoosa KF, Paul RJ, et al. Antithetic regulation by beta-adrenergic receptors of Gq receptor signaling via phospholipase C underlies the airway beta-agonist paradox. *J Clin Invest* 2003; 112: 619–626.
37. Sutherland ER, Martin RJ. Airway inflammation in chronic obstructive pulmonary disease: comparison with asthma. *J Allergy Clin Immunol* 2003; 112: 819–827.
38. Miranda C, Busacker A, Balzar S, Trudeau J, Wenzel SE. Distinguishing severe asthma phenotypes: role of age at onset and eosinophilic inflammation. *J Allergy Clin Immunol* 2004; 113: 101–108.
39. Kenyon NJ, Louie S. Asthma. In: Gershwin ME and Naguwa SM, eds. *Allergy and Immunology Secrets*. 2nd ed. St. Louis, MO, Elsevier Mosby, 2005, pp. 91–108.
40. Meurs H, Maarsingh H, Zaagsma J. Arginase and asthma: novel insights into nitric oxide homeostasis and airway. *Trends Pharmacol Sci* 2003; 24: 450–455.
41. Morris CR, Poljakovic M, Lavrisha L et al. Decreased arginine bioavailability and increased serum arginase activity in asthma. *Am J Respir Crit Care Med* 2004; 170: 148–153.
42. Woolcock AJ, Read J. Improvement in bronchial asthma not reflected in forced expiratory volume. *Lancet* 1965; 2: 1323.
43. Enright PL. The diagnosis and management of asthma is much tougher in older patients. *Curr Opin Allergy Clin Immunol* 2002; 2: 175–181.
44. Sin DD, Man J, Sharpe H, et al. Pharmacological management to reduce exacerbations in adults with asthma: a systematic review and meta-analysis. *JAMA* 2004; 292: 367–376.
45. Storms W, Chervinsky P, Ghannam AF, et al. A comparison of the effects of oral montelukast and inhaled salmeterol on response to rescue bronchodilation after challenge. *Respir Med* 2004; 98: 1051–1062.
46. Sims EJ, Jackson CM, Lipworth BJ. Add-on therapy with montelukast or formoterol in patients with the glycine-16 beta2-receptor genotype. *Br J Clin Pharmacol.* 2003; 56: 104–111.
47. Varga EM, Nouri-Aria K, Till SJ, Durham SR. Immunomodulatory treatment strategies for allergic diseases. *Curr Drug Targets Inflamm Allergy* 2003; 2: 31–46.
48. Barnes PJ. New drugs for asthma. *Nat Rev Drug Discov* 2004; 3: 831–844.
49. Abramson MJ, Bailey MJ, Forbes AB, Walters EH. How well do doctors know their patients with severe asthma? *Intern Med J* 2003; 33: 557–565.
50. Abdulwadud OA, Abramson MJ, Forbes AB, Walters EH. The relationships between patients' related variables in asthma: implications for asthma management. *Respirology* 2001; 6: 105–112.

51. Green RH, Brightling CE, McKenna S, et al. Asthma exacerbations and sputum eosinophil counts: a randomised controlled trial. *Lancet* 2002; 360: 1715–1721.

52. Drazen JM, Boccuzzi SJ, Wogen J, et al. Adherence to prescribed treatment for asthma. *Am J Respir Crit Care Med* 2000; 161: A402.

53. Salpeter SR, Ormiston TM, Salpeter EE. Meta-analysis: respiratory tolerance to regular β2-agonist use in patients with asthma. *Ann Intern Med* 2004; 140: 802–813.

54. Lazarus SC, Boushey HA, Fahy JV, et al. Long-acting beta2-agonist monotherapy vs continued therapy with inhaled corticosteroids in patients with persistent asthma: a randomized controlled trial. *JAMA* 2001; 285: 2583–2593.

55. Szefler SJ, Martin RJ, King TS, et al. Significant variability in response to inhaled corticosteroids for persistent asthma. *J Allergy Clin Immunol* 2002; 109: 410–418.

56. Barnes PJ, Ito K, Adcock IM. Corticosteroid resistance in chronic obstructive pulmonary disease: inactivation of histone deacetylase. *Lancet* 2004; 363: 731–733.

57. Salpeter S, Ormiston T, Salpeter EE. Cardioselective beta-blockers for reversible airway disease. *Cochrane Database Syst Rev* 2002; 1: CD002992.

58. Wolfenden LL, Diette GB, Skinner EA, et al. Gaps in asthma care of the oldest adults. *J Am Geriatr Soc* 2002; 50: 877–883.

6

The Patient With Asthma in the Emergency Department

Donna Kinser, MD

KEY POINTS

- Peak expiratory flow meters aid in assessing and following the progress of acute asthma patients in conjunction with history, examination, and pulse oximetry.
- Mild asthma attacks should be treated with albuterol by nebulizer or metered-dose inhlaer with holding chamber.
- Moderate to severe asthma attacks should be treated with larger doses of albuterol, ipratropium bromide, and corticosteroids (CSs), usually by the oral route.
- The CS dose does not need to be supra-high range.
- Very severe asthma attacks should be treated with continuous high-dose albuterol, ipratropium bromide, and CSs, usually by the intravenous route, plus intravenous magnesium.

From: *Current Clinical Practice: Bronchial Asthma:*
A Guide for Practical Understanding and Treatment, 5th ed.
Edited by: M. E. Gershwin and T. E. Albertson © Humana Press Inc., Totowa, NJ

- Other options for difficult situations include heliox, ketamine, and noninvasive positive pressure ventilation.
- Determination of disposition is more feasible after the first phase of treatment than at the time of initial presentation.
- Discharge from the emergency department should involve appropriate discharge medications, teaching of action plan, and follow-up arrangements.

INTRODUCTION

Patients of all ages present to the emergency department (ED) with respiratory distress and wheezing. Initial evaluation entails assessing the severity of the respiratory distress and developing a working diagnosis of the cause.

Asthma may present as a new problem, and the first diagnosis will need to be established in the ED. However, in the majority of cases, the patient will be aware of the underlying diagnosis of asthma and will communicate it in the field or at triage. This simplifies the initial categorization of the problem and treatment approach, and the emergency practitioner can focus on identifying a triggering cause or complicating condition. However, occasionally asthma is used as a catch-all term, so the clinician should consider the possibility of another type of disease process, and sometimes other disease entities present with features of asthma exacerbation and will need to be distinguished.

Asthma is a common condition that accounts for approx 2 million ED visits each year in the United States. Because it involves paroxysmal spasmodic narrowing of the bronchial airways and inflammation of the bronchi, it is not surprising that patients experience sudden symptoms requiring prompt medical attention. Although improved medication regimens and step-up treatment plans have been successful in decreasing ED visits, in certain centers, acute asthma may still comprise 10% of all ED visits.

ASSESSING THE SEVERITY OF RESPIRATORY DISTRESS

Rapid initial assessment is required for the expert provision of emergency services. The universal concept of ABC—airway, breathing, and circulation—must be applied to the patient with severely symptomatic asthma. In respiratory failure, ventilatory support needs to precede detailed history and physical examination.

The presenting appearance of the patient provides key information (*see* Table 1). Mental status changes or indications of extreme fatigue, such as diaphoresis and recumbent position, are ominous signs. Limited ability to speak, assuming the tripod position, and using accessory muscles are worrisome signs. Vital signs showing low blood pressure, pulse rate, or respiratory rate are indications for immediate resuscitative intervention. Vital signs showing high blood pressure, pulse rate, or respiratory rate are usually indications for aggressive emergency treatment.

Pulse oximetry provides a guide regarding adequacy of oxygenation. Values below 91–92% for room air are cause for concern. Typically, however, the patient with a more serious condition is administered supplemental oxygen as an urgent treatment, and it is the pulse oximetry on oxygen that is assessed and followed in the ED.

Auscultation of the chest gives information regarding the presence, type, and nature of the breath sounds, plus the quality and symmetry of aeration. Bronchospasm is evaluated by degree of wheezing and airflow. Prolongation of the expiratory phase

Table 1
Primary Assessment

Signs of a severe asthma attack in an adult

Appearance of exhaustion
Decrease in consciousness
Diaphoresis
Hunched sitting position with arms supporting torso (tripod)
Limited ability to speak
Use of accessory muscles
Cyanosis
Respiratory rate more than 30/min

Signs of a severe asthma attack in an infant

Use of accessory muscles
Supraclavicular and intercostal retractions
Nasal flaring
Paradoxical breathing
Cyanosis
Respiratory rate more than 60/min

reflects severity of acute asthma. In mild bronchospasm, the inspiration–expiration ratio may be 1:1; in severe bronchospasm, the ratio may be 1:3.

However, studies have indicated that the practitioner cannot fully accurately assess degree of airway obstruction and distress through clinical examination alone. Therefore, use of indices derived from a forced exhalation by the patient into a measurement apparatus has become a standard technique in EDs. Most commonly, a peak expiratory flow meter is used and yields the index of peak expiratory flow rate (PEFR); less commonly, a spirometer is employed and yields the index of forced expiratory volume in 1 s (FEV_1). The advantages of this approach include objectivity and a numerical result to follow, ideally with a comparison to historical baseline being possible. PEFR less than 50% is regarded as representing a moderately severe attack, and PEFR less than 35% of predicted is regarded as representing a severe attack. Unfortunately, a parameter such as PEFR is not obtainable in all patients. Testing cannot be performed by the patients with more severe symptoms, and often testing is not performed reliably by a subset of patients because of ability or effort. Also, children younger than 4–5 yr of age cannot be expected to perform this type of maneuver.

An arterial blood gas (ABG) is a consideration for patients in whom there is incongruity between clinical impression and other clinical information. The other main use of the ABG is to follow patients who are close to needing ventilatory support. If an ABG is collected as a routine test, it usually shows a respiratory alkalosis. Normal or increased CO_2 implies severe disease, although the converse is not necessarily true. Hypercarbia is unlikely, unless marked airflow obstruction exists. Metabolic acidosis should be recognized as a marker of very severe disease.

Certain historical information is helpful in gauging the seriousness of the attack and has implication for prognosis and response to therapy. Usually the information is gained bit by bit, as allowed by the patient's condition and treatment course. Of relevance are the types and doses of medications the patient has been using, the current constellation of symptoms, and any exposures. Comorbid conditions, such as heart disease, propensity

Table 2
Categorization of Severity of Asthma Episode: Quick Clinical
Information and Tests to Use

History	Physical examination	Clinical parameters
Breathlessness	Vital signs	Pulse oximetry
Duration of symptoms	Skin	Peak expiratory flow rate
Prior intubation for asthma	Lung examination	
Medications	Level of alertness	

for barotrauma or atelectasis, and substance abuse, may be important. If the patient has previously been intubated for asthma exacerbation, there is an almost 20-fold increase in likelihood this will be required again (1). Although older case–control studies using retrospectively collected data suggest that excess use of short-acting β-agonists was a risk factor, more recent information suggests that patterns of use may be a marker for more severe asthma rather than causal or severe attacks (2). Most patients have worsening of asthma symptoms for a 2- to 7-d period; however, a subset of approx 10% have onset of the attack in less than 6 h but tend to respond rapidly to treatment.

In summary, numerous pieces of information can be gathered and assimilated quickly in the ED for use in preliminarily categorizing the severity of the presenting asthma attack. Mild, moderate, and severe categories can be assigned based on the degree of normality or abnormality of the responses and measurements (see Table 2). Although this information correlates only loosely with ultimate outcome and disposition for the severe episode, it provides the basis for decision making for initial level of monitoring and treatment intensity.

DIAGNOSIS

In the ED, typically the clinician uses a prior diagnosis of asthma or makes the presumptive diagnosis. The ED physician should be able to rely on the prior diagnosis in the following circumstances: patient has a history of bronchospasm from childhood that has been responsive to asthma medications; patient has a positive prior methacholine challenge test. In most other circumstances, the diagnosis would be presumptive, based on evidence for asthma and lack of evidence for other disease processes. In patients with a significant smoking history, an emphysematous disease, such as chronic obstructive pulmonary disease (COPD), may be likely.

TRIGGERING AND/OR COMPLICATING FACTORS

Many patients with asthma are able to recognize their own triggers (see Table 3). These may have been identified through experience or specific testing. Triggers may include exposure to allergens, such as from grasses, trees, weeds, dust, mite, cockroach, fungi, and animals. They may also include exposure to irritants, such as smoke, chemical products, or occupational hazards. Asthma exacerbation may be induced by exercise or exposure to cold. It may be induced by use of aspirin or β-blocking drugs.

Patients with underlying asthma may have an exacerbation when there is a complicating problem, such as infection, pneumothorax, or arrhythmia. In many settings, the most common precipitant of asthma exacerbation is infection with a respiratory viral

Table 3
Potential Events Antecedent to Asthma Attack

Asthma triggers and exacerbating factors
Infection
Exposures
Allergens
Aspirin
Cold temperature
Exercise
Irritants
Alteration in medications
Out of medications
Change in medications
Steroid dose reduction
Other pulmonary or cardiac conditions

pathogen, *Mycoplasma pneumoniae* or *Chlamydia pneumoniae*. Bronchospasm frequently increases with active sinusitis.

The clinician must consider that the basis for the acute exacerbation may be medication noncompliance, medication change, or steroid dose reduction.

DIFFERENTIAL DIAGNOSIS

Other medical conditions can be confused with asthma. Misdiagnoses may be present in 1% of general asthma admissions and 10% of intensive care unit admissions.

Upper airway obstruction may masquerade as lower airway obstruction. Especially in pediatric patients, common conditions to be considered include rhinitis and sinusitis and less common conditions to be considered include epiglottitis and retropharyngeal abscess. Foreign body may be present in the upper airway or one of the larger lower airways. Angioedema may occur and cause upper airway obstruction.

In the pediatric population, croup and certain congenital and acquired anatomical problems may contribute to large airway obstruction. Obstruction in the small and large lower airways are features of acute infections, such as bronchiolitis and *Chlamydia trachomatis*, and chronic underlying diseases, such as cystic fibrosis, bronchopulmonary dysplasia, and α-1 antiprotease deficiency. The differential diagnosis of wheezing in pediatric patients should also include aspiration, as a result of gastroesophageal reflux or swallowing disorders, and primary cardiac conditions resulting in congestive heart failure (CHF).

In the adult population, the differential diagnosis includes COPD, bronchiectasis, endobronchial lesions, pneumonia, pulmonary emboli, and cardiogenic and noncardiogenic pulmonary edema. Examples of other conditions associated with wheezing include anaphylaxis and carcinoid syndrome.

Glottic dysfunction may be a form of a conversion reaction and is characterized by the paradoxical adduction of the vocal cords. Although clinical features may include hypoxemia and hypercapnia-like asthma, the blood gas pattern is that of central alveolar hypoventilation, and there may be stridolous or halting breathing over the neck. Although direct vocal cord visualization for dysfunctional movement and/or ventilation scanning to confirm a normal distribution can be done in the ED, frequently the patient is treated presumptively for asthma and laryngeal assessment is deferred.

Table 4
Predicted Peak Expiratory Flow Rate for Adults and Children

Table of predicted peak expiratory flow for age and height: adult (L/min)

Age (yr)	Women (height)					Men (height)				
	55"	60"	65"	70"	75"	60"	65"	70"	75"	80"
20	390	423	460	496	529	554	602	649	693	740
30	380	413	448	483	516	532	577	622	664	710
40	370	402	436	470	502	509	552	596	636	680
50	360	391	424	457	488	486	527	569	607	649
60	350	380	412	445	474	463	502	542	578	618
70	340	369	400	432	461	440	477	515	550	587

Table of predicted peak expiratory flow for height: children

Height	39"	43"	47"	51"	55"	59"	63"	67"	71"	75"
L/min	110	160	210	260	320	370	420	475	530	570

Adapted from refs. *2a* and *2b*.

TESTING IN THE ED

Patients with mild to moderate acute asthma exacerbation need little in the way of specialized testing. Vital signs and pulse oximetry are conventional standard pieces of information. If the exacerbation is more than mild or mild but not responsive to initial intervention, then measurement of PEFR is indicated, with sequential checks over time if the initial value is significantly below expected baseline (*see* Table 4). An alternative would be the performance of pulmonary function tests (PFTs) or spirometry, but this equipment is generally not available in EDs and the extra information gathered is typically not germane for emergency care.

When complicating conditions are being considered, additional information through diagnostic testing is warranted. A complete blood count and differential may be helpful to look for eosinophilia. Elevation of the white blood cell count may suggest infection but also may simply be a nonspecific marker of stress or may reflect catecholamine or steroid treatment. Measurement of electrolytes, blood urea nitrogen, and creatinine may be helpful to assess for hydration status and may be important preparatory information for certain treatment interventions, such as diuretics, or for certain types of diagnostic testing, for example those using radiocontrast media. If applicable, theophylline level should be done.

Chest radiograph (CXR) is an option for the first presentation of bronchospasm but would not be expected to show more than hyperinflation. A CXR is indicated when other conditions are suspected, such as pneumothorax/pneumomediastinum, CHF, pneumonia, bullous disease, and fibrotic or interstitial disease. A CXR is usually done if the patient is being admitted to the hospital.

Electrocardiogram (EKG) in asthma may show sinus tachycardia and right heart strain. EKG is important when there is a question of dysrhythmia or cardiac ischemia. In older patients with suspected or known cardiovascular disease, and EKG should be a routine test when there is a presentation of shortness of breath, with or without chest pain. Similarly, if high-quality, rapid turn-around time cardiac enzyme testing is available, this also should be done on the patient at risk for cardiac ischemia presenting with shortness of breath. If B-type natruretic peptide testing is available, this result may help diagnose an exacerbation of CHF when a patient may have an exacerbation of CHF, asthma, or both. Evaluation for pulmonary embolus may revolve around chest computed tomography (CT) scanning. This type of radiological evaluation also helps characterize many other lung conditions. Sinusitis is frequently a clinical diagnosis in the ED, but with the availability of CT scanning, the sinuses can be more accurately assessed and treatment based on more objective criteria.

The question of the need for cultures in patients with wheezing often is raised in the ED. Sputum cultures are generally not needed for bronchitis. The variable quality of the submitted specimens and the obligatory slow turn-around time do not make them cost-effective for decision making in the ED. When antibiotic therapy is indicated for bronchitis, the choice of drug is typically empiric. Sputum cultures generally also are not needed for community-acquired pneumonia that will be treated on an outpatient basis. For patients who will be treated in the hospital, however, the admitting physician's preference probably will be for sputum cultures to be obtained, as well as blood cultures.

In the pediatric population, viral testing is a consideration. Bronchiolitis, a viral infection of the bronchioles, is usually seen in children younger than 2 yr old. Respiratory syncytial virus (RSV) is the most common etiology, occurring November to March, although other etiologies include parainfluenza and *Mycoplasma*. Antigen tests of nasal washings may detect RSV and be helpful in the management of high-risk patients.

TREATMENT OF THE MILD ASTHMA ATTACK

If a patient presents with the features of a mild exacerbation of asthma, the first-line medication is albuterol (Ventolin®, Proventil®, metered-dose inhaler [MDI] with or Salbutamol®). A mild attack is confirmed when the patient experiences a prompt and near-complete response with resolution of wheezing, cough, and/or shortness of breath.

Delivery of the albuterol may be by nebulizer or holding chamber. Studies of adults and older children with acute asthma have shown that both modalities are effective in providing particles of the optimal 1- to 5-μ size to the lower airways *(3)*. This translates to no significant difference in terms of rate of hospital admission, length of time spent in the ED, or PEFR. The comparable efficacy of the MDI with holding chamber vs the nebulizer has also been demonstrated for the more severely affected patients with FEV_1 less than 30% of predicted. There is no significant difference in heart rates between the two methods, although less medication accumulates in the oropharynx if the holding chamber is used rather than the nebulizer.

Nebulizer dosage for adults is 2.5 mg albuterol (0.5 mL of 0.5% solution) in 2–3 mL of saline given one to three times during a 1- to 2-h interval. Pediatric dosage is 0.15 mg/kg albuterol solution given in a similar manner. Premixed nebules can be used instead. Mode of delivery is typically via a medication reservoir attached to a pipe-like mouthpiece, but for infants and young children, a facemask device can be employed. Oxygen or compressed air at 6–9 L/min, from wall outlet or tank, is connected by tubing to drive the nebulization.

Alternatively, an MDI may be used in conjunction with a spacer device or holding chamber to deliver the albuterol. The standard for the MDI is 90 μg albuterol per actuation. The dose is six to eight puffs into the spacer for inhalation by the patient. Dosing frequency can be every 30–60 min.

A patient who has a mild exacerbation and responds well to the initial therapy generally does not require additional time in the ED. There is no advantage to giving larger quantities of albuterol once pulmonary mechanics approach the lower limit of normal.

TREATMENT OF THE MODERATE-TO-SEVERE ASTHMA ATTACK

These patients have more pronounced respiratory distress. Supplemental oxygen is typically provided, with the decision making based on clinical experience and pathophysiology rather than randomized controlled trials or systematic review. Prompt treatment with albuterol, 2.5–5.0 mg, three times in 1 h, is customary.

Ipratropium bromide (Atrovent®) is usually also given with the first and subsequent treatments, 0.25–0.50 mg nebulized. If the MDI with spacer approach is being used, four to eight puffs of ipratropium are intermixed with the albuterol. Ipratropium has a relatively slow onset of action, with its peak in 60–90 min. Although the benefits of ipratropium are still a matter of debate, studies have been interpreted to indicate that this medication provides additive benefit to short-acting β-agonists by marginally increasing PEFR and by reducing hospitalization rates in adult and pediatric populations with severe asthma (4,5). The addition of a single dose of inhaled anticholinergic agent to albuterol improves lung function but does not influence admission rate.

An alternative to the inhaled bronchodilator medications is to use the subcutaneous route. Historically, epinephrine has been given to reverse bronchospasm, at the dose of 0.01 mg/kg of 1:1000, not to exceed 0.3–0.5 mg. Epinephrine can be repeated every 5–20 min for a total of approximately three doses. Epinephrine is an effective treatment, but it can cause side effects such as tachycardia, hypertension, and tremulousness. In patients with cardiac disease, deaths have been attributed to the use of epinephrine. In pregnant patients, it may contribute to uterine vessel spasm. Terbutaline is one of the newer moderately short-acting β-2 agonist bronchodilators, and compared to epinephrine, it generates fewer side effects. It may be given in the dose of 0.25 mg subcutaneously for adults and repeated in 15–30 min. If it is possible to use inhaled medications, however, it is the preferable route because it is more direct. Oral preparations of albuterol and terbutaline are available but have little clinical applicability in the ED.

Albuterol is a racemic mixture of (R)- and (S)- isomers. The (R)-albuterol has the bronchodilating properties, whereas the (S)-form has preferential pulmonary retention, a longer half-life, and possible proinflammatory effects (6). The pure (R)-form, levalbuterol (Xopenex®), induces bronchodilation on a 4:1 ratio compared with albuterol and induces systemic side effects on a 2:1 ratio compared with albuterol (7). The ultimate balance of cost, beneficial bronchodilatory effect, and adverse side effects for levalbuterol vs albuterol has yet to be defined, but in a patient susceptible to side effects and anticipated to require a large dose, levalbuterol may be the preferable alternative.

CSs are part of the treatment plan for patients with moderate exacerbation of asthma. They are used to counter airway inflammation and hasten resolution of the asthma exacerbation. Because they act through ligand-dependent activation of receptors, gene regulation, and new protein synthesis, clinical benefits are likely to occur gradually, over 6–12 h. Treatment algorithms typically suggest giving systemic steroids to patients who do not respond rapidly to β-agonist use alone. The decision can usually be made in

30–60 min, once a dose of 5 to 10 mg of nebulized albuterol or an equivalent has been given. In the emergency setting, the practitioner may wish to factor in the timing and dose of treatment with β-agonists in the ambulance and/or the intensity of rescue treatment the patient has employed before the visit. A meta-analysis to define the benefit of treating patients with acute asthma with systemic steroids within an hour of presenting to the ED has concluded that it reduces the need for hospital admission for adult patients (number needed to treat of eight) and for pediatric patients (NNT of three) *(8)*. A systematic review found that systemic CSs (oral or intramuscular) given at the start of an acute asthma exacerbation also reduced the number of relapses requiring additional care and reduced the subsequent use of β2-agonists *(9)*.

Adult patients who appear stable and likely to improve on therapy are given an oral dose. This route is regarded as equally effective when compared to the iv route *(10)*.

A meta-analysis has indicated that low, medium, or high dosing of methylprednisolone in the first 24 h (≤80 mg, >80 mg, and ≤360 mg, and > 360 mg, respectively), showed a similar therapeutic advantage *(11)*. In the United States, the standard approach is 60 mg of prednisone for the adult patient. In other parts of the world, it is 30 to 40 mg of prednisolone. For pediatric patients in the ED, choices include prednisone or prednisolone 2 mg/kg by mouth or intravenous methylprednisolone 2 mg/kg if more easily accomplished than the oral route. Although reference manuals often recommend repeat dosing every 6 h, high and frequent doses do not confer a therapeutic advantage.

At discharge, a typical dose of oral CSs for adult patients is 0.5–1 mg/kg/d for 5–10 d and for pediatric patients is 1 mg/kg twice a day for 4 d. A randomized controlled trial has compared tapering of prednisolone over a week against abrupt cessation and found that once asthma control was achieved, prednisolone could be stopped without tapering *(12)*. Several trials have investigated the replacement of oral CSs with inhaled CSs (ICSs) at the time of discharge. Although there is some evidence that high-dose ICS therapy alone may be as effective as oral CS therapy prescribed for patients with mild asthma, this is not firmly proven, and the approach has not been tested in patients with severe asthma *(13)*.

In the past giving ICSs during an acute asthma exacerbation was contraindicated. The reasoning was that components of the inhaled preparation might be irritative and cause increased cough or bronchospasm. This is not believed to be of clinical importance at this time, and in fact, the direct delivery to the airways is regarded as a potential advantage. Several randomized controlled trials have been conducted to explore a potential role for ICSs in acute asthma, especially in the pediatric population because this route simplifies delivery and spares systemic steroids. A meta-analysis has combined review of (1) studies that investigated systemic steroids with and without ICSs and of (2) studies that investigated ICSs vs placebo, and the meta-analysis found that patients treated with ICSs were less likely to be admitted to the hospital and tolerated the treatment well but showed only small improvements in PEFRs such that they were unlikely to be clinically significant *(14)*. Overall, the immediate effect of ICSs in acute asthma is marginal, and there is insufficient evidence that ICSs alone are as effective as systemic steroids.

For patients who do not respond to or are not able to take standard emergency treatment medications, intravenous aminophylline, at 5–6 mg/kg bolus and then 0.6–0.9 mg/kg/h is a consideration. As an older and well-studied approach, it is not clearly an added benefit to albuterol plus ipratropium plus steroids, and it is difficult to use because of the narrow therapeutic window before toxic side effects such as nausea/vomiting, seizure. Therefore, it is considered a second-line alternative.

For patients who are suboptimally responding to standard emergency treatment medications, the addition of a leukotriene-modifying agent, such as montelukast (Singulair), should be considered. These oral agents are generally prescribed for the treatment of mild asthma in patients who are reluctant to take ICS or as add-on therapy for patients who remain symptomatic on ICS. Because studies have shown that urinary leukotrienes are elevated in acute asthma, it has been theorized that early initiation of a leukotriene-modifying agent may quiet the process of inflammation and provide an extra edge to allow recovery sooner. A study with iv montelukast has shown a prompt incremental improvement, suggesting at least a component of immediate reversal of bronchospasm *(15)*. However, guiding information is not currently available regarding a role for an oral dose of a leukotriene-modifying agent in the ED treatment of moderately severe asthma.

TREATMENT OF THE VERY SEVERE ASTHMA ATTACK

Patients who are having a very severe asthma attack are in obvious respiratory distress and require the full resources of the ED. These patients should be placed on monitors for continuous recording of the rhythm strip and pulse oximetry and for frequent recording of the blood pressure. If end-tidal air stream CO_2 monitoring is available, it could be used in this situation. This technology allows breathing through a sampling probe and measurement of the dCO_2/dt. Because the result correlates with PEFR, it may provide a rapid, noninvasive, effort-independent measure of bronchospasm *(16)*.

Supplemental oxygen should be provided, typically at the highest percentage available, waiving concern regarding CO_2 narcosis if there is existing significant hypoxia. Intravenous access should be established, preferably at two sites. Intravenous fluids will be needed in most pediatric patients and should be considered for adult patients.

If the patient can cooperate, albuterol by nebulizer should be initiated immediately. A dose of 15–20 mg may be given as a continuous treatment over 1 h. Per randomized controlled trials, in adults with more severe airflow obstruction, continuous nebulizer treatment improves outcome more than intermittent treatment. One study, looking at a subgroup of patients with more severe asthma, has shown increased PEFR at 120 min and lower hospitalization rates *(17)*.

Subcutaneous terbutaline or epinephrine, if not contraindicated, would be alternatives if the inhaled route were unavailable or failing. In general, though, this approach will not change the course of the patient who is not responding to inhaled high-dose albuterol. Intravenous β-agonists have been tried in difficult situations. Randomized controlled trials have produced conflicting evidence regarding whether the intravenous route or the inhaled route is more efficacious; there is agreement that the intravenous route is associated with more adverse effects, for example, tachycardia and hypokalemia *(18,19)*. The conclusion of a meta-analysis was that evidence is lacking to support the use of intravenous β2-agonists in ED patients with severe acute asthma, except possibly for those patients for whom inhaled therapy is not feasible *(20)*.

In addition to intense β-agonist treatment, ipratropium should be given, for example, 0.5 mg by nebulization initially and then repeated at 0.25 mg. In a study of patients who received 2880 µg of albuterol and 504 µg of ipratropium or placebo by MDI plus spacer for 3 h, the subgroup of those with more severe obstruction (FEV_1 <30% predicted) and long duration of symptoms before ED presentation (>24 h) had a particularly favorable response to the addition of ipratropium bromide in terms of improvement in FEV_1 and decrease in admission rate *(21)*.

CSs should be given early in the severe attack, even with the realization that there will be a lag time before effect. This ensures the benefit at the earliest possible time. The intravenous route is the one of choice because the patient is generally too compromised to reliably take and absorb oral medications. A typical medication and dose would be methylprednisolone (Solu-Medrol®) 80–125 mg intravenously.

Broad-spectrum antibiotics are often given early, after cultures, for definite or suspected infection.

The most extreme stages of severe acute asthma are respiratory failure, cardiopulmonary arrest, and death. Emergency medicine is in search of special approaches for the patient with severe bronchospasm and near-fatal asthma. Magnesium and ketamine are two supplemental medication treatments that have been investigated for effectiveness. Respiratory care options, such as use of heliox and noninvasive positive pressure support, have also been examined.

Magnesium Sulfate

Per meta-analysis review, single-dose intravenous magnesium is regarded as likely to be beneficial in patients with acute severe asthma, that is, those with a presenting FEV_1 of less than 25–30% of predicted *(22)*. A typical adult dose is 2 g over 20 min, although higher doses and faster rates have been safely employed. The pediatric dose is 25–100 mg/kg over 1 h, up to 2 g. The typical scenario is administration within 60 min of arrival after a poor response to initial bronchodilators. The benefit that can be anticipated several hours later is an improvement of 10% in predicted FEV or 50 L/min in PEFR, and a decrease in admission rate. No significant adverse effects are associated with intravenous treatment in this dose range. Magnesium's mechanism of action may have to do with calcium antagonism and bronchial smooth muscle relaxation, reducing the neutrophilic burst associated with the inflammatory response in asthma, and/or potentiation of β2-agonist effects.

Studies have explored the adjunctive use of magnesium sulfate by the nebulized route. One randomized controlled trial compared 2.5 mg of albuterol plus 3 mL of saline against 2.5 mg of albuterol plus 3 mL of isotonic magnesium sulfate through a nebulizer; peak flows at 10 min and 20 min after treatment showed more improvement compared with baseline in the albuterol–magnesium group *(23)*. In another study, a randomized double-blind placebo-controlled trial, an enhanced bronchodilator response with isotonic magnesium as an adjuvant to nebulized albuterol for patients with presenting FEV_1 of less than 50% predicted was demonstrated at 90 min *(24)*. In a prospective, randomized, double-blinded study of the management of children with mild to moderate asthma, the addition of magnesium to albuterol provided short-term benefits *(25)*. The accumulating evidence lends credence to a bronchodilatory effect of magnesium but does not yet define the relative role compared to other standard interventions, such as treatment with an anticholinergic agent or CSs.

Ketamine

Ketamine (Ketalar®) is a dissociative anesthetic agent that acts on the cortex and limbic system. Structurally derived from phencyclidine and introduced into clinical practice in the 1970s, it is used as an induction agent before the administration of general anesthesia. It also had a role in sedation for short but painful procedures. Scientific research has demonstrated a bona fide bronchodilatory effect as a direct smooth muscle relaxant, and it may also act by increasing circulating catecholamines and/or inhibiting vagal outflow.

Clinical case reports have indicated a value as a bronchodilator in severe asthma. However, ketamine has several precautionary aspects: it is not safe in pregnancy and it is contraindicated in several medical conditions, such as elevated intracranial pressure, hypertension, thyrotoxicosis, angina, and CHF. Furthermore, it increases bronchial secretions and it has the propensity to cause dysphoria. A beneficial effect of ketamine in severe asthma remains to be definitively proven. In a small randomized placebo-controlled trial, at subanesthetic doses sufficiently low to avoid dysphoria (0.1 mg/kg bolus and 0.5 mg/kg/h infusion for several hours), no benefit was demonstrated compared to standard therapy in terms of increased bronchodilatory effect or decreased hospital admission rate (26). Nonetheless, case reports continue to suggest that there is some benefit from ketamine at higher doses in patients requiring mechanical ventilation, with alleviation of bronchospasm and improved oxygenation. For induction, the adult dose is 1.0–2.0 mg/kg intravenously, and the pediatric dose can be the same.

Heliox

Heliox is the mixture of helium and oxygen. Because of its low density and its ability to reduce turbulent airflow, it has been tried as a therapeutic option for various upper and lower airway conditions. Evidence-based guidelines for use are sparse. Although administering heliox is relatively cumbersome and costly, there are no significant side effects associated with it, so heliox is regarded as a reasonable alternative for trial in the following conditions: mechanical upper airway obstruction; postoperative stridor; severe exacerbations of COPD, particularly in conjunction with noninvasive ventilation (see "Noninvasive Positive Pressure Ventilation"); and in asthma complicated by impending respiratory failure and refractory to standard therapy. Early use of this intervention may help reduce the work of the respiratory muscles and forestall fatigue. The highest ratio of helium to oxygen that will maintain oxygen saturation higher than 90% should be used, for example, 80:20 or 70:30, because beneficial effects are theoretically proportional to the percentage of helium in the inhaled gas. Any clinical benefit is likely to be apparent early and, in the case of asthma treatment, may later be overshadowed by the accumulation of therapeutic benefits from standard therapy. However, recent meta-analysis of randomized controlled trials of heliox for treating patients who have acute asthma and are not intubated did not encourage its use. In fact, the reviewers concluded that existing evidence does not provide support for the administration of helium–oxygen mixtures to patients in the ED with moderate to severe asthma (27). More research is needed, and it would be especially helpful to know if heliox can aid in averting tracheal intubation and mechanical ventilation.

If the clinician decides to use heliox, the practical set up is as follows. A commercial mixture of helium and oxygen is used, available in a portable cylinder, often as 79% helium and 21% oxygen. Administration is best via a non-rebreathing face mask to minimize mixing of heliox with room air. For patients in whom there is a concern regarding hypoxia, supplemental oxygen can be provided via nasal cannulas, although this tends to increase the density of the gas mixture and possibly negates any clinical benefit. It should be noted that peak flow readings vary depending on the viscosity of the gas being delivered, and the relatively lower density of heliox would be expected to result in a higher peak flow compared to air unless standardization is done.

Noninvasive Positive Pressure Ventilation

Noninvasive positive pressure ventilation (NPPV), also known as noninvasive pressure support ventilation (NIPSV), represents the delivery of mechanically assisted breaths via a device that is external to the body, such as a tightly fitting nasal or facial mask, rather than an internal artificial airway. It is also referred to as bilevel pressure ventilation (BiPAP), based on the name of the ventilator commonly used, produced by Respironics, Murrysville, PA. Studies have shown that the technique is efficacious in acute respiratory failure related to exacerbations of COPD, acute cardiogenic pulmonary edema, and hypoxemic respiratory failure. In patients with symptomatic asthma, continuous positive airway pressure (CPAP) delivered by mask decreases airway resistance and the work of breathing but does not improve gas exchange. In COPD with acute respiratory failure, adding intermittent positive pressure ventilation to mask CPAP, for example, inspiratory pressure of 15 cm H_2O and expiratory pressure of 4 cm H_2O, provides the component of correction in gas exchange abnormalities. Improvements in pH and pCO_2 within 1.5–2 h are predictive of the eventual success of NPPV, and if they do not occur, intubation should be considered. Barotrauma is uncommon, modest air leaks are common but not prohibitive, and adverse hemodynamic effects are unusual. Nosocomial pneumonia and sinusitis are decreased compared with patients who are intubated.

The role of NPPV in asthma is not defined; the number of studies addressing its use in patients with asthma with severe respiratory distress is limited. One case series reported an encouraging experience when NPPV was used in 17 patients with asthma with hypercapnic acute respiratory failure; all survived, and 15 did not require intubation (28). In view of such reports and the success with NPPV in conditions such as respiratory failure resulting from COPD or owing to cardiogenic pulmonary edema, emergency physicians and respiratory therapists have been inclined to convey the technique to patients with asthma in severe respiratory distress. When applied with prudence, it obviates intubation in some patients. Of note, one study has shown a relative benefit for patients with FEV_1 less than 60% of predicted treated with bilevel NPPV: after 3 h, the treated patients had a 50% or more improvement of FEV_1 from baseline and reduced hospitalization rates compared with controls (29). Nonetheless, the use of NPPV in patients with severe asthma is currently regarded as experimental therapy and awaits additional study.

MANAGEMENT OF RESPIRATORY FAILURE IN SEVERE ASTHMA

Intubation and mechanical ventilation can be a life-saving management approach for patients with severe bronchospasm, although it has associated risks. The risks include hypotension, barotrauma, infection, and myopathy.

If the patient is in extremis, intubation is performed immediately according to the dictum of ABCs—airway, breathing, and circulation. If the patient's status is borderline, often a trial of aggressive interventions is conducted, however, at the same time preparing for the possibility of intubation. Patients with slowing or weakening respiratory pattern and persistent bronchospasm require intubation. Patients who have mental status changes and inability to cooperate with therapy, whether on the basis of hypoxia and/or carbon dioxide build-up, should be intubated. Patients who are severely symptomatic and working hard to breathe for an extended period must be intubated to relieve fatigue.

Rapid-sequence intubation is the standard approach for these patients. It must be conducted expeditiously because of the patient's lack of reserve. If ketamine is not used, then etomidate or another sedating agent would be used, plus succinylcholine or other neuromuscular blocking agents. An oral endotracheal tube is placed, trying to maximize diameter to minimize airflow obstruction and enhance secretion removal. Generally, nasal awake intubations are not attempted because the patient is unable to cooperate. Once the patient is intubated, longer acting sedative agents should be used, and possibly paralytic agents, although prolonged use of neuromuscular blocking agents and CSs is associated with myopathy *(30)*.

The practitioner must be aware of certain strategies to deal with potential consequences of mechanical ventilation. There may be a drop in blood pressure. Intravenous fluids should be administered and the patient evaluated for tension pneumothorax. If pneumothorax is present, the chest must be vented with a needle and later with placement of a chest tube. The possibility of auto-PEE needs to be considered; it may be empirically treated by removing the patient from the ventilator for a period. For the risk of barotrauma, evidence is accumulating that the policy of permissive hypercapnia should be pursued. Cohort studies and case reports suggest fewer deaths occur when respiratory acidosis is managed with tolerance and intravenous bicarbonate if pH is less than 7.2 than by aggressive ventilation employing high pressures to keep carbon dioxide levels in the normal range.

Although not suitable for ED care, general anesthesia, as with isoetharine, is effective for patients with high pressures. The emergency practitioner should be aware of this option and consider arranging transfer of the patient to the operative setting where the rooms are properly vented.

Some of the special strategies for treating severe asthma before intubation, can be considered for initiation or continuation in the postintubation period. These include infusion of magnesium, infusion of ketamine, and use of heliox.

ADVERSE RESPONSES TO MEDICATION TREATMENTS

Albuterol is the mainstay of therapy for patients with acute asthma exacerbation. Commonly reported mild adverse effects associated with frequent dosing include tachycardia, tremor, and headache. If continuous high-dose albuterol is administered by nebulizer, tremor occurs in approx 20% of patients *(31)* A known effect of albuterol is shift of potassium into cells with the result of hypokalemia by laboratory measurement. Although preexisting hypokalemia should be corrected, aggressive replenishment of potassium during albuterol therapy is not recommended. Albuterol in high doses may cause arrhythmias. It is difficult to sort out this propensity because the patients may have hypoxia and concomitant acid–base abnormalities. There are rare reports of lactic acidosis with albuterol administration.

The most common adverse events associated with inhaled ipratropium included tremor, agitation, vomiting, increase in pulse, dry mouth, palpitations, chest pain, back pain, nervousness, headache, nausea, and dizziness. However, many of the reported side effects are minor and occur during administration of ipratropium for more than 12 wk rather than in the setting of the acute treatment of asthma.

Table 5
Adverse Effects of Systemic Corticosteroids

Organ system	Adverse effect
Dermatological	Skin thinning/purpura, alopecia, acne, hirsutism, striae
Eye	Posterior capsular cataract, elevated intraocular pressure
Cardiovascular	Hypertension, dyslipoproteinemia, premature atherosclerotic disease
Gastrointestinal	Gastritis, peptic ulcer disease, pancreatitis, steatohepatitis, visceral perforation
Renal	Hypokalemia, fluid volume shifts
Genitourinary, reproductive	Amenorrhea, infertility, intrauterine growth retardation
Bone	Osteoporosis, avascular necrosis
Muscle	Myopathy
Neuropsychiatric	Euphoria/dysphoria/psychosis, insomnia, akathisia, pseudo tumor cerebri
Endocrine	Diabetes mellitus, hypothalamic–pituitary–adrenal insufficiency
Infectious disease	Heightened risk of infection

Systemic CSs have a large number of known adverse effects (*see* Table 5). An important issue is how much systemic effect inhaled steroids cause, particularly for the growing pediatric patient. Studies of the newer agents, such as fluticasone, indicate that there is rapid breakdown and currently no known significant systemic effects.

ADVERSE ASTHMA RESPONSES TO NONASTHMA MEDICATIONS

The practitioner must be aware that certain medications are contraindicated or relatively contraindicated in patients with acute or latent bronchospasm. β-blockers are in this category. Although the newer agents are more β-selective and less likely to provoke bronchospasm than older medications, such as propranolol, for high-risk patients, β-blockers should be avoided.

Patients with aspirin allergy or with the syndrome of asthma, nasal polyposis, and aspirin sensitivity should not be given aspirin. There is an approx 20% cross-reactivity with nonsteroidal anti-inflammatory drugs (NSAIDs). For patients presenting with acute coronary syndrome, the main alternative would be clopidogrel (Plavix®), which has supplanted ticlopidine (Ticlid®) after reports of a better safety profile.

DISPOSITION OF THE PATIENT WITH ASTHMA

Managing acute episodes of asthma in the ED involves relieving troublesome symptoms as rapidly and cost effectively as possible. Care paths or practice guidelines can aid in this endeavor, as long as the algorithms are simple and logical.

The emergency practitioner will be making the decision regarding disposition of the patient to home, into the hospital, or into an intermediary care unit (often termed observation units for patients who are unlikely to require more than 24 h of treatment). At the time of presentation, it can be projected that more than 75% of patients presenting with severe exacerbation will require admission and less than 30% of patients presenting with nonsevere exacerbation will require admission. Certainly, patients with persisting severe asthma exacerbations will need to be admitted and those with easily correctable mild to moderate exacerbations will be sent home. Those in the intermediate group typically need to be treated and reassessed to make the determination regarding admission.

Some features of the patient's case may heighten the caution required in the disposition decision. Frequent ED visits, frequent hospitalizations, frequent intensive care unit admissions, and prior intubation should weight the decision more toward admission. Duration of symptoms for more than 2 d is associated with a higher admission rate, perhaps because potentially reversible bronchospasm has been complicated by bronchial edema, tenacious secretions, mucous plugging, and atelectasis.

For the patients who are being discharged, a period of observation off of bronchodilating agents should be done as an indication that there would not be early significant relapse. Also, testing the patient's ability to ambulate without development of significant dyspnea or hypoxia should be done in borderline cases.

Provisions must be made for the patient to have medications, typically inhaled bronchodilators and a burst of oral steroids. Discussion regarding avoidance of triggers should be undertaken. The patient should be provided with a peak expiratory flow meter and instructed regarding its best use. The patient's asthma should be categorized per the National Institutes for Health guidelines and long-term therapy directed accordingly. Outpatient follow-up needs to be arranged and highly encouraged.

A systematic review has indicated that education of adults about asthma to facilitate self-management reduces risk of hospital admission, unscheduled visits to the doctor, and days missed at work; best results were seen in patients who had written care plans *(32)*. Although there is acknowledged importance to teaching proper inhaler technique, holding chamber use, recognition of asthma triggers, and rationale for medications, the minority of ED departments have formal asthma education programs *(33)*.

PREDICTING RESPONSE TO THERAPY

Early identification of patients with acute asthma who should be hospitalized and at what level of care would be helpful for the management of ED resources. It is not unusual for patients to be treated for 4–24 h before a disposition decision is made. Additionally, because a substantial number of patients who are discharged from an ED suffer relapse and require a repeat visit within 2–14 d, variously reported as 10–40%, it would also be helpful to prospectively identify this group.

Many studies have investigated methodology for predicting outcome. There is general agreement that for the majority of patients presenting with acute asthma, there is not a single universal parameter in the initial history, physical examination, or bedside testing that accurately categorizes the patient as a good responder or poor responder to conventional therapy. Also, multivariate formulas based on initial information have not proven to be accurate predictors for all-comers.

The data gathered at a time of reevaluation, for example, in 1 h, is more helpful. A key feature for adults revolves around the PEFR measured after initial treatment with inhaled albuterol and systemic CSs. Although it is difficult to make generalizations, PEFR of less than 40% of predicted seems correlated with need for hospitalization or need for subsequent treatment after discharge, particularly if combined with either the determination of use of accessory muscles or the PEFR variation of less than 60 L *(34)*. However, the caveat is that although many patients can be accurately judged as likely suitable for discharge or likely requiring admission, there are also many patients who fall between the defining parameters for an index. Also, PEFR as a percentage of predicted is a somewhat difficult parameter for the emergency practitioner to apply, because some patients with asthma have significant fixed airflow obstruction even during asymptomatic periods. The baseline personal best PEFR for the patient may be the more relevant comparison, but often this is not available in the acute setting. In the pediatric population, especially in those younger patients who are not able to perform peak expiratory flow meter testing, clinical assessment is important. A score based on the three clinical findings of wheezing, prolonged expiration, and work of breathing—assessed at presentation, after 1 h of treatment, and at the time of disposition—seems helpful in discriminating among those patients in need and not in need of hospital admission (35).

PREDICTING FATAL OR NEAR-FATAL EPISODES

Death from acute asthma episodes is reported in less than 0.1% of patients with asthma. Approximately half die out of the hospital and half in the hospital. Although the impression is that death occurs suddenly, regarding the in-hospital cases, the majority of patients have had symptoms for more than 12 h.

Near fatality has been viewed as the occurrence of respiratory arrest and/or coma necessitating emergency tracheal intubation and mechanical ventilation, and the condition is distinguished from those patients who are electively intubated because of fatigue. Despite research efforts, clinically infallible predictors of patients who are at risk for fatal or near-fatal episodes of asthma have not been identified because the associations are not sensitive or specific. Risk factors occur too frequently in the general asthma population and too infrequently in subpopulations who are at risk for a fatal or near-fatal episode to allow precise application. Patient characteristics include lack of understanding or misinterpretation of the seriousness of the symptoms, poor medical compliance, and coincident psychiatric illness and/or drug abuse. Statistically, such patients are likely to have repeated hospitalizations, multiple ED visits, and history of respiratory failure. Conversely, retrospective surveys indicate that 15–30% of asthma deaths occur in patients with only mild asthma. Histopathological findings suggest that the type of acute asthma that leads to death may be a unique entity. However, until more information is available to explain why some patients with asthma die of a potentially reversible disease, outpatient chronic asthma management must teach proficiency in the use of bronchodilator rescue therapy and emphasize universal availability. Acute ED management needs to focus on rapid and proficient evaluation and intervention.

CONCLUSION

The full spectrum of acute asthma is addressed in the ED, from mild to life-threatening exacerbations, straightforward to complicated presentations, and good responses to poor responses to treatment. For all asthma cases, the goal is to practice evidence-based medicine. For the patients who are unstable, the special expertise required in the ED relates to timing and application of infrequently used techniques.

REFERENCES

1. Turner MT, Noertjojo K, Vedal S, et al. Risk factors for near-fatal asthma: a case control study in patients hospitalized with acute asthma. *Am J Respir Crit Care Med* 1998; 157: 1804–1809.
2. Rea H, Garrett J, Lanes S, Birmann B, Kolbe J. The association between asthma drugs and severe life-threatening attacks. *Chest* 1996; 110: 1446–1451.

2a. Leiner GC, Abramowitz S, Small MJ, Stenby VB, Lewis WA. Expiratory peak flow rate. Standard values for normal subjects. *Am Rev Resp Dis* 1963; 88: 644–651.

2b. McElroy, SP. *Pediatric Emergency Medicine: The Essentials.* Boston, MA, Health Emergency Publishing, 2004.

3. Cates CC, Bara A, Crilly JA, Rowe BH. Holding chambers versus nebulisers for beta-agonist treatment of acute asthma. *Cochrane Database Syst Rev* 2003; (3): CD000052.

4. Rodrigo G, Rodrigo C, Burschtin O. Ipratropium bromide in acute adult severe asthma: a meta-analysis of randomized controlled trials. *Am J Med* 1999; 107: 363–370.

5. Plotnick LH, Ducharme FM. Acute asthma in children and adolescents: should inhaled anticholinergics be added to beta-2 agonists? *Am J Respir Med* 2003; 2: 109–115.

6. Page CP, Morley J. Third-generation beta-agonists: changing of the guard, contrasting properties of albuterol stereoisomers. *J Allergy Clin Immunol* 1999; 104: S31–S41.

7. Nowak R. Single-isomer levalbuterol: a review of the acute data. *Curr Allergy Asthma Rep* 2003; 3: 172–178.

8. Rowe BH, Spooner C, Ducharme FM, Bretzlaff JA, Bota GW. Early emergency department treatment of acute asthma with systemic corticosteroids. *Cochrane Database Syst Rev* 2001; 1: CD0021178.

9. Rowe BH, Spooner CH, Duchrame FM, Bratzlaff JA, Bota GW. Corticosteroids for preventing relapse following acute exacerbations of asthma. *Cochrane Database Syst Rev* 2000; 3: CD000195.

10. Ratto D, Alfaro C, Sipsey J, Glovsky MM, Sharma OP. Are intravenous corticosteroids required in status asthmaticus? *JAMA* 1988; 260: 527.

11. Manser R, Reid D, Abramson H. Corticosteroids for acute severe asthma in hospitalized patients. *Cochrane Database Syst Rev* 2000; (2): CD001740.

12. O'Driscoll BR, Kalra S, Wilson M, et al. Double-blind trial of steroid tapering in acute asthma. *Lancet* 1993; 341: 324–327.

13. Edmonds ML, Camargo CA Jr, Brenner BE, Rowe BH. Replacement of oral corticosteroids with inhaled corticosteroids in the treatment of acute asthma following emergency department discharge: a meta-analysis. *Chest* 2002; 121: 1798–1805.

14. Edmonds ML, Camargo CA Jr, Pollack CV Jr, Rowe BH. The effectiveness of inhaled corticosteroids in the emergency department treatment of acute asthma: a meta-analysis. *Ann Emerg Med* 2002; 40: 145–154.

15. Camargo CA Jr, Smithline HA, Malice MP, Green SA, Reiss TF. A randomized controlled trial of intravenous montelukast in acute asthma. *Am J Respir Crit Care Med* 2003; 167: 528–533.

16. Yaron M, Padyk P, Hutsinpiller M, Cairns CB. Utility of the expiratory capnogram in the assessment of bronchospasm. *Ann Emerg Med* 1996; 28: 403–407.

17. Rudnitsky GS, Eberlein RS, Schoffstall JM, et al. Comparison of intermittent and continuously nebulized albuterol for treatment of asthma in an urban emergency department. *Ann Emerg Med* 1993; 22: 1842–1846.

18. Cheong B, Reynolds SR, Rajan G, Ward MJ. Intravenous β-agonist in acute severe asthma. *Br Med J* 1988; 297: 448–450.

19. Salmeron S, Brochard L, Mal H, et al. Nebulized versus intravenous albuterol in hypercapneic acute asthma. A multi-center, double blind, randomized study. *Am J Respir Crit Care Med* 1994; 149: 1466–1470.

20. Travers AH, Rowe BH, Barker S, Jones A, Camargo CA Jr. The Effectiveness of IV beta-agonists in treating patients with acute asthma in the emergency department: a meta-analysis. *Chest* 2002; 122: 1116–1118.

21. Rodrigo GJ, Rodrigo C. First-line therapy for adult patients with acute asthma receiving multiple dose protocol of ipratropium bromide plus albuterol in the emergency department. *Am J Respir Crit Care Med* 2000; 161: 1862–1868.

22. Rowe BH, Bretzlaff JA, Bourdon C, Bota GW, Camargo CA Jr. Magnesium sulfate for treating acute asthmatic exacerbations of acute asthma in the emergency department. *Cochrane Database Syst Rev* 2000; 3: CD001490.

23. Nannini LJ, Pendino JC, Corna RA, Mannarino S, Quispe R. Magnesium sulfate as a vehicle for nebulized salbutamol in acute asthma. *Am J Med* 2000; 108: 193–197.

24. Hughes R, Goldkorn A, Masoli M, et al. Use of isotonic nebulised magnesium sulphate as an adjuvant to salbutamol in treatment of severe asthma in adults: randomised placebo-controlled trial. *Lancet* 2003; 361: 2114–2117.

25. Mahajan P, Haritos D, Rosenberg N, Thomas R. Comparison of nebulized magnesium sulfate plus albuterol to nebulized albuterol plus saline in children with acute exacerbations of mild to moderate asthma. *J Emerg Med* 2004; 27: 21–25.

26. Howton JC, Rose J, Duffy S, Zoltanski T, Levitt MA. Randomized, double-blind, placebo-controlled trial of intravenous ketamine in acute asthma. *Ann Emerg Med* 1996; 27: 170–175.

27. Rodrigo G, Pollack C, Rodrigo C, Rowe BH. Heliox for nonintubated acute asthma patients. *Cochrane Database Sys Rev* 2003; 4: CD002884.

28. Meduri CF, Cook TR, Turner RE, Cohen M, Leeper KV. Noninvasive positive pressure ventilation in status asthmaticus. *Chest* 1995; 110; 767–774.

29. Soroksky A, Stav D, Shpirer I. A pilot prospective, randomized, placebo-controlled trial of bilevel positive airway pressure in acute asthmatic attack. *Chest* 2003;123: 1018–1025.

30. Behbehani NA, Al-Mane FD, Yachkova Y, Pare PD, FitzGerald JM. Myopathy following mechanical ventilation for acute severe asthma: the role of muscle relaxants and corticosteroids. *Chest* 1999; 115: 1627–1631.

31. Shrestha M, Bidadi K, Gourlay S, Hayes J. Continuous vs intermittent albuterol, at high and low doses, in the treatment of severe acute asthma in adults. *Chest* 1996; 110: 42–47.

32. Gibson PG, Coughlan J, Wilson AJ, et al. Self-management education and regular practitioner review for adults with asthma. *Cochrane Database Syst* Rev 2000; 3: CD001117.

33. Emond S, Reed C, Graff L, Clark S, Camargo C. Asthma education in the emergency department. *Ann Emer Med* 2000; 36: 204–211.

34. Mallmann F, Fernandes AK, Avila EM, et al. Early prediction of poor outcome in patients with acute asthma in the emergency room. *Braz J Med Biol Res* 2002; 35: 39–47.

35. Gorelick MH, Stevens MW, Schultz TR, Scribano PV. Performance of a novel clinical score, the Pediatric Asthma Severity Score (PASS), in the evaluation of acute asthma. *Acad Emerg Med* 2004; 11: 10–18.

7

Severe Asthma

From ICU to Discharge

Brian M. Morrissey, MD, *Nicholas J. Kenyon,* MD,
and Timothy E. Albertson, PhD, MD, MPH

CONTENTS

KEY POINTS

- The in-hospital mortality rate for all patients with asthma is less than 1%, but for patients with near-fatal asthma who require intubation, the mortality rate may be as high as 5%.
- Near-fatal asthma refers to a life-threatening asthma attack that requires ventilatory support; status asthmaticus refers to an asthma attack that does not readily respond to aggressive standard treatment.
- β-agonists remain the main pharmacotherapy in status asthmaticus and near-fatal asthma (NFA).
- African-Americans, women, and the elderly are at increased risk of fatal asthma.
- Controlled modes of ventilation that allow for a prolonged expiratory time are favored in patients with NFA.

From: *Current Clinical Practice: Bronchial Asthma:*
A Guide for Practical Understanding and Treatment, 5th ed.
Edited by: M. E. Gershwin and T. E. Albertson © Humana Press Inc., Totowa, NJ

- General anesthesia by either intravenous infusion or gas inhalation are therapeutic options for the patients with the most severe asthma.
- Coordination of discharge and follow-up care can safely reduce length of hospital stay.

INTRODUCTION

Status asthmaticus (SA) and near-fatal asthma (NFA) are common medical emergencies faced by critical care physicians. SA is defined as an acute, severe asthma exacerbation that does not respond readily to initial intensive therapy, whereas NFA refers loosely to a SA attack that progresses to respiratory failure. Timely evaluation and treatment in the clinic, emergency room, or, ultimately, the intensive care unit (ICU) can prevent the morbidity and mortality associated with respiratory failure. Intensivists must be skilled in managing patients with asthma with respiratory failure and knowledgeable about the few but potentially serious complications associated with mechanical ventilation. Bronchodilator and anti-inflammatory medications remain the standard therapies for managing patients with SA and NFA in the ICU. Patients with NFA who are on mechanical ventilation require modes that allow for prolonged expiration and reverse the dynamic hyperinflation associated with the attack. Several adjuncts to mechanical ventilation, including heliox, general anesthesia, and extracorporeal carbon dioxide removal, can be used as life-saving measures in extreme cases.

TRIAGE OF PATIENTS TO THE ICU

Most patients with asthma requiring hospital admission do not need ICU-level care. The majority of hospitalized patients with asthma improve while in the emergency department and warrant observation on a ward for a few days to ensure continued improvement. In an analysis of nearly 30,000 hospital admissions for acute asthma, 10.1% required admission to the ICU and 2.1% required intubation and mechanical ventilation (1). Patients who have been intubated averaged 4.5 extra days in the hospital and more than $11,000 in additional costs as compared with asthma admissions to non-ICU beds. Absolute criteria for triaging patients with acute, severe asthma are lacking; existing guidelines recommend that patients with peak expiratory flow rate (PEFR) less than 200 L/min, a pulsus paradoxus more than 15 mmHg, use of accessory muscles of respiration or a less than 10% improvement in PEFR be monitored in an ICU (2), but data supporting these recommendations are scant. Clearly, worrisome patients—with a worsening respiratory or metabolic acidosis—should be transferred to an intensive care setting.

EPIDEMIOLOGY OF FATAL ASTHMA

Death from asthma is relatively uncommon in this country (5000–6000 cases per year in the United States in the 1990s), but approx 100,000 asthma deaths per year occur worldwide (3). It has been suggested that from 1 to 7% of people with severe asthma will die each year of their disease, and perhaps 17% of those who survive NFA attacks will eventually succumb to asthma (4).

Mortality rates for patients with NFA who require mechanical ventilation vary from 0 to 22% in reported series during the last three decades (5,6), but the rate is probably less than 5% in most settings. In general, morbidity and mortality of hospitalized patients with SA have decreased significantly, and much of the credit results from timely assessment

Table 1
Risk Factors for Fatal Asthma

History of near-fatal asthma	Female gender
African-American ethnicity	Psychiatric illness
Elderly	Blunted perception of dyspnea
Poverty	β-agonist use (long-/short-acting)
Short duration of attack ("Brittle asthma") *(66)*	

and treatment by out-of-hospital providers and better ICU care *(7)*. Hospital care for asthma is not without problems, of course; patients have died because of inadequate initial observation and treatment *(8)* and therapeutic measures may cause debilitating complications.

RISK FACTORS FOR FATAL ASTHMA

The single largest risk factor for fatal asthma is a history of NFA (*see* Table 1). One study found a 16-fold increased risk of asthma death for patients with a history of NFA. Other factors correlate with fatal asthma. Psychiatric illness, for example, is consistently associated with an increased risk of fatal asthma *(9)*. Similarly, persistent smoking carries a twofold increased risk of death in patients with asthma. Another often reported risk factor for fatal asthma is frequent short-acting β_2-agonist use *(10)*. In a case–control study, the use of short-acting β_2-agonists conferred a two- to threefold increased risk per bronchodilator canister per month *(10)*.

Patients with SA and NFA may have blunted perceptions of dyspnea. In one study, 11 patients with severe asthma had blunted ventilatory responses and lower Borg dyspnea scores compared to patients with mild asthma when exposed to hypoxic conditions, suggesting that these patients were unable to recognize their deterioration and impending respiratory failure *(11)*.

Demographics

The majority of adult patients seen in asthma referral clinics are women *(12)*, and this is in contrast to the pediatric population where boys are more prevalent. Furthermore, the age-adjusted mortality rates are significantly higher for women (2.5 vs 1.9/100,000 population), as they are for blacks (3.6 vs 1.2/100,000), Hispanics, and the elderly *(13)*. Why women comprise 60–80% of adult patients with severe asthma is unclear. Genetic predisposition, hormonal effects, and increased prevalences of vocal cord dysfunction and gastroesophageal reflux disease may be contributors in women.

Genetics

Gene polymorphisms are factors in the pathophysiology of severe asthma and possibly fatal asthma. Several studies have outlined the effect of the Gly-16 polymorphism of the β_2-adrenoreceptor. Patients who are homozygous for Gly-16 undergo desensitization and downregulation of this β-receptor response; this genotype is more prevalent in the acute, severe asthma population *(14,15)*. In addition, certain polymorphisms for interleukin-4 and its receptor correlate loosely with SA *(16)*. Other factors that may play a role in predisposition to SA are transforming growth factor-β *(17)* and 5-lipoxygenase activating protein *(18)*.

Psychosocial and Socioeconomic Factors

Poverty and poor access to medical care correlate with increased risk for fatal asthma. For example, 21% of all asthma deaths among young people in the late 1980s occurred in the inner cities of Chicago and New York *(19)*. Several hypotheses have been proposed to explain the correlation between socioeconomic status and fatal asthma. Certainly, one of the most important is that poor patients have inadequate medical care. Risk factors for death from asthma include lack of appropriate anti-inflammatory controller medication, limited self-management skills, increased exposures to air pollution and indoor allergens (house, dust, dust mite, and cockroach), dietary factors, and drug abuse.

Stress

The effect of psychosocial stress on asthma has been demonstrated in several studies. One recent study demonstrated a strong correlation between worsening airway inflammation after antigen challenge during a week of intensive examinations among a university cohort *(20)*. In the European Network for Understanding the Mechanisms of Severe Asthma (ENFUMOSA) study *(21)*, men with severe asthma reported that stress was a common trigger for exacerbations. Psychiatric illness has also consistently been associated with an increased risk of fatal asthma *(9)*.

PATHOPHYSIOLOGY OF NEAR-FATAL AND FATAL ASTHMA

Acute, severe asthma leads to hypoxemia via lung hyperinflation and regional ventilation/perfusion (V/Q) alterations. Studies of patients presenting to the emergency department with severe asthma attacks using multiple inert gas elimination techniques have shown a bimodal blood flow pattern with a significant portion of the cardiac output perfusing poorly ventilated lungs. Again, a host of inflammatory mediators have been implicated in potentiating this abnormality. Platelet-activating factor, for example, is an important culprit. Inhaled platelet-activating factor induces V/Q mismatching and decreases arterial oxygenation in patients with stable asthma *(22)* by eliciting a capillary leak phenomenon *(23)*. Other local and systemic mediators most likely act at the alveolar–capillary interface in SA to generate the profound V/Q abnormalities. Further research in this area is ongoing.

Carbon dioxide retention does not usually develop in SA until the forced expiratory volume in 1 s (FEV_1) is less than 30% of predicted, and one large meta-analysis of patients with severe asthma found that only 13% had partial pressure of oxygen ($PaCO_2$) values more than 45 mmHg *(3)*. Increased physiological dead space associated with the V/Q abnormalities and alveolar hypoventilation secondary to respiratory fatigue both lead to hypercarbia and a heightened respiratory drive.

Asthma is a spectrum of disease, and research efforts have attempted to delineate specific biomarkers that might differentiate NFA from milder forms of asthma. Marked airway thickening and a brisk infiltration of neutrophils into the airways are consistent findings in NFA. In cases of fatal asthma, bronchial thickening is 25–300% greater than normal airways, whereas in patients with NFA this is less dramatic *(24)*. More recently, Lamblin and colleagues found significantly increased numbers of neutrophils and levels of the neutrophil chemoattractant, interleukin-8, in bronchoalveolar lavage fluid in patients with asthma who require mechanical ventilation compared to patients with milder asthma *(25)*. In addition, increased matrix metalloproteinases, presumably triggered by neutrophil-mediated epithelial cell injury, were found in the bronchoalveolar lavage fluid in patients with severe asthma *(3)*. In contrast, Wenzel and colleagues found that the presence of both eosinophils and neutrophils in transbronchial biopsy specimens, rather than neutrophils alone, correlated with the number of NFA events in severe asthma (i.e., patients requiring at least 10 mg of prednisone daily more than 75% of the year) *(26)*. Currently, the association between specific inflammatory cell types and NFA is not clearly defined.

Two other pathological features of interest in NFA and fatal asthma are mucous cell hyperplasia and smooth muscle hypertrophy. The contributions of mucous cell metaplasia and mucous secretion are debated. Clearly, in many cases of fatal asthma and SA, mucous plugging with airway cast formation is a critical factor *(27)*. Airway samples in fatal asthma often reveal a marked infiltration of the mucous glands by mast cells and neutrophils *(28)* (*see* Fig. 3). Smooth muscle hyperplasia is prominent in the larger generation airways, and this has been documented in cases of fatal asthma *(29)*. Excess growth of these myocytes leads to a web-like binder around the airways that is hypercontractile to stimuli. Several inflammatory mediators have been implicated as potential triggers of the smooth muscle hypertrophy, including histamine and T-helper 2 cytokines.

CLINICAL EVALUATION ON ADMISSION TO THE ICU

SA is a medical emergency, and patients with SA who are not intubated and are admitted to the ICU require urgent assessment and timely institution of therapy. Patients with signs of respiratory failure (a decreased level of consciousness, shallow respirations, central cyanosis or other signs of profound fatigue) should be endotracheally intubated urgently. Most patients, however, who are examined and reassessed by the intensivist during the first hours in the ICU do not require mechanical ventilation.

Much of the relevant physical examination of a patient with SA can be obtained from the vital signs and by observation (*see* Table 4). The most worrisome patients will often be sitting upright, tachypneic, wheezing and have sternocleidomastoid contraction with respiration. Brenner and colleagues showed a strong correlation between patient position and accessory muscle use and a reduction in PEFR and PaO_2 *(30)*. In general, however, physical findings in SA gage the work of breathing rather than the degree of airway obstruction.

The vital signs of a patient with SA will consistently include respiratory rates more than 30 breaths/min and heart rates more than 120 beats/min *(31)*. Blood pressure can fluctuate depending on the degree of hemodynamic embarrassment owing to high intrathoracic pressures. The most worrisome patients are hypotensive because of dehydration and marked lung hyperinflation with impaired cardiac filling. Safe endotracheal intubation in these patients is often a challenge. Perhaps more useful than blood pressure is the pulsus paradoxus. Mountain and Sahn found that patients with SA who are hypercapnic had an increased mean pulsus paradoxus (23 mmHg) compared to patients with acute asthma who were normocapnic (14 mmHg) *(32)*. It should be remembered that as respiratory failure progresses, a drop in pulsus paradoxus to near-normal readings may be seen. The remainder of the physical examination should look for possible mechanical complications of SA. Pneumomediastinum and pneumothorax may be identified by observing a deviated trachea, palpating subcutaneous emphysema, or auscultating asymmetric breath sounds or a Hamman's mediastinal crunch.

Assessment of Airway Obstruction

The intensivist should order a PEFR or spirometry in the patient with SA who is not intubated, if it was not done recently in the emergency room. Patients who are severely compromised will be unable to perform the test properly, so it should be deferred. Patients with SA typically have PEFR readings less than 25% predicted *(33)* and FEV_1 less than 20% predicted *(34)*. In one study of 86 patients presenting with acute, severe asthma, an FEV_1 reading of less than 1 L (<25% predicted) or a PEFR less than 200 L/min (<30% predicted) identified all patients with hypercarbia ($PaCO_2$ >42 mmHg) or severe hypoxemia (PaO_2 <60 mmHg) *(35)*. Reductions in PEFR to less than 33% of normal is considered life-threatening. One advantage to performing spirometry with a full-flow volume loop is that is can diagnose asthma mimics, such as vocal cord dysfunction or a tracheal tumor, that may be admitted to the ICU in extremis.

Arterial Blood Gas Measurement

In patients with SA who are in the ICU, arterial blood gases (ABGs) provide important information in terms of respiratory reserve, metabolic disturbances, and degree of hypoxemia. Respiratory alkalosis is the most common abnormality found during asthma exacerbations *(36)*, but as PEFR and FEV_1 drop to less than 30% of predicted, hypercarbia and respiratory acidosis develop *(35)*. Furthermore, concomitant lactic acidosis occurs in up to 28% of patients with SA with elevated $PaCO_2$ levels *(36)*. The lactate production presumably stems from overload of the thoracic cage muscles and tissue hypoxia. ABGs should be obtained early in the ICU course of patients with SA.

Chest Radiography

As with ABGs, chest radiographs (CXRs) are not routinely performed in all patients with SA patients in the emergency room. Abnormal CXR findings other than hyperinflation or subsegmental atelectasis in all asthma exacerbations is less than 5% *(37)*. Complications from barotrauma in patients with SA, however, are sufficiently prevalent to justify routine CXRs in this population. A review of 54 admission CXRs on hospitalized patients with asthma found that 20 (34%) were believed to have major abnormalities that warranted attention *(38)*. Most of these major abnormalities were focal infiltrates, and only one patient had a pneumothorax. In the ICU population with asthma, routine CXRs are clinically useful.

Other

Few other studies need be obtained in evaluating patients with SA in the ICU. Electrocardiograms in middle-aged patients or those with suspected ischemic heart disease are standard. Screening laboratory chemistries may reveal hypokalemia related to aggressive β_2-agonist use or abnormalities in sodium and glucose, suggesting concomitant illness. A complete blood count could reveal signs of an acute infectious process, but this will be infrequent. In general, specific laboratory tests and studies should be ordered only if other diagnoses or contributing factors are being considered.

INITIAL ICU MANAGEMENT

As with most patients in the ICU, treatment of patients with SA continues in parallel with their ongoing assessment and diagnostic evaluation. Timely intervention is necessary if intubation and mechanical ventilation are to be avoided. The cornerstones of SA treatment are oxygen, bronchodilators, corticosteroids, and, if necessary, ventilatory support.

Oxygen

Modest hypoxemia is common in severe asthma exacerbations, but a PaO_2 less than 55 mmHg is rare *(2)*. Supplemental oxygen should be administered to improve the hypoxia caused by V/Q mismatch, airway plugging, and atelectasis; oxygen therapy may ameliorate some of the symptoms of air hunger. In the majority of patients with SA, fraction of oxygen (FiO_2) levels of 30–50% will correct the hypoxemia; failure to do so should prompt investigation for pulmonary parenchymal or vascular disease. One hundred percent oxygen may increase $PaCO_2$ levels by 5–6 mmHg and, infrequently, may suppress the respiratory drive in patients with SA *(39)*. Physicians should refrain from routinely administering unnecessarily high oxygen concentrations without close patient monitoring.

Bronchodilators

The cornerstone of acute asthma management, bronchodilators, have several modes of delivery, mechanisms action, and potential complications. Delivery of the short-acting β-agonist albuterol by intermittent inhalation is the most common therapy for acute asthma. Although delivery of short-acting β-agonists by dry powder, nebulization, or meter dose inhalation is effective in severe acute asthma *(40)*, each modality offers distinct advantages. Delivery by nebulization provides adequate drug delivery in a range of clinical settings: the infant by mask delivery, the adolescent with tachypnea, or even the intubated patient with respiratory failure. Nebulized delivery may decrease some of the adverse effects (e.g., tachycardia) as compared with oral or systemic delivery. Delivery by metered-dose inhaler with the use of a spacer has also been effectively employed in acute settings but is often more cumbersome, particularly in the patient who is anxious or uncomfortable. In the patient who is calm and cooperative, delivery of β-agonist by metered-dose inhaler may provide more rapid and efficacious delivery to the airways. In the patient who is acutely ill with SA or NFA, aerosol delivery remains the mode of choice.

Delivery by continuous nebulization may offer distinct advantages to intermittent dosing. Even with similar per-hour dosing (e.g., 0.5–1.0 mg/h vs 2.5 mg every 2–4 h) continuous nebulization, in some studies, shows a more rapid clinical improvement with a decreased medical personnel workload than intermittent administration *(28,40–42)*. The addition of heliox as a carrier gas may also improve drug delivery in SA *(43)*.

Future roles for levalbuterol (levo isomer of albuterol)—a rapid-onset, more-selective form of albuterol or formoterol, a rapid-onset, long half-life inhaled powder, may be found, but at this time neither has been adequately tested in the acute severe asthma setting to recommend their routine use. Alternatively, systemic delivery (e.g., subcutaneous terbutaline) may offer a more reliable dosing in the patient who is profoundly ill or pregnant. Systemic β-receptor antagonism using subcutaneous epinephrine can be effective and may forestall respiratory failure in selected cases, but there is potential for significant adverse cardiovascular effects. Epinephrine, with its significant α adrenergic stimulation, may initially reduce edema by decreasing blood flow but can also promote delayed airway edema and should be used with extreme caution in patients with coincident cardiac disease.

The most common side effects of β-agonists are tachycardia and jitteriness. Serious cardiac dysrhythmias are uncommon when using selective β-agonists. Salpeter reports an attributable heart rate increase of just more than 9 bpm *(45)*. The decreases in serum potassium levels—on average 0.36 mmol/L—do not usually warrant intervention *(45)*.

Although anticholinergics were once a mainstay of asthma therapy, they currently play only a small role. The addition of an inhaled anticholinergic (ipratropium, 0.5 mg/q 6 h) may speed recovery in pediatric cases of severe acute asthma, but the benefits for adults are less certain *(44)*.

Methylxanthines

The methylxanthines, theophylline and aminophylline, are less specific bronchodilators, and some evidence that show they improved diaphragmatic contractility may be of use in the failing patient *(43)*. Nonetheless, given the higher risk of adverse cardiac events, narrow therapeutic dosing windows, and lack of proven additional efficacy, these are not commonly used.

Other Therapies

Magnesium by intravenous infusion (as high as 2 g for 20–60 min) has proved to be safe as adjunctive therapy in acute asthma. In the case of severe acute asthma, there is little convincing evidence of better outcomes, but some believe it provides benefit over standard therapy *(46)*. In the ICU patient with SA or NFA who is being closely monitored, supplemental magnesium has little downside.

Inhaled heparin and inhaled furosemide have been proposed as immune-modulating adjunctive therapies in the treatment of asthma *(47)*. The few clinical trials using heparin (inhaled or intravenous) show a decrease in hyperresponsiveness when used as a pretreatment. No discernible respiratory benefit has been shown in the patient with acute asthma. Inhaled furosemide has shown mixed results. As with heparin, pretreatment decreases hyperresponsiveness and some case series' data show that in refractory cases of acute asthma, inhaled furosemide was associated with a clinical improvement *(47)*.

Noninvasive Ventilation

Noninvasive mask ventilation (NIV) or continuous positive airway pressure ventilation may be attempted in select patients with severe asthma attacks in the ICU. NIV decreases morbidity and mortality in chronic obstructive pulmonary disease, but data are limited in asthma. NIV decreases the need for mechanical ventilation in some patients with asthma with acute respiratory acidosis *(48)*; however, it should not be used in patients who are in respiratory distress, patients with altered level of consciousness, or patients with hemodynamic instability and impending cardiorespiratory arrest. Patients who deteriorate while on NIV should be promptly intubated and placed on mechanical ventilation.

INTUBATION

The decision to endotracheally intubate and mechanically ventilate a patient with SA may be made urgently but, preferably, is made electively in patients who are failing to respond to treatment and are fatiguing (*see* Table 2).

Intubation and initiation of mechanical ventilation of patients with NFA is challenging and must be performed by skilled intensivists or anesthesiologists. Hypotension

Table 2
Indications for Intubation

Absolute	Relative
Cardiorespiratory arrest	Hypercarbia
Decreased level of consciousness	Worsening acidosis
Inability to care for patient appropriately	Clinical signs of fatigue
	Failure to improve with therapy
Hypopneas	

(20–40% of cases) *(49)*, arrhythmias, barotrauma, laryngospasm, worsening bronchospasm, aspiration, and seizures will be encountered in the periintubation period in patients with NFA *(31)*. Excessive bag ventilation should be avoided because of the risk of pneumothorax. While patients are awake, nasotracheal intubations may be preferred in these tenuous patients; orotracheal artificial airways are preferred for prolonged management. Orotracheal tubes of at least 8.0 mm diameter significantly decrease inspiratory airway resistance and allow for suctioning of secretions and bronchoscopy. The proper use of sedatives and neuromuscular-blocking agents (NMBA) are important in aiding intubation and initiating mechanical ventilation in these patients. A full understanding of their onset, duration of actions, and side effects is required and is discussed in "Adjuncts to Standard Mechanical Ventilation."

Physiology and Mechanical Ventilation

Patients with NFA who require intubation and ventilation have high airway resistance and significant distal airway mucous plugging that lead to obstruction of airflow during expiration. Severe airflow obstruction that has developed over days causes significant dynamic hyperinflation and increased intrathoracic pressures at the end of expiration (intrinsic positive end expiratory pressure [$PEEP_i$]). The inspiratory capacity of the patient with NFA is reduced as the residual volume of the lung steadily increases and the patient breathes near the limits of their total lung capacity (*see* Fig. 1). At these lung volumes, there is a mechanical disadvantage of the respiratory muscles as the diaphragm flattens, the thoracic muscle fibers stretch, and dead space increases. Overall, the patient with severe asthma has high ventilatory demands and is at a significant mechanical disadvantage to breathe. Fatigue in these patients is inevitable, but surprisingly, many patients with this physiology improve and do not require intubation.

Patients with NFA may worsen in the hours immediately after intubation. Hypotension often results from a combination of sedative and NMBAs in the setting of high intrathoracic pressures. Intravascular volume supplementation before and immediately after intubation can prevent this expected complication. Furthermore, ventilation may be compromised further if sedation is inadequate in the patient who is awakening from anesthesia or if the initial ventilator settings provide excessive minute ventilation. In either situation, dynamic hyperinflation and gas exchange worsen and barotrauma may result.

PNEUMOTHORAX

The occurrence of life-threatening pneumothorax with asthma is rare. High intrathoracic pressure and hyperinflation are believed to lead to parenchymal or distal airway injury. In the case of pneumomediastinum, "trapped" air tracks along the bronchial tree

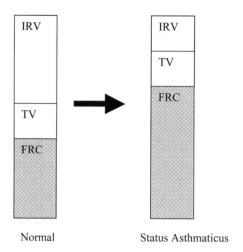

Fig. 1. Effect of dynamic hyperinflation on lung volumes—normal and SA. FRC, functional residual capacity; TV, tidal volume; IRV, inspiratory reserve volume.

Table 3
Suggested Initial Ventilator Settings

Modes	Synchronized, Intermittent Mandatory Ventilation (SIMV) and Pressure-Control Ventilation (PCV)
Rate	8–12 breaths/min
Tidal volume	6–8 mL/kg ideal body weight
Minute ventilation	8–10 L/min
Inspiratory to expiratory ratio (I:E)	1:3–1:4
Plateau pressure	Less than 35 cm H_2O
Positive-end expiratory pressure (PEEP)	Less than 5 cm H_2O
FiO_2	100%

to the confluence of the pulmonary and mediastinal reflections where small rents or tears allow communication to the mediastinum. Pneumothoraces may arise through rents in the parenchyma caused by subsegmental overdistension distal to mucous plugs or severe airway inflammation.

In the patient who is mechanically ventilated, pneumothoraces warrant tube thoracostomy for decompression and prevention of tension pneumothorax. When mediastinal air is present, cardiac tamponade, albeit rare, should be considered and would warrant intervention.

SETTING THE VENTILATOR

The intensivist must pay close attention to the ventilator parameters in patients with SA who are newly intubated (see Table 3). Junior or in-training physicians err frequently in setting the initial ventilator variables in patients with severe asthma. Errors occur because physicians attempt to correct the hypercarbia and acidemia too quickly and fail to recognize the extent of the dynamic hyperinflation. The key goal at this time is to maximize the time for expiration and target a low minute ventilation strategy.

Table 4
Physical Findings in Severe Asthma

Finding	What it is	What it means	Reference
Pulsus paradoxus	Respiratory induced systolic blood pressure variation (abnormal more than 15 mmHg)	Wide intrathoracic pressure variation causing variable ventricular filling	67
Hamman's crunch	Crackles heard with cardiac cycle	Pneumomediastinum	68
Paradoxical respirations	Abdominal retraction during inspiratory effort	Respiratory failure, respiratory diaphragm exhaustion	69
Respiratory alternans	Abdominal efforts alternate with rib-cage efforts	Respiratory failure, inspiratory muscle fatigue	69

A low minute ventilation strategy (8–10 L/min) aims to permit time for expiration, decrease air trapping, and reduce PEEP$_i$. The ICU physician should accept a moderate degree of hypercapnia with this strategy, and PaCO$_2$ levels less than 100 mmHg are usually well tolerated in the first day (32,50). One exception to this is in patients who have suffered a cardiorespiratory arrest at the time of presentation. In these patients, PaCO$_2$ levels should be normalized, if possible, to prevent cerebral vasodilatation and cerebral edema.

Controlled modes of ventilation are favored over support modes when initiating mechanical ventilation. Patients have an impressive drive to breathe because of the elevated PaCO$_2$ levels and acidemia and may require deep sedation initially to breathe synchronously with the controlled modes. Two common modes of ventilation used in this setting are synchronized intermittent mandatory ventilation (SIMV) and pressure-controlled ventilation. Pressure-controlled ventilation is favored by some intensivists in this setting because peak airway pressures do not vary as they do in volume-control modes but minute ventilation is less tightly controlled.

A relatively low minute ventilation of 8–10 L/min can be achieved by targeting tidal volumes of 7–10 mL/kg of body weight and a respiratory rate of 10–14 breaths/min. The inspiratory to expiratory ratio in the respiratory cycle should be between 1:2 and 1:4. In SIMV, inspiratory flow rates of 100 L/min allow for a prolonged expiratory phase. Plateau pressures should remain less than 35 cm H$_2$O to prevent barotrauma, and the set PEEP should be 0–5 cm H$_2$O initially. The inspiratory FiO$_2$ should be decreased from a level of 1.0 over the first several hours. If patients with NFA continue to require a FiO$_2$ more than 0.55, the intensivist should search for a concomitant process, such as pneumonia or pulmonary embolism.

On these initial ventilator settings—with aggressive bronchodilator and steroid therapy—airway resistance and lung compliance will improve during the first 24 h and hypercapnia will correct easily. The average duration of intubation in most studies of NFA is 3 d (48,51); some patients, however, prove refractory to standard medical therapy and ventilator support. Three adjuncts to standard mechanical ventilation that have been explored in severe asthma include general anesthesia, inhaled helium–oxygen mixtures, and extracorporeal CO$_2$ removal.

Table 5
Example Drug Dosing in Severe Asthma

Class	Agent	Typical adult dosing
β-agonists	Albuterol	2.5 mg q 2–4 h by nebulizer
		x.x mg/h by continuous nebulization
	Levabuterol	0.63mg–1.25 mg q 2–4 h by nebulizer
	Terbutaline	0.25 mg subcutaneously up to two doses separated by 15–30 min
Anticholinergics	Ipratropium	0.5 mg by nebulizer q 4 h
Andrenergics	Epinephrine	0.2–0.5 mg subcutaneously (0.2–0.5 mL of 1:1000) up to three doses separated by 20 min subcutaneously
Corticosteroids	Prednisone	1–2 mg/kg/d po
	methylprednisolone	2 mg/kg q 4–6 h intravenously

ADJUNCTS TO STANDARD MECHANICAL VENTILATION

General Anesthesia

The inhaled general anesthetics (halothane, sevoflurane, and isoflurane) and inravenous anesthetics (ketamine and propofol) have been used in SA cases with continued clinical decline, despite mechanical ventilation and aggressive bronchodilator therapy. The rationale for general anesthesia is to further promote bronchodilation, decrease metabolic demand, and eliminate ventilator patient dyssynchrony.

Anesthetic gases are modestly potent, rapidly acting bronchodilators and pulmonary vasodilators (52). A beneficial effect with decreased airway pressures and improved gas exchange should be evident within several hours. If no effect is seen in this time period, it is unlikely to work. Finding a ventilator that can handle anesthetic gases (e.g., the Siemens Servo 900) is problematic, and, overall, this rescue modality has become less popular with the use of other bronchodilating intravenous sedatives, such as propofol and ketamine.

Propofol is a unique anesthetic agent with an effectively short biological half-life. As with gas anesthesia, propofol affords bronchodilation in addition to the beneficial anesthetic properties. Potential adverse effects include hypotension on initial administration and metabolic acidosis (propofol infusion syndrome) with prolonged use (53).

Ketamine, a dissociative anesthetic, has been successfully used for severe asthma in both children and adults. Ketamine can cause bronchorrhea and bronchodilation—both of which may be beneficial in NFA. The potential serious adverse effects of hypertension and tachycardia must be considered before dosing and during use. Ketamine's notorious dysphoria and hallucinations are usually managed with coincident benzodiazepine administration.

NMBAs are often used during tracheal intubation and allow for complete control during mechanical ventilation. However, NMBAs do not promote bronchodilation, nor do they treat the airway inflammation associated with asthma. The use of NMBAs in patients with asthma should be minimized or avoided altogether when possible. Other more efficacious modes of therapy often obviate the need for NMBAs. When used in combination with corticosteroids, NMBAs are associated with relatively high risk of drug-induced prolonged weakness (54,55). The risk of prolonged weakness is correlated with dose and duration of NMBA and corticosteroids (56). All NMBAs are implicated *(57)*. Patients with NMBA myopathies may take months to recover normal muscle function *(58)*.

Helium–Oxygen

A helium:oxygen gas (heliox) mixture of 70:30 or 80:20 decreases resistance to airflow in obstructed large airways because helium is not as dense as nitrogen and may provide better drug delivery. It is an excellent option in upper airway obstruction and can be useful in SA. When used in the emergency department in SA, heliox may improve PEFR faster than standard therapy, decrease the pulsus paradoxus, and help prevent the need for intubation in some patients *(59)*. In some instances, heliox can improve ventilation in patients with NFA who are intubated *(60)*. Oxygen requirements need to be less than 30% FiO_2 for this modality to be tried. Unfortunately, most ventilators are not calibrated for heliox gas. Still, it remains an option for patients with NFA who continue to worsen on the ventilator.

Extracorporeal Techniques

Perhaps the last intervention that can prove life-saving in patients with NFA with worsening gas exchange and acidemia is extracorporeal CO_2 removal. This technique mirrors that of the more common extracorporeal membrane oxygenation in that patients are placed on bypass to provide gas exchange *(61)*. Numerous reports document the success of this life-saving technique in patients with severe asthma on mechanical ventilation and should be considered, if available and appropriate.

Sedation

The used of sedatives in patients with asthma has a long history of use. William Osler describes his use in the 1892, *The Principles and Practice of Medicine*:

> *In a child with very severe attacks, resisting all the usual remedies, the treatment by chloroform gave immediate and permanent relief.... The sedatives antispasmodics... belladonna, henbane, stramonium and lobelia, may be given in solution or used in the form of cigarettes.*

Most patients with acute asthma will benefit from anxiolysis and those with NFA require sedation. Reducing the anxiety of air-hunger and illness may allow for better delivery of medical care, decrease ventilation requirements, and even obviate the need of mechanical ventilation. Short-acting benzodiazepines (e.g., midazolam or lorazepam) allow for careful titration to effect with subsequent continuous or scheduled bolus delivery. Although standardized administrations are not established, it is reasonable to adopt a daily interruption strategy as tested by Kress *(62)*. Dosing is initiated incrementally and interrupted daily. The length of stay and length of time on ventilator are decreased using this method.

LIBERATION FROM THE VENTILATOR, TRACHEOTOMY

The majority of intubated patients with NFA will be liberated from mechanical ventilation with a mean time to extubation of 3.5 d. Once the patient's airway resistance decreases, airway obstruction improves, and hypercarbia resolves, the patient can be switched to a spontaneous support mode of ventilation. Patients who are unlikely to tolerate extubation can be identified by performing a spontaneous breathing trial of 30–60 min on a continuous positive airway pressure of 5 cm H_2O or a T-piece with supplemental oxygen *(63)*. Patients require close observation immediately postextubation for worsening bronchospasm and can usually be transferred out of the ICU after 24 h.

Tracheotomy will be required in few patients with NFA. Patients with NFA who have concomitant conditions, such as brain injury from an out-of-hospital arrest or lung injury from ventilator-associated pneumonia, may require prolonged ventilator support and are more apt to have a tracheotomy performed. The optimal time to perform tracheotomy in patients with NFA is not well defined, but the timing should not differ significantly from that of other patients with acute on chronic lung injury. The mortality rates for NFA patients requiring mechanical ventilation longer than 3 wk appears worse than that of chronic obstructive pulmonary disease and adult respiratory distress syndrome.

TRANSITION OUT OF THE ICU AND DISCHARGE

Within 12–24 h of reversal of respiratory failure or liberation from mechanical ventilation, most NFA of SA cases may be cared for outside of an ICU setting. Medications previously administered parenterally may be changed to oral dosing. Acute corticosteroid therapy is typically administered for 5–7 d. Further dosing is adjusted based on the prior-to-admission asthma status and level of therapy. Educating the patient about and implementing a stepped up asthma management plan similar to those recommended by the national guidelines should be initiated before discharge, and reinforcement of an updated asthma action plan provides for safe and successful discharge (as outlined in Chapter 5). Hospital discharge requires stabilization of asthma symptoms, demonstrated tolerance of current asthma therapy, and confirmation of outpatient postdischarge plan. With these elements assured, it is not necessary for full resolution of asthma symptoms before discharge *(64)*. Lim and others have found that with careful patient education and reliable discharge plans patients may have a shorter length of stay without an increased readmission rate *(64,65)*.

SUMMARY

Once recognized, severe asthma and NFA are clearly life-endangering diagnoses. Early diagnosis of high-risk individuals, through recognition of the physical signs of progressive respiratory decline and institution of aggressive therapy, may forestall respiratory failure and the need for mechanical support. Once respiratory failure occurs, successful patient management includes the careful use of mechanical ventilation, which may require long expiratory times and permissive hypercapnia. Pharmacotherapy, in addition to β-agonists and corticosteroids, with sedatives or even general anesthetics offers further techniques to improve impaired respiratory physiology. After clinical improvement is established, patients will need to maintain a higher level of asthma care to help decrease recurrences of SA and NFA.

REFERENCES

1. Pendergraft TB, Stanford RH, Beasley R, et al. Rates and characteristics of intensive care unit admissions and intubations among asthma-related hospitalizations. *Ann Allergy Asthma Immunol* 2004; 93(1): 29–35.
2. Corbridge TC, Hall JB. The assessment and management of adults with SA. *Am J Respir Crit Care Med* 1995; 151: 1296–1316.

3. McFadden ER Jr, Hejal R. Asthma. *Lancet* 1995; 345: 1215–1220.
4. Sly RM. Increases in deaths from asthma. *Ann Allergy* 1984; 53(1): 20–25.
5. Lee KH, Tan WC, Lim TK. Severe asthma. *Singapore Med J* 1997; 38: 238–240, 243.
6. Scoggin CH, Sahn SA, Petty TL. SA. A nine-year experience. *JAMA* 1977; 238: 1158–1162.
7. Mansel JK, Stogner SW, Petrini MF, Norman JR. Mechanical ventilation in patients with acute severe asthma. *Am J Med* 1990; 89: 42–48.
8. Shugg AW, Kerr S, Butt WW. Mechanical ventilation of paediatric patients with asthma: short and long term outcome. *J Paediatr Child Health* 1990; 26: 343–346.
9. Miller TP, Greenberger PA, Patterson R. The diagnosis of potentially fatal asthma in hospitalized adults. Patient characteristics and increased severity of asthma. *Chest* 1992; 102: 515–518.
10. Spitzer WO, Suissa S, Ernst P, et al. The use of beta-agonists and the risk of death and near death from asthma. *N Engl J Med* 1992; 326: 501–506.
11. Kikuchi Y, Okabe S, Tamura G, et al. Chemosensitivity and perception of dyspnea in patients with a history of near-fatal asthma. *N Engl J Med* 1994; 330: 1329–1334.
12. Sears MR, Greene JM, Willan AR, et al. A longitudinal, population-based, cohort study of childhood asthma followed to adulthood. *N Engl J Med* 2003; 349: 1414–1422.
13. Serafini U. Can fatal asthma be prevented? A personal view. *Clin Exp Allergy* 1992; 22: 576–588.
14. Holloway JW, Dunbar PR, Riley GA, et al. Association of beta2-adrenergic receptor polymorphisms with severe asthma. *Clin Exp Allergy* 2000; 30: 1097–1103.
15. Taylor DR, Kennedy MA. Genetic variation of the beta(2)-adrenoceptor: its functional and clinical importance in bronchial asthma. *Am J Pharmacogenomics* 2001; 1: 165–174.
16. Burchard EG, Silverman EK, Rosenwasser LJ, et al. Association between a sequence variant in the IL-4 gene promoter and FEV(1) in asthma. *Am J Respir Crit Care Med* 1999; 160: 919–922.
17. Rosenwasser LJ. Promoter polymorphism in the candidate genes, IL-4, IL-9, TGF-beta1, for atopy and asthma. *Int Arch Allergy Immunol* 1999; 118: 268–270.
18. Koshino T, Takano S, Kitani S, et al. Novel polymorphism of the 5-lipoxygenase activating protein (FLAP) promoter gene associated with asthma. *Mol Cell Biol Res Commun* 1999; 2: 32–35.
19. Weiss KB, Gergen PJ, Crain EF. Inner-city asthma. The epidemiology of an emerging US public health concern. *Chest* 1992; 101(6 Suppl): 362S–367S.
20. Liu LY, Coe CI, Swenson CA, et al. School examinations enhance airway inflammation to antigen challenge. *Am J Respir Crit Care Med* 2002; 165: 1062–1067.
21. The ENFUMOSA cross-sectional European multicentre study of the clinical phenotype of chronic severe asthma. European Network for Understanding Mechanisms of Severe Asthma. *Eur Respir J* 2003; 22: 470–477.
22. Felez MA, Roca J, Barbera JA, et al. Inhaled platelet-activating factor worsens gas exchange in mild asthma. *Am J Respir Crit Care Med* 1994; 150: 369–373.
23. Rodriguez-Roisin R. Acute severe asthma: pathophysiology and pathobiology of gas exchange abnormalities. *Eur Respir J* 1997; 10: 1359–1371.
24. James AJ. Relationship between airway thickness and airway hyperresponsiveness. In AG Stewart, ed. *Airway Wall Remodelling in Asthma*. Boca Raton, CRC Press, 1997, pp. 1–27.
25. Lamblin C, Gosset P, Tillie-Leblond I, et al. Bronchial neutrophilia in patients with noninfectious SA. *Am J Respir Crit Care Med* 1998; 157: 394–402.
26. Wenzel SE, Szefler SJ, Leung DY, et al. Bronchoscopic evaluation of severe asthma. Persistent inflammation associated with high dose glucocorticoids. *Am J Respir Crit Care Med* 1997; 156(3 Pt 1): 737–743.
27. Saetta M, Di Stefano A, Rosina C, Thiene G, Fabbri LM. Quantitative structural analysis of peripheral airways and arteries in sudden fatal asthma. *Am Rev Respir Dis* 1991; 143: 138–143.
28. Carroll NG, Mutavdzic S, James AL. Increased mast cells and neutrophils in submucosal mucous glands and mucus plugging in patients with asthma. *Thorax* 2002; 57: 677–682.
29. Ebina M, Yaegashi H, Takahashi T, Motomiya M, Tanemura M. Distribution of smooth muscles along the bronchial tree. A morphometric study of ordinary autopsy lungs. *Am Rev Respir Dis* 1990; 141(5 Pt 1): 1322–1326.
30. Brenner BE, Abraham E, Simon RR. Position and diaphoresis in acute asthma. *Am J Med* 1983; 74: 1005–1009.
31. FitzGerald JM, Hargreave FE. The assessment and management of acute life-threatening asthma. *Chest* 1989; 95: 888–894.
32. Mountain RD, Sahn SA. Clinical features and outcome in patients with acute asthma presenting with hypercapnia. *Am Rev Respir Dis* 1988; 138: 535–539.

33. Martin JG, Shore S, Engel LA. Effect of continuous positive airway pressure on respiratory mechanics and pattern of breathing in induced asthma. *Am Rev Respir Dis* 1982; 126: 812–817.

34. McFadden ER Jr, Lyons HA. Arterial-blood gas tension in asthma. *N Engl J Med* 1968; 278: 1027–1032.

35. Nowak RM, Tomlanovich MC, Sarkar DD, Kvale PA, Anderson JA. Arterial blood gases and pulmonary function testing in acute bronchial asthma. Predicting patient outcomes. *JAMA* 1983; 249: 2043–2046.

36. Mountain RD, Heffner JE, Brackett NC Jr, Sahn SA. Acid-base disturbances in acute asthma. *Chest* 1990; 98: 651–655.

37. Sherman S, Skoney JA, Ravikrishnan KP. Routine chest radiographs in exacerbations of chronic obstructive pulmonary disease. Diagnostic value. *Arch Intern Med* 1989; 149: 2493–2466.

38. White CS, Cole RP, Lubetsky HW, Austin JH. Acute asthma. Admission chest radiography in hospitalized adult patients. *Chest* 1991; 100: 14–16.

39. Society BT. Guidelines on the management of asthma. *Thorax.* 1993; 49: S1–S24.

40. Raimondi AC, Schottlender J, Lombardi D, Molfino NA. Treatment of acute severe asthma with inhaled albuterol delivered via jet nebulizer, metered dose inhaler with spacer, or dry powder. *Chest* 1997; 112: 24–28.

41. Rodrigo GJ, Rodrigo C. Continuous vs intermittent beta-agonists in the treatment of acute adult asthma: a systematic review with meta-analysis. *Chest* 2002; 122: 160–165.

42. Shrestha M, Bidadi K, Gourlay S, Hayes J. Continuous vs intermittent albuterol, at high and low doses, in the treatment of severe acute asthma in adults. *Chest* 1996; 110: 42–47.

43. Kress JP, Noth I, Gehlbach BK, et al. The utility of albuterol nebulized with heliox during acute asthma exacerbations. *Am J Respir Crit Care Med* 2002; 165: 1317–1321.

44. Peterson GM, Boyles PJ, Bleasel MD, Vial JH. Ipratropium treatment of acute airways disease. *Ann Pharmacother* 2003; 37: 339–344.

45. Salpeter SR, Ormiston TM, Salpeter EE. Cardiovascular effects of beta-agonists in patients with asthma and COPD: a meta-analysis. *Chest* 2004; 125: 2309–2321.

46. Rowe BH, Bretzlaff JA, Bourdon C, Bota GW, Camargo, CA Jr. Magnesium sulfate for treating exacerbations of acute asthma in the emergency department. *Cochrane Database Syst Rev* 2000; (2): CD001490.

47. Niven AS, Argyros G. Alternate treatments in asthma. *Chest* 2003; 123: 1254–1265.

48. Afessa B, Morales I, Cury JD. Clinical course and outcome of patients admitted to an ICU for SA. *Chest* 2001; 120: 1616–1621.

49. Williams TJ, Tuxen DV, Scheinkestel CD, Czarny D, Bowes G. Risk factors for morbidity in mechanically ventilated patients with acute severe asthma. *Am Rev Respir Dis* 1992; 146: 607–615.

50. Mutlu GM, Factor P, Schwartz DE, Sznajder JI. Severe SA: management with permissive hypercapnia and inhalation anesthesia. *Crit Care Med* 2002; 30: 477–480.

51. Zimmerman JL, Dellinger RP, Shah AN, Taylor RW. Endotracheal intubation and mechanical ventilation in severe asthma. *Crit Care Med* 1993; 21: 1727–1730.

52. Marshall BE, Longnecker DE. General anesthetics. In AG Goodman, Rall TW, Nies AS, Taylor P, eds. *The Pharmacological Basis of Therapeutics* (8th ed.). New York, Pergamon Press, 1984; pp. 285–310.

53. Vasile B, Rasulo F, Candiani A, Latronico N. The pathophysiology of propofol infusion syndrome: a simple name for a complex syndrome. *Intensive Care Med* 2003; 29: 1417–1425.

54. Griffin D, Fairman N, Coursin D, Rawsthorne L, Grossman JE. Acute myopathy during treatment of SA with corticosteroids and steroidal muscle relaxants. *Chest* 1992; 102: 510–514.

55. Road J, Mackie G, Jiang TX, Stewart H, Eisen A. Reversible paralysis with SA, steroids, and pancuronium: clinical electrophysiological correlates. *Muscle Nerve* 1997; 20: 1587–1590.

56. Shee CD. Risk factors for hydrocortisone myopathy in acute severe asthma. *Respir Med* 1990; 84: 229–233.

57. Leatherman JW, Fluegel WL, David WS, Davies SF, Iber C. Muscle weakness in mechanically ventilated patients with severe asthma. *Am J Respir Crit Care Med* 1996; 153: 1686–1690.

58. Gooch JL. Prolonged paralysis after neuromuscular blockade. *J Toxicol Clin Toxicol* 1995; 33: 419–426.

59. Kass JE, Terregino CA. The effect of heliox in acute severe asthma: a randomized controlled trial. *Chest* 1999; 116: 296–300.

60. Gluck EH, Onorato DJ, Castriotta R. Helium-oxygen mixtures in intubated patients with SA and respiratory acidosis. *Chest* 1990; 98: 693–698.

61. Cooper DJ, Tuxen DV, Fisher MM. Extracorporeal life support for SA. *Chest* 1994; 106: 978–979.
62. Kress JP, Pohlman AS, O'Connor MF, Hall JB. Daily interruption of sedative infusions in critically ill patients undergoing mechanical ventilation. *N Engl J Med* 2000; 342: 1471–1477.
63. Meade M, Guyatt G, Cook D, et al. Predicting success in weaning from mechanical ventilation. *Chest* 2001; 120(6 Suppl): 400S–404S.
64. Lim TK, Chin NK, Lee KH, Stebbings AM. Early discharge of patients hospitalized with acute asthma: a controlled study. *Respir Med* 2000; 94: 1234–1240.
65. Ebbinghaus S, Bahrainwala AH. Asthma management by an inpatient asthma care team. *Pediatr Nurs* 2003; 29: 177–183.
66. Kallenbach JM, Frankel AH, Lapinsky SE, et al. Determinants of near fatality in acute severe asthma. *Am J Med* 1993; 95: 265–272.
67. Rebuck AS, Tomarken JL. Pulsus paradoxus in asthmatic children. *Can Med Assoc J* 1985; 112: 710–711.
68. Hamman L. Spontaneous mediastinal emphysema. *Bull Johns Hopkins Hosp* 1939; 64: 1–21.
69. Cohen CA, Zagelbaum G, Gross D, Roussos C, Macklem PT. Clinical manifestations of inspiratory muscle fatigue. *Am J Med* 1982; 73: 308–316.

8 Complementary/Alternative Therapies in Asthma

Andrea Borchers, PhD, Carl L. Keen, PhD, and M. Eric Gershwin, MD

KEY POINTS

- Up to almost 60% of patients with asthma use some sort of complementary and alternative medicine therapy.
- There is insufficient evidence to make recommendations for the incorporation of acupuncture into the treatment or management of asthma.
- There are insufficient data to determine whether homeopathy is a valid adjunctive therapy in the management of asthma.
- Breathing exercises may improve symptom scores and quality-of-life measures, but evidence for their effectiveness in improving lung function is still inconclusive.
- Muscle relaxation shows some promise in improving lung function, but the available evidence on relaxation techniques is limited.
- There is insufficient evidence to support the use of chiropractic spinal manipulation and other manual therapies in the treatment of asthma.
- The authors suggest a healthy well-balanced diet with high intake of fruits and vegetables rich in antioxidant vitamins, flavonoids, and minerals; there is not enough evidence to recommend supplementation with antioxidant vitamins or selenium for patients with asthma.

From: *Current Clinical Practice: Bronchial Asthma:*
A Guide for Practical Understanding and Treatment, 5th ed.
Edited by: M. E. Gershwin and T. E. Albertson © Humana Press Inc., Totowa, NJ

- The authors also suggest supplementation with magnesium in the subset of patients with asthma with low intracellular levels of this mineral.
- Supplementation with certain n-3 fatty acids and the n-6 fatty acid γ-linolenic acid reduces markers of inflammation in patients with asthma, but there is little evidence of a beneficial effect on lung function or asthma control.
- There is as yet no conclusive evidence of effectiveness in the treatment of asthma for any botanical.
- *Do ask* your patients whether and what botanicals they use, and *do tell* your patients about the potential risk of allergies, toxicities, and herb–drug interactions associated with many herbal compounds.

INTRODUCTION

Complementary and alternative medicine (CAM) can be defined as a group of diverse medical and health care systems, practices, and products that are not presently considered to be part of allopathic medicine. The National Center for Complementary and Alternative Medicine (NCCAM) has proposed grouping CAM therapies into five categories (*see* Table 1).

According to surveys conducted in the United States and other Western countries, the prevalence of CAM use in the general population ranges between 10 and almost 50%, with some of the variability attributable to different definitions of what constitutes CAM therapies. Generally, the proportion of patients with asthma reporting CAM use is even higher (27–59%). The reasons for the widespread CAM use among patients with asthma and other chronic diseases are incompletely understood but include the perceived ineffectiveness of pharmaceutical regimens and fear of the side effects frequently associated with them. Nonetheless, patients generally use CAM approaches as complementary, rather than as alternative, therapies. Because of the high prevalence of CAM usage among patients with asthma, physicians treating these patients should be knowledgeable about the various CAM therapies available and the evidence regarding their efficacy and safety. This chapter contains an overview of the CAM approaches most commonly used by patients with asthma, which differ among countries and populations, but generally include acupuncture, homeopathy, manual therapies, relaxation and breathing exercises, and nutritional and botanical supplements. Note that all of the available randomized, controlled trials (RCTs) have evaluated CAM treatments as adjunctive therapies.

ACUPUNCTURE

Acupuncture is one of several treatment approaches that are part of traditional Chinese medicine (TCM), an alternative medical system with a tradition going back several millennia. In TCM, acupuncture is used to correct disturbances in the flow of Qi. Qi, a crucial concept in TCM, is often translated as life force or energy but is a concept that also encompasses material attributes. Qi is channeled through 12 primary and 8 "extraordinary" meridians, which contain approx 360 acupuncture points. Chinese acupuncturists make use of numerous diagnostic techniques to determine the nature of the disturbance and choose the appropriate acupuncture points. The traditional method of acupuncture consists of rapidly inserting a long thin needle through the skin, then manipulating it manually and withdrawing it slowly. Other mechanisms of manipulation include heat, pressure, friction, suction, and electric stimulation.

Table 1
Types of Complementary and Alternative Medicine (CAM) Therapies

Type of CAM	Description	Examples
Alternative medical systems	Philosophies of medicine that integrate theory and practice; many of them evolved earlier than allopathic medicine and are based on different concepts of health, disease, diagnosis, and therapy	Traditional Chinese medicine Ayurveda Homeopathy Naturopathy
Mind–body interventions	Various techniques designed to enhance the mind's capacity to affect bodily function and symptoms (Note that some techniques have become mainstream, e.g., patient support groups and cognitive-behavioral therapy.)	Meditation Prayer Mental healing Therapies using creative outlets (art, music, and dance)
Biologically based therapies	Involve substances found in nature, such as botanicals, foods, and vitamins	Certain dietary interventions Most dietary supplements
Manipulative and body-based methods	Methods based on manipulation and/or movement of one or more body parts	Chiropractic manipulation Massage[a]
Energy therapies Biofield	Approaches intended to affect energy fields that purportedly surround and penetrate the human body. Some forms of energy therapy manipulate biofields by applying pressure and/or manipulating the body by placing the hands in, or through, these fields	qi gong Reiki Therapeutic touch
Bioelectromagnetic	Therapies involving the unconventional use of electromagnetic fields	Pulsed fields Magnetic fields Alternating or direct current fields

[a]Further example listed by NCCAM is osteopathic manipulation. In the United States, however, osteopathic medicine is not practiced by CAM practitioners but by doctors of osteopathic medicine (DOs), i.e., physicians who receive the same 4-yr medical school training as medical doctors, except that special emphasis is placed on the osteopathic philosophies and practices.

(Modified From the National Center for Complementary and Alternative Medicine [NCCAM] Web Site, http://nccam.nih.gov)

The design of clinical trials of acupuncture is challenging. The classical TCM approach is to tailor the choice of acupuncture points to each patient. In contrast, it is common western practice to use a formula approach, in which the same acupuncture points are stimulated in all patients. Although this approach may lend itself more readily to clinical trials, it will always be open to the criticism that failure to individualize therapy must inevitably result in lack of response. In addition, it is necessary to consider and control for a large number of parameters, including the number and location of the points used for the true and sham acupuncture treatments, type and duration of needle insertion and manipulation, and achievement of dachi (de qui), a tingling or irradiating sensation after needling that is believed to indicate effectiveness. Furthermore, blinding can only be partial in any RCT of acupuncture because the acupuncturist knows whether he or she is giving real or sham acupuncture.

There are several investigations of the effects of acupuncture on immune parameters in patients with asthma, using either a formula approach and sham treatment of the same points as a control or acupuncture according to the principles of TCM with the control group treated at points not specific for asthma. The observed effects included alterations in the percentages of leukocytes and leukocyte subsets and increases in lymphocyte proliferation and the production of several cytokines. Some of these changes were also noted in patients who received sham acupuncture. A reduction in peripheral blood and sputum eosinophil concentrations and a decrease in interleukin (IL)-6 and IL-10 suggest that acupuncture could have anti-inflammatory and anti-allergic effects. However, the neutrophil respiratory burst also significantly increased. In addition, acupuncture can stimulate the secretion of certain cytokines that are already overproduced by patients with asthma and are implicated in the pathology of the disease (e.g., IL-4 and IL-8). This suggests that acupuncture could have proinflammatory or proallergic effects, and detrimental effects have indeed been described in some studies.

A Cochrane systematic review on the use of acupuncture in chronic asthma identified 11 RCTs (involving a total of 324 patients) that met the inclusion criteria (1). There were no statistically significant or clinically relevant differences in lung function parameters between real and "sham" acupuncture, but subjective symptoms were significantly improved in two of the trials. In some of the studies, the control groups received acupuncture at true acupuncture points believed not to affect asthma. This may, however, have resulted in therapeutic benefit and may have masked at least some of the effect of needling at asthma-specific acupuncture points. The conclusion of the Cochrane review was that the existing data do not allow recommendations for the incorporation of acupuncture into the treatment or management of asthma (1). Further research is needed and should address the problems encountered in previous RCTs and explore the usefulness of acupuncture in patients with less well-controlled disease than were included in the existing trials.

With appropriate precautions and in the hands of qualified practitioners, acupuncture is rarely associated with major adverse events, although cases of pneumothorax causally related to acupuncture have been reported and other serious adverse events possibly or likely caused by acupuncture have also been described. Nonserious adverse events after acupuncture include needling pain, hematoma, bleeding, orthostatic problems, forgotten needles, local skin irritation, and, occasionally, exacerbation of symptoms.

HOMEOPATHY

Homeopathy is a Western CAM system that was developed approx 200 yr ago by the German physician Samuel Hahnemann (1755–1843). It is based on two basic concepts: the "simile principle" and the dilution principle. These principles summarize the theory that a substance that produces specific symptoms of an illness or disease in a healthy person can, when given in minute quantities, induce a self-healing response in a patient suffering from this illness. Remedies containing small quantities of a particular substance are obtained by repeatedly diluting the original solution, called the mother tincture. The extent of dilution varies, but the final extract frequently contains few, if any, of the original molecules. According to homeopathic thinking, such highly diluted extracts not only retain some form of biological activity but also become more potent. In addition to physical examination and laboratory work, case taking involves an extensive interview with the purpose of obtaining an account by the patient of the totality of his or her physical, mental, and emotional symptoms. The choice of the homeopathic remedy is based on the totality of symptoms and is, by definition, individualized.

In addition to classical homeopathy, three other types of homeopathy, namely clinical and complex homeopathy and isopathy, have been developed. Clinical homeopathy uses the same remedy in patients presenting with similar signs and symptoms. In complex homeopathy, the patient is treated with a fixed combination of several homeopathic remedies developed for a specific condition. Isopathy or homeopathic immunotherapy uses dilutions of allergens.

A recently updated Cochrane review of homeopathy for chronic asthma included six placebo-controlled double-blind clinical trials of varying quality, assessing the effect of various types of homeopathy in addition to usual care in a total of 556 patients (2). The results from some of the smaller trials suggest a significant difference in favor of homeopathy between the active treatment and placebo groups in lung function measurements, such as peak expiratory flow rate (PEFR) and forced vital capacity (FVC), and also in medication use. In contrast, more adequately powered and better reported studies did not find significant differences between the two groups in lung function measurements, medication use, symptom scores, and quality-of-life scores. In particular, the only trial using classical individualized homeopathy (provided by three nonmedically trained classical homeopaths with at least 10 yr of experience) did not find a significant effect of homeopathy on the quality of life as the primary outcome measure or on lung function as one of the secondary outcome measures. The quality-of-life scales used in this study may not have been sensitive enough to detect changes, and the percentage of predicted PEFR at baseline essentially left no room for improvement. In addition, children from the active treatment and the placebo groups could attend up to six consultations with a homeopath, who not only prescribed the homeopathic remedy, but also could provide other advice, such as dietary recommendations. It may have been attributable to the effects of these intensive consultations that an improvement of PEFR by 15% or more and a decrease in inhaler use were seen in similar numbers of children in both groups.

In conclusion, there are as yet not enough data available to reliably assess whether homeopathy constitutes a valid adjunctive therapy in the management of asthma, and further rigorously controlled trials are needed (2). Future studies should address the effect of the "package of care," i.e., the extensive consultations that form part of classical homeopathy.

BREATHING EXERCISES AND RELAXATION TECHNIQUES

Emotional stress can precipitate or exacerbate acute and chronic asthma, and several physical or mental relaxation therapies have been studied in patients with asthma, including progressive relaxation, biofeedback training, autogenic training, hypnotherapy, and transcendental meditation. According to a systematic review, the overall methodological quality of the 15 identified RCTs was poor, and only 9 trials appropriately compared treatment and control groups (3). Only two of five RCTs on progressive muscle relaxation alone or in conjunction with mental relaxation showed a statistically significant effect on lung function. This was, however, considered to be clinically relevant in only one study (an 18% increase in forced expiratory volume in 1 s [FEV_1]). A large (252 children) study comparing hypnosis and relaxation and breathing exercises found a statistically significant but clinically irrelevant increase of 4.3% in FEV_1 only in the hypnosis group. In two trials on biofeedback-induced facial relaxation, no significant or meaningful effect on lung function was observed, but asthma severity was significantly decreased in one of the studies. The conclusion was that evidence for the effectiveness of relaxation techniques in the management of asthma was still largely lacking, but muscle relaxation had shown some promise in improving lung function. A more extensive review of biofeedback techniques in asthma, either directly targeting respiratory resistance or using the indirect technique of facial muscle relaxation, also concluded that there was little evidence for the usefulness of biofeedback in the treatment of asthma (4). In a study not yet included in either of the reviews (also suffering from lack of methodological details), patients with asthma receiving heart rate variability biofeedback were able to reduce their medication use to a significantly greater extent than patients in the placebo biofeedback or the waiting-list control groups (5). Airway resistance also decreased significantly.

A recent double-blind RCT compared Sahaja yoga sessions and a control intervention consisting of relaxation and cognitive behavior therapy-like exercises in 59 patients with moderate to severe asthma (6). At the end of the treatment period, the yoga groups had a significantly greater improvement in airway hyperresponsiveness to methacholine than the control group. Both interventions were associated with considerable improvements in asthma-related quality-of-life scores, and the difference between the groups was only marginally significant.

Yoga includes breathing exercises as a component of physical, as well as mental, relaxation techniques, and trials assessing mainly the breathing techniques of yoga are part of a Cochrane review of breathing exercises or breathing retraining in asthma (7). The various interventions are based on widely differing concepts regarding the pathophysiology of asthma and the precise role of breathing retraining in the treatment of asthma. The Buteyko technique, developed in Russia by Konstantin Buteyko, is based on the premise that asthma is mainly caused by hypocapnia resulting from hyperventilation and that control of the disease can be improved and medication use reduced by techniques that decrease minute ventilation and increase carbon dioxide levels. The deep diaphragmatic breathing technique is similarly aimed at correcting hyperventilation and hypocapnia, thereby providing symptom relief and allowing the reduction of medication. It has been suggested that this may be particularly beneficial in patients with asthma with dysfunctional breathing, who may constitute up to one-third of adults with asthma.

The Cochrane review on breathing exercises in asthma included seven RCTs involving a total of 292 subjects (7). Aside from a significant improvement in PEFR in one of the studies using yoga training, breathing retraining was not associated with significant changes in this or other measures of lung function (FEV_1 or FVC). Two studies (one yoga, one Buteyko) reported a significant reduction in bronchodilator use, and there was a significant decrease in inhaled steroid use in another study of Buteyko. Quality of life improved in two studies, one assessing an adaptation of Buteyko and the other using diaphragmatic breathing exercises in patients with dysfunctional breathing as determined by Nijmegen scores. Another RCT undergoing assessment for inclusion in the Cochrane review compared Buteyko breathing, the use of a Pink City Lung exerciser to mimic yoga breathing exercises (pranayama), and a placebo device of this exerciser in a total of 90 patients with asthma. Lung function measures and bronchial reactivity were not significantly affected by any of the treatments. Symptom scores and bronchodilator use were reduced only in the Buteyko group.

The authors of the Cochrane review concluded that the evidence was as yet insufficient to make recommendations concerning the use of breathing exercises for asthma *(7)*. Because of the decreases in medication use and the improvements observed in symptom scores and quality-of-life measures, further studies seem warranted, particularly because up to one-third of patients with asthma report the use of breathing exercises. The safety of these techniques remains to be evaluated.

CHIROPRACTIC SPINAL MANIPULATION/MANUAL THERAPY

Chiropractics is based on the theory that spinal joint dysfunction, or vertebral subluxation, directly or indirectly affects the nervous system, thereby possibly disturbing the function of organs and tissues and compromising overall health. An important therapeutic procedure is therefore the manipulation of this vertebral subluxation.

The only three RCTs of manual therapy in asthma that are at least of moderate methodological quality compared chiropractic spinal manipulation with simulated treatment in a total of 158 patients (127 children) *(8)*. None of the studies demonstrated an effect on objective measures of lung function. Substantial improvements in quality-of-life and symptom scores, as well as reduction in the use of β-agonists, were reported after both active and simulated treatment without significant differences between the two groups. Thus, there is insufficient evidence to support the use of manual therapies in the treatment or management of asthma.

DIETARY SUPPLEMENTS

Vitamins and Minerals Involved in Antioxidant Defense

OBSERVATIONAL STUDIES

There have been considerable changes in dietary patterns in recent decades, and the incidence of asthma has markedly increased during the same period. This has led to speculations that alterations in the intake of certain dietary constituents may contribute to the growing incidence of asthma.

In particular, the intake of fresh fruits and vegetables has decreased, and the results of a majority of epidemiological studies suggest that low intake of these foods is associated with wheezing and decreased lung function *(9,10)*. Numerous observational studies have focused on the contribution of antioxidants to this protective effect of fruit and vegetable consumption, including vitamin C, vitamin E, carotenoids, and also selenium (Se) as an essential cofactor of the antioxidant enzyme glutathione peroxidase (GSH-Px).

In most cross-sectional studies of the general population, greater vitamin C intake has been associated with improved lung function (measured as FEV_1) and decreased risk of bronchial hyperreactivity and wheezing *(10–12)*. Results concerning the association of vitamin E intake and lung function are inconsistent, with some studies showing a protective effect and others detecting no association *(11)*. In 2566 Californian children, low dietary vitamin E intake was associated with decreased lung function (FEV$_1$ between 25 and 75% or FVC) *(9)*.

The relationship between asthma and the intake of vitamins C and E, carotenoids, and Se is even less clear *(11,12)*. Several recent analyses of National Health and Nutrition Examination Survey (NHANES) III data for children and adults found little evidence for an association between low vitamin C intake and self-reported asthma. Data from the Nutrition and Health Survey in Taiwan (NAHSIT) indicated a marginally significant association between the lowest quartile of vitamin C intake and the risk of physician-diagnosed asthma in 1166 Taiwanese adolescents.

The only prospective study using diagnosed asthma as an endpoint is the Nurses' Health Study, with data on almost 78,000 women *(13)*. Asthma incidence over a 10-yr period was not significantly affected by dietary vitamin C and was positively associated with the use of vitamin C supplements. Dietary vitamin E was inversely associated with 6-yr, but not 10-yr, risk of asthma, with recent consumption having greater importance than vitamin E intake at baseline. Vitamin E intake from supplements alone was associated with increased asthma risk. A possible explanation for the positive association between supplemental vitamin C and vitamin E is that nurses who are at high risk of developing asthma started taking these supplements because of publications indicating benefits from increased antioxidant consumption.

Lower plasma/serum levels of antioxidant vitamins and Se have been reported in patients with asthma compared with healthy controls, although the overall results are conflicting *(12)*. NHANES III data for more than 16,500 adults did not reveal significant differences in serum ascorbate, α-tocopherol, carotenoids, or Se concentrations between patients with current asthma compared with those who had never been diagnosed with asthma. Only when subjects with current and former asthma were combined did a decrease in their serum vitamin C concentrations become statistically significant. In contrast, two recent analyses of data from NHANES III for children found serum levels of ascorbate, carotenoids, and Se, but not vitamin E, to be significantly associated with self-reported diagnosis of asthma. Importantly, a standard deviation decrease in serum ascorbate, β-carotene, or Se was associated with a decrease in prevalent asthma by 20, 10, and 10%, respectively. Only serum Se showed a strong positive association with FEV$_1$.

Compared with healthy controls, the bronchoalveolar lavage (BAL) and bronchial wash of adult patients with mild asthma contain significantly reduced concentrations of vitamins C and E. Together with increased levels of oxidized glutathione, this indicates that asthmatic airways are exposed to increased oxidative stress and increased consumption of antioxidants, which is consistent with the pro-oxidative effects of inflammation. In addition to low antioxidant vitamin concentrations, patients with asthma are frequently characterized by decreased activities of the antioxidant enzymes platelet GSH-Px and superoxide dismutase, driving the balance even further toward a prooxidative state.

INTERVENTION STUDIES

These observations provide an important rationale for assessing the effect of antioxidant supplementation in patients with asthma. Additional reasons for supplementation with vitamin C are afforded by its direct effects on smooth muscle and its ability to accelerate histamine metabolism and modulate prostaglandin production. However, the results obtained with ascorbic acid supplementation in patients with asthma are conflicting and largely disappointing. Only 8 of 16 identified studies met the inclusion criteria for a recently updated Cochrane review on vitamin C supplementation in asthma *(14)*. Four of the included trials investigated the acute effects of a one-time dose of ascorbic acid, and two of these studies involved patients with exercise-induced asthma. Because of the diversity in the design of these studies and the outcomes they measured, no overall conclusions could be reached and the evidence was deemed insufficient to recommend vitamin C supplementation for patients with asthma. The results from the largest of the trials (201 patients of whom 95 were supplemented with vitamin C) indicated that supplementation with 1 g/d of vitamin C for 16 wk did not have a clinically meaningful effect on various lung function parameters, symptom scores, or bronchodilator use *(15)*.

These findings contradict those of epidemiological studies suggesting an inverse correlation between vitamin C intake and lung function or asthma prevalence. This could indicate that vitamin C intake is a marker of a healthier diet or even a healthier lifestyle overall. Such a healthier diet could be characterized by a higher intake of flavonoids, which are found in many of the same foods as ascorbic acid. Flavonoids are a class of polyphenolic compounds, many of which exhibit not only strong antioxidant but also immunomodulatory activities. Intake of certain flavonoids was inversely associated with asthma incidence in a cross-sectional study of more than 10,000 Finnish subjects *(16)*. It is also possible that supplementation with a single antioxidant is insufficient to provide significant benefit in patients with asthma.

The antioxidant function of tocopherol in the lung is likely to be of lesser significance than that of ascorbate, but vitamin E may affect asthma symptoms via its interactions with vitamin C or by several other mechanisms, including suppression of eicosanoid production and neutrophil migration and inhibition of immunoglobulin E synthesis.

In a recent double-blind, placebo-controlled RCT, however, supplementation with 500 mg/d of natural vitamin E for 6 wk did not provide any benefit to patient with mild to moderate asthma in terms of lung function, symptom scores, or bronchodilator use *(17)*.

The Se content of plant-derived foods depends on the Se concentration in the soil, which varies among different geographical regions. This results in large regional variation in Se intake, with adequate amounts provided by the typical diet in the United States, but low dietary intake in areas with low soil content, such as Scandinavia and certain regions of China.

Because Se is an essential cofactor of GSH-Px, Se intake and status influence the activity of this enzyme, which plays a vital role in the defense against oxidative stress. Another as yet poorly characterized Se-containing protein inhibits lipid peroxidation. Lipid hydroperoxides are initial metabolites of lipoxygenases and can enhance their own formation by stimulating lipoxygenase activity. Increased defense against oxidative stress, reduced lipoxygenase activity, and, possibly, alterations in the profile of inflammatory mediators produced via the cyclooxygenase pathway are all mechanisms by which Se may influence inflammatory processes in asthma.

To date, there has been only one small RCT ($N = 20$) investigating the effects of Se supplementation in patients with asthma *(18)*. It reported significant improvement in a composite score in patients receiving 100 µg of sodium selenite for 14 wk, compared with the placebo group. However, the objective individual components of this score (changes in vital capacity, FEV_1, histamine challenge, and PEFR) did not change significantly from the preintervention to the postintervention period. This study was conducted in Sweden, where soil Se content and Se intake are suboptimal. It remains unclear, therefore, whether Se supplementation results in some improvement only in patients with low Se status or could provide some benefit even in Se-replete patients.

Most of the antioxidant supplementation studies enrolled small numbers of patients, and these patients generally had mild or moderate asthma and had been on a stable medication regimen without experiencing exacerbations for several months. It may have been impossible to see significant effects on lung function in patients whose asthma is so well controlled. Because some of the vitamins are believed to act not only as antioxidants but also as anti-inflammatory agents, assessment of markers of inflammation and of anti-inflammatory medication use may have revealed significant differences. Instead, some of the studies specifically excluded patients who were able to decrease, or had to increase, their medication. Furthermore, the intervention period was short in a majority of these trials. In addition, the published results of most of the crossover studies—at least on vitamin C—do not contain any mention of a washout period. All of these factors represent potential reasons for the ineffectiveness of antioxidant supplementation.

It is also possible that supplementation with a single antioxidant is insufficient for patients with asthma to obtain a significant benefit. To date, the effect of supplementation with a combination of antioxidants on lung function has only rarely been assessed in patients with asthma and only in conjunction with exposure to either experimentally or naturally high levels of ozone and other environmental pollutants.

Supplementation with a combination of vitamins C and E provided some protection from decreases in lung function and from increases in inflammatory mediators during periods of exposure to high levels of ozone *(19,20)*, but this may have been simply attributable to the correction of an underlying vitamin E deficiency in one investigation *(19)*. The other study was small and neglected to provide data on serum vitamin levels according to the severity of asthma, although supplementation was protective mainly in the subgroup with severe asthma. The effectiveness of supplementation is likely to depend greatly on the overall antioxidant status of serum and BAL, because other components of the antioxidant defense, e.g., urate and antioxidant enzymes, may compensate for the lack of antioxidant vitamins in patients with asthma. In patients with asthma with high levels of exposure to environmental pro-oxidants in addition to those arising from the inflammatory processes of asthma itself, these other defense systems and mechanisms may also be overwhelmed. It is in this group of patients with asthma that increased intake of antioxidants is likely to be of particular importance. This is further supported by the finding of a much stronger inverse association between serum antioxidant levels and asthma prevalence in children exposed to second-hand smoke compared with those who lived in nonsmoking households *(21)*.

In view of the rather conflicting data from supplementation trials, the recommendation should probably be to consume a healthy and well-balanced diet of foods rich in various vitamins and flavonoids rather than to use supplements. This may, however, not always be possible if a food or food group (e.g., nuts, many of which are one of the best sources of vitamin E) is associated with asthma exacerbations in atopic subjects.

Magnesium

An association between higher magnesium (Mg) intake and improved lung function and decreased risk of airway hyperreactivity has been reported in several observational and case–control studies in adults and children *(12)*. Lower Mg status was found in patients with asthma compared with healthy controls and was associated with a significantly higher number of hospitalizations for acute asthma exacerbations. Furthermore, a marked decrease in intracellular Mg concentrations has been observed during acute asthma exacerbations. That none of these findings are entirely consistent among studies may be explained by the observation that only a subset of patients with asthma (30–40%) exhibits Mg deficiency. Another explanation is provided by the use of different indicators of Mg status. It has been suggested that plasma or serum Mg does not accurately reflect Mg status and that intracellular (erythrocyte or leukocyte) free or ionized Mg constitute better indices. The intravenous Mg load is time-consuming but appears to represent an accurate method.

Low Mg status may contribute to the inflammation of asthma by increasing the release of proinflammatory mediators, such as leukotriene B_4, IL-1, IL-6, and tumor necrosis factor and/or by increasing the production and cytotoxicity of reactive oxygen species. Mg supplementation of 17 patients with asthma resulted in significantly decreased symptom scores, but lung function was not significantly improved *(22)*. In a recent study involving a total of 201 (99 in the Mg arm) patients with asthma who took at least one dose of inhaled corticosteroids daily, supplementation with 450 mg/d of Mg amino chelate for 16 wk did not significantly affect lung function, responsiveness to methacholine, or symptom scores *(15)*.

Nonetheless, supplementation is indicated in those patients with low intracellular Mg concentrations. There is no evidence that large oral intake of Mg is harmful, except in people with impaired renal function; however, high Mg intake can cause osmotic diarrhea. This does not seem to occur at levels of supplementation of 400 mg/d or less.

Essential Fatty Acids

OBSERVATIONAL STUDIES

Among the dietary changes that have occurred during the same period as the dramatic rise in the incidence of atopy and asthma is an increased intake of linoleic acid and other *n*-6 polyunsaturated fatty acids (PUFAs) and a corresponding alteration in the ratio of *n*-6:*n*-3 fatty acids. Because of their respective effects on cell membrane fluidity and the production of eicosanoids, *n*-6 PUFAs are considered to be detrimental in asthma, whereas *n*-3 PUFAs are believed to have beneficial effects.

An important source of *n*-3 PUFAs is fish, particularly fatty fish, and high dietary fish intake was associated with improved lung function in several studies in the general population *(11,23)*. The evidence regarding fish consumption and respiratory disease is less consistent, with some studies showing that it provided protection from airway hyperresponsiveness, wheeze, and asthma in children and adults, whereas others were unable to detect a significant association. Most notably, in the large prospective Nurses' Health Study, intake of *n*-3 fatty acids was not significantly associated with the 10-yr incidence of asthma, and intake of linoleic acid did not confer increased risk *(13)*. A case–control study of dietary fatty acid intake of adults in the United Kingdom found the odds ratio for asthma to be increased with higher intake of the *n*-3 PUFAs, eicosapentaenoic acid (EPA), and docosahexaenoic acid, adjusted for body mass index and energy intake *(24)*. This might be explained by reverse causation, i.e., subjects increasing their intake of fish after becoming aware of its potential protective effects.

A recent analysis of dietary intake data for Australian adolescents did not find a consistent association between *n*-3 PUFA intake or the *n*-6:*n*-3 ratio and asthma *(25)*. Certain *n*-6 fatty acids were associated with one or more definitions of asthma, the most consistent association being observed with dihomo γ-linolenic (GLA) acid. When erythrocyte membrane fatty acid composition was analyzed, the proportion of docosahexaenoic acid was not significantly different between cases and controls and EPA was undetectable in most participants. Of note, the membrane levels of *n*-6 linoleic acid were significantly higher in asthma cases compared with controls, and adjustment for potential confounders did not greatly alter the strength of the association. In a case–control study of 335 Australian children, no significant association was detected between higher ratios of *n*-6:*n*-3 fatty acid intake and risk of current asthma in univariate analysis *(26)*. The association became significant, however, after adjusting for energy and antioxidant intake, BMI, and several demographic, environmental, and other factors potentially influencing the incidence of asthma.

INTERVENTION STUDIES

Dietary essential long-chain PUFAs are incorporated into cell membranes as phospholipids, which can become substrates for the synthesis of eicosanoids via the cyclooxygenase and lipoxygenase enzymatic pathways. Eicosanoids, i.e., prostaglandins and leukotrienes, can be proinflammatory or anti-inflammatory depending on the fatty acid precursor. *n*-3 Fatty acids, but also GLA (an *n*-6 fatty acid), competitively inhibit the conversion of arachidonic acid into proinflammatory mediators and themselves yield products that exhibit anti-inflammatory activities in several experimental systems. Note that leukotriene antagonists, such as zileuton, are effective in the treatment of some patients with asthma but can be associated with substantial toxicity. Therefore, less toxic alternatives would be highly desirable.

A Cochrane review on supplementing patients with asthma with marine *n*-3 fatty acids concluded that the results of the nine RCTs that satisfied the inclusion criteria provided little evidence for a beneficial effect on lung function and asthma control but also no evidence for any risk associated with such supplements *(27)*. In an RCT not yet included in that review, supplementation with 100 mg/d of *n*-3 PUFA in the form of a lipid extract of New Zealand green-lipped mussel, *Perna canaliculus*, was associated with a significantly greater decrease in daytime wheeze and increase in morning PEFR compared with the placebo group *(28)*. Evening PEFR, FEV_1, $β_2$-agonist use, and night awakenings were not significantly affected.

GLA supplementation can produce significant improvements in patients with rheumatoid arthritis *(29)*, but the few randomized, controlled intervention trials conducted in patients with asthma have yielded disappointing results, with no improvement in lung function or asthma symptom scores. In rheumatoid arthritis, clinically relevant improvements were generally only seen in those studies using a dose of at least 1.4 g/d of GLA supplemented for a period of 6–12 mo. In most RCTs with patients with asthma, considerably lower doses were administered for shorter periods. In a recent double-blind, placebo-controlled RCT, however, supplementation with 2.0 g of GLA/d for 12 mo also did not significantly affect asthma scores, although it was associated with a significant reduction in leukotriene B_4 synthesis by polymorphonuclear leukocytes (30). Supplementation with a combination of GLA and the n-3 PUFA EPA for 4 wk also significantly decreased stimulated whole blood leukotriene biosynthesis in another RCT involving 43 patients with asthma (31). No effects on asthma control were reported.

A primary prevention study tested the efficacy of a high dietary and supplemental intake of n-3 fatty acids in children at high risk of developing asthma and allergy (32). Interim data for the first 18 mo of life indicated that the diet intervention reduced the prevalence of wheeze ever and wheeze lasting for more than 1 wk but did not significantly affect atopy and doctor's diagnosis of asthma. At the age of 3 yr, n-3 fatty acid supplementation was associated with a significant reduction in the prevalence of cough in atopic, but not among nonatopic, children (33). The prevalence of wheeze itself or asthma as defined by patterns of wheeze was not significantly different between the active diet and control groups.

Botanicals

Web sites and popular books on herbal remedies recommend numerous botanicals or individual plant constituents for the relief of asthma symptoms, including thyme, fennel, cayenne (*Capsicum frutescens*), *Ginkgo biloba*, *Lobelia inflata*, licorice (*Glycyrrhiza glabra* or *Glycyrrhiza uralensis*), stinging nettle (*Urtica dioica*), *Tylophora indica*, *Boswellia serrata*, butterbur (*Petasites hybrides*), and flavonoids, such as quercetin and genistein. In addition, one finds recommendations of various TCM formulas and their Japanese (Kampo) counterparts, which contain combinations of up to 12 botanicals. Ephedra is a constituent of many of these formulas, and there are still numerous Web sites that recommend ephedra extract (*Ephedra sinica* or ma huang) for the treatment of asthma. Importantly, the Food and Drug Administration prohibited the sale of dietary supplements containing ephedrine alkaloids and advised consumers to stop taking ephedra products because of the severe toxicities caused by them (http://vm.cfsan.fda.gov/~dms/ds-ephed.html).

Many of the recommended botanicals have not been examined in any clinical trials, some only as part of TCM or Kampo formulae. A systematic review of botanical treatments for asthma indicated that most of the 17 RCTs it identified were of moderate to poor methodological quality (34). This renders their results difficult to interpret and makes it difficult to arrive at firm conclusions concerning the usefulness of the studied botanicals in the treatment of asthma. Table 2 summarizes the results of double-blind, placebo-controlled trials contained in that review and several others that have been published since then.

It is encouraging that the methodological quality and the reporting of the methods and results of such trials are improving. This is particularly obvious in a recent study from Japan that evaluated treatment of 100 children with mild to moderate asthma with encapsulated dried powder of Mai-Men-Dong-Tang, a TCM formula consisting of *Ophiopogon japonicus*, American Ginseng (*Panax quinquefolium L.*), *Pinellia ternata*, licorice (*G. uralensis*), and *Tridax procumbens* Linn (35). Treatment with either 40 or 80 mg/kg/d of this formula was not associated with major adverse events or toxicities and resulted in significantly greater increases in FEV_1 and decreases of symptom scores compared with placebo. Although these results await independent confirmation, particularly in adults, they suggest that Mai-Men-Dong-Tang could be a valid adjunctive treatment for patients with mild to moderate asthma.

Table 2
Double-Blind, Placebo-Controlled RCTs With Botanicals

Treatment	Duration of treatment	Characteristics of randomized, controlled trials	n	Results	Reference
Tylophora indica	16 d–12 wk in 5 trials	3 P 2 C	593	Inconclusive: ranging from no significant effect to significantly greater percentage of treated patients with improvement in forced expiratory volume in 1 s (FEV$_1$) of ≥15% and significant improvement in symptoms and reduction in medication usage	34 review
Boswellia serrata	6 wk	P	80	Significant increase in FEV$_1$	34 review
Ginkgo biloba liquor	8 wk	P	61	Significantly greater, clinically relevant increase in FEV$_1$ compared to placebo group	34 review
Ivy leaves for 3 d	3 d	C (washout 3–5 d)	24	Significant improvement in airway resistance	34 review
Saiboku-to (TJ-96)	4 wk	C (washout 4 wk)	33 adults (42 ± 7 yr)	No significant change in FEV$_1$; significant improvement in bronchial responsiveness and symptom scores; significant decreases in inflammatory parameters (blood and sputum eosinophils and serum and sputum eosinophilic cationic protein)	38

Agent	Duration	Design	n	Results	Reference
Eucalyptol (1.8-cineol, the major monoterpene of eucalyptus oil)	12 wk	P	32	Significantly greater steroid-sparing effect compared with placebo	39
Mai-Men-Dong-Tang (composed of five botanicals)	4 mo	P with 3 groups receiving one of 2 doses of mMMDT or placebo	100 children (5–18 yr)	Significantly greater increases in FEV_1 at both doses compared with placebo; Significantly greater decreases in symptom scores; No significant changes in total or dust-mite specific immunoglobulin E; No major adverse events or toxicities as assessed by liver and kidney function measurements and blood tests	35
Propolis (honey bee resin)	2 mo	P	46	Significantly improved lung function (19% forced vital capacity, 30% FEV_1, 30% peak expiratory flow rate, and 41% FEV_{25-75}), paralleled by significant decreases in the serum concentration of proinflammatory mediators, including eicosanoids and cytokines (IL-1, IL-6, IL-8, and tumor necrosis factor-α), and intercellular adhesion molecule-1	40
Butterbur (*Petasites hybrides*)	1 wk	C (washout 1 wk)	16	Significant improvement in bronchial responsiveness (adenosine 5′-monophosphate PC_{20})	41

P, parallel; C, crossover; mMMDT, modified Mai-Men-Dong-Tang.

Table 3
Reasons for Adverse Events Caused by Botanical Supplements

1. Ingestion of higher than recommended doses either intentionally or inadvertently because of greater potency than indicated on the product label
2. Deliberate or accidental substitution of botanicals, with the substitutes being toxic
3. Contamination with heavy metals (reported particularly in Ayurvedic and Traditional Chinese medicine [TCM] remedies) or pesticide residues
4. Admixture of pharmaceuticals (detected in a variety of TCM remedies)
5. Toxic substances produced by molds and fungi on improperly stored or processed raw plant material
6. Herb–drug and herb–herb interactions

SAFETY OF BOTANICALS

Many consumers consider botanical remedies to be safe simply because they are "natural." Yet, numerous herbal preparations can cause allergies and serious toxicities, including hepatotoxicity, nephrotoxicity, and death (36). Table 3 lists reasons for adverse reactions other than outright toxicities of the botanical itself.

Some major adverse events are attributable to herb–drug interaction, in which numerous botanicals have been implicated (37). These include several that are recommended by CAM practitioners for use in asthma or are constituents of TCM asthma remedies, such as *G. biloba*, licorice (*G. glabra* or *G. uralensis*), *Panax ginseng*, and chili pepper (source of capsaicin). Some constituents of these plants can alter the pharmacokinetics or pharmacodynamics of pharmaceuticals by either enhancing or inhibiting their absorption and/or metabolism or by exerting similar or additive effects.

It is difficult to determine the actual incidence of adverse events resulting from herb–drug interactions because existing case reports often lack sufficient information to establish causality, but considerable underreporting of such events is highly likely. In a US survey, almost 20% of individuals taking prescription medication reported the concurrent use of at least one botanical product and/or a high-dose vitamin supplement. This suggests that as many as 15 million adults in the United States could be at risk of adverse interactions between such compounds.

Information on herb–herb interactions is almost completely lacking. This is particularly worrisome because increasing numbers of commercially available dietary supplements, including many multivitamin/mineral supplements, contain various combinations of botanicals.

Patients frequently do not inform their physician of their usage of botanical or other supplements but will generally do so if asked specifically. In view of the allergic reactions, toxicities, and drug interactions associated with many botanicals, physicians should inquire about the intake of botanical supplements and be able to inform their patients of potential risks associated with them. Table 4 lists Web sites that provide information on many aspects of dietary supplements, particularly safety issues.

SUMMARY AND CONCLUSION

Interpretation of the existing evidence for all forms of CAM therapy discussed here is hampered by the methodological flaws and small sample sizes of many of the RCTs assessing them, the short intervention and observation periods, and the numerous

Table 4
Web Sites Providing Information on Composition and Safety Aspects of Dietary Supplements

	Organization	Web Address	Type of information contained in the website
Free access	Center for Food Safety and Applied Nutrition, Food and Drug Administration (FDA)	http://vm.cfsan.fda.gov/~dms/supplmnt.html	Definition of dietary supplements, labeling requirements, and other regulatory and industry information.
	National Center for Complementary and Alternative Medicine (NCCAM), National Institutes of Health (NIH)	http://nccam.nih.gov	Safety information and warnings. Adverse events associated with dietary supplements should be reported to the FDA using the instructions provided on this site. Advisories and warnings on potential toxicities and interactions with pharmaceuticals of individual products or product categories; also information about ongoing trials.
	Agricultural Research Service, US Department of Agriculture	http://www.ars-grin.gov/duke	Information on the chemical composition of botanicals.
	HerbMed	http://www.herbmed.org	Information on 40 botanical compounds, including available evidence of their efficacy from clinical and observational studies. Investigations on pharmacodynamics, adverse effects/toxicities, and drug interactions is also listed.
Subscriber access	HerbMedPro	http://www.herbmed.org	Information as in HerbMed for another 128 botanicals.
	Consumer Lab	http://www.consumerlab.com	Reports on independent laboratory testing of different brands of dietary supplements, including comparisons of potency; also information on recalls and warnings regarding individual products or product categories.

outcome measures used, which precludes the combination of results in meta-analyses. The available data suggest that several types of CAM therapy provided subjective benefit to the patients. There is, however, insufficient evidence of effectiveness in improving objective measures of lung function for recommending any of them for the treatment of asthma. The relationship between objective physiological measures of asthma and patients' perception of their symptoms and asthma-related health status is complex, this perception being influenced by psychosocial and emotional factors that are independent of the severity of their disease. Therefore, the significant improvements in symptom and quality-of-life scores associated with several of the CAM treatments (and some of the control strategies involving extensive simulated therapies) should not be neglected. They may reflect an improved sense of control and enhanced coping ability in these patients.

REFERENCES

1. McCarney RW, Brinkhaus B, Lasserson TJ, Linde K. Acupuncture for chronic asthma. *Cochrane Database Syst Rev* 2003; Issue 3: CD000008.
2. McCarney RW, Linde K, Lasserson TJ. Homeopathy for chronic asthma. *Cochrane Database Syst Rev* 2003; Issue 4: CD000353.pub2.
3. Huntley A, White AR, Ernst E. Relaxation therapies for asthma: a systematic review. *Thorax* 2002; 57: 127–131.
4. Ritz T, Dahme B, Roth WT. Behavioral interventions in asthma: biofeedback techniques. *J Psychosom Res* 2004; 56: 711–720.
5. Lehrer PM, Vaschillo E, Vaschillo B, et al. Biofeedback treatment for asthma. *Chest* 2004; 126: 352–361.
6. Manocha R, Marks GB, Kenchington P, Peters D, Salome CM. Sahaja yoga in the management of moderate to severe asthma: a randomised controlled trial. *Thorax* 2002; 57: 110–115.
7. Holloway E, Ram FS. Breathing exercises for asthma. *Cochrane Database Syst Rev* 2004; Issue 1: CD001277.
8. Balon JW, Mior SA. Chiropractic care in asthma and allergy. *Ann Allergy Asthma Immunol* 2004; 93: S55–S60.
9. Gilliland FD, Berhane KT, Li YF, et al. Children's lung function and antioxidant vitamin, fruit, juice, and vegetable intake. *Am J Epidemiol* 2003; 158: 576–584.
10. Forastiere F, Pistelli R, Sestini P, et al. Consumption of fresh fruit rich in vitamin C and wheezing symptoms in children. SIDRIA Collaborative Group, Italy (Italian Studies on Respiratory Disorders in Children and the Environment). *Thorax* 2000; 55: 283–288.
11. Smit HA, Grievink L, Tabak C. Dietary influences on chronic obstructive lung disease and asthma: a review of the epidemiological evidence. *Proc Nutr Soc* 1999; 58: 309–319.
12. Fogarty A, Britton J. The role of diet in the aetiology of asthma. *Clin Exp Allergy* 2000; 30: 615–627.
13. Troisi RJ, Willett WC, Weiss ST, et al. A prospective study of diet and adult-onset asthma. *Am J Respir Crit Care Med* 1995; 151: 1401–1488.
14. Ram FS, Rowe BH, Kaur B. Vitamin C supplementation for asthma. *Cochrane Database Syst Rev* 2004; Issue 3: CD000993.
15. Fogarty A, Lewis SA, Scrivener SL, et al. Oral magnesium and vitamin C supplements in asthma: a parallel group randomized placebo-controlled trial. *Clin Exp Allergy* 2003; 33: 1355–1359.
16. Knekt P, Kumpulainen J, Jarvinen R, et al. Flavonoid intake and risk of chronic diseases. *Am J Clin Nutr* 2002; 76: 560–568.
17. Pearson PJK, Lewis SA, Britton J, Fogarty A. Vitamin E supplements in asthma: a parallel group randomised placebo controlled trial. *Thorax* 2004; 59: 652–656.
18. Hasselmark L, Malmgren R, Zetterström O, Unge G. Selenium supplementation in intrinsic asthma. *Allergy* 1993; 48: 30–36.
19. Romieu I, Sienra-Monge JJ, Ramírez-Aguilar M, et al. Antioxidant supplementation and lung functions among children with asthma exposed to high levels of air pollutants. *Am J Respir Crit Care Med* 2002; 166: 703–709.

20. Trenga CA, Koenig JQ, Williams PV. Dietary antioxidants and ozone-induced bronchial hyper-responsiveness in adults with asthma. *Arch Environ Health* 2001; 56: 242–249.
21. Rubin RN, Navon L, Cassano PA. Relationship of serum antioxidants to asthma prevalence in youth. *Am J Respir Crit Care Med* 2004; 169: 393–398.
22. Hill J, Micklewright A, Lewis S, Britton J. Investigation of the effect of short-term change in dietary magnesium intake in asthma. *Eur Respir J* 1997; 10: 2225–2229.
23. Schwartz J. Role of polyunsaturated fatty acids in lung disease. *Am J Clin Nutr* 2000; 71 Suppl: 393S–396S.
24. Broadfield EC, McKeever TM, Whitehurst A, et al. A case-control study of dietary and erythrocyte membrane fatty acids in asthma. *Clin Exp Allergy* 2004; 34: 1232–1236.
25. Woods RK, Raven JM, Walters EH, Abramson MJ, Thien FCK. Fatty acid levels and risk of asthma in young adults. *Thorax* 2004; 59: 105–110.
26. Oddy WH, de Klerk NH, Kendall GE, Mihrshahi S, Peat JK. Ratio of omega-6 to omega-3 fatty acids and childhood asthma. *J Asthma* 2004; 41: 319–326.
27. Thien FCK, Woods R, De Luca S, Abramson MJ. Dietary marine fatty acids (fish oil) for asthma in adults and children. *Cochrane Database Syst Rev* 2002; Issue 2: CD001283.
28. Emelyanov A, Fedoseev G, Krasnoschekova O, et al. Treatment of asthma with lipid extract of New Zealand green-lipped mussel: a randomised clinical trial. *Eur Respir J* 2002; 20: 596–600.
29. Little C, Parsons T. Herbal therapy for treating rheumatoid arthritis. *Cochrane Database Syst Rev* 2003; 3: last substantive amendment August 2000.
30. Ziboh VA, Naguwa S, Vang K, et al. Suppression of leukotriene B4 generation by ex-vivo neutrophils isolated from asthma patients on dietary supplementation with gammalinolenic acid-containing borage oil: possible implication in asthma. *Clin Dev Immunol* 2004; 11: 13–21.
31. Surette ME, Koumenis IL, Edens MB, et al. Inhibition of leukotriene biosynthesis by a novel dietary fatty acid formulation in patients with atopic asthma: a randomized, placebo-controlled, parallel-group, prospective trial. *Clin Ther* 2003; 25: 972–979.
32. Mihrshahi S, Peat JK, Marks GB, et al. Eighteen-month outcomes of house dust mite avoidance and dietary fatty acid modification in the Childhood Asthma Prevention Study (CAPS). *J Allergy Clin Immunol* 2003; 111: 162–168.
33. Peat JK, Mihrshahi S, Kemp AS, et al. Three-year outcomes of dietary fatty acid modification and house dust mite reduction in the Childhood Asthma Prevention Study. *J Allergy Clin Immunol* 2004; 114: 807–813.
34. Huntley A, Ernst E. Herbal medicines for asthma: a systematic review. *Thorax* 2000; 55: 925–929.
35. Hsu CH, Lu CM, Chang TT. Efficacy and safety of modified Mai-Men-Dong-Tang for treatment of allergic asthma. *Pediatr Allergy Immunol* 2005; 16: 76–81.
36. Ernst E. Harmless herbs? A review of the recent literature. *Am J Med* 1998; 104: 170–178.
37. Fugh-Berman A, Ernst E. Herb-drug interactions: review and assessment of report reliability. *Br J Clin Pharmacol* 2001; 52: 587–595.
38. Urata Y, Yoshida S, Irie Y, et al. Treatment of asthma patients with herbal medicine TJ-96: a randomized controlled trial. *Respir Med* 2002; 96: 469–474.
39. Juergens UR, Dethlefsen U, Steinkamp G, et al. Anti-inflammatory activity of 1.8-cineol (eucalyptol) in bronchial asthma: a double-blind placebo-controlled trial. *Respir Med* 2003; 97: 250–256.
40. Khayyal MT, el-Ghazaly MA, el-Khatib AS, et al. A clinical pharmacological study of the potential beneficial effects of a propolis food product as an adjuvant in asthmatic patients. *Fundam Clin Pharmacol* 2003; 17: 93–102.
41. Lee DK, Haggart K, Robb FM, Lipworth BJ. Butterbur, a herbal remedy, confers complementary anti-inflammatory activity in asthmatic patients receiving inhaled corticosteroids. *Clin Exp Allergy* 2004; 34: 110–114.

III | SPECIAL CLINICAL PROBLEMS

9 The Pregnant Patient With Asthma

Arif M. Seyal, MD

KEY POINTS

- The course of asthma during pregnancy is variable; it may improve, worsen, or remain unchanged.
- In general, women with severe asthma before pregnancy are more likely to experience worsening of their symptoms during pregnancy.
- Diagnosis of asthma can be confirmed by the demonstration of reversible airway obstruction by pulmonary function test.
- Methacholine challenge test and skin testing should be deferred until after childbirth.
- Avoidance of trigger factors and discontinuation of smoking are particularly beneficial during pregnancy because better control of asthma symptoms can be achieved while reducing the reliance on pharmacotherapy.
- Pharmacological management of bronchial asthma during pregnancy is not substantially different from the asthma management in patients who are not pregnant.

From: *Current Clinical Practice: Bronchial Asthma:*
A Guide for Practical Understanding and Treatment, 5th ed.
Edited by: M. E. Gershwin and T. E. Albertson © Humana Press Inc., Totowa, NJ

- When indicated, systemic corticosteroids should be used for the treatment of acute asthma exacerbation during pregnancy.
- Although ongoing immunotherapy can be continued at a reduced dosage schedule, it should not be initiated during pregnancy.
- Open communication between the patient and her physician will improve the patient's understanding of her asthma care plan and overall outcome.

INTRODUCTION

Bronchial asthma is among the most common chronic respiratory problems to complicate pregnancy. It is estimated that approx 4% of pregnancies may be affected by asthma (1). Clinically, asthma may manifest itself as a spectrum of disorders, ranging from infrequent intermittent wheezing to chronic severe asthma causing substantial disability. Uncontrolled asthma during pregnancy is associated with various maternal and fetal complications. A pregnant mother with asthma presents a unique challenge for the medical consultant because at any given time both mother and fetus are involved. Status of asthma symptoms control, maternal oxygenation, and asthma therapy affects both parties. When asthma is treated in the mother, there is a salutary effect on the fetal environment as well. Undertreatment of asthma during pregnancy is a major problem because of an unsubstantiated fear of fetal effects from maternal pharmacological therapy of asthma. The report of the National Asthma Education Program Working Group on Asthma and Pregnancy (1) emphasizes that proper control of asthma during pregnancy will improve maternal health and fetal well-being and significantly diminish perinatal morbidity and mortality.

CHANGES IN THE MATERNAL RESPIRATORY SYSTEM PHYSIOLOGY IN PREGNANCY

Physiological changes in the maternal respiratory and cardiovascular systems during pregnancy influence fetal oxygenation and acid–base status (see Table 1). There is an increase in minute ventilation up to approx 50% in late pregnancy, compared with a nonpregnant state (2). This is the result of progesterone-induced stimulation of respiratory drive and an increase in the tidal volume (3,4). These changes are responsible for alveolar hyperventilation and hypocapnia, with an arterial carbon dioxide pressure to lower than 35 mmHg. This relative hypocarbia (serum bicarbonate 18–22 mmol/L) leads to a rise in maternal arterial pH, thus causing mild respiratory alkalosis. The rise in pH because of respiratory alkalosis is blunted by increased renal excretion of bicarbonate. Baseline arterial blood gas values during pregnancy are presented in Table 2. Respiratory rate is relatively unchanged during pregnancy. Therefore, tachypnea during pregnancy (respiratory rate >20 bpm) is an abnormal finding and should be further investigated. Normal partial pressure of oxygen (PO_2) ranges from 106 to 108 mmHg during the first and second trimesters but decreases to 95–100 mmHg in the third trimester of pregnancy (5). A late pregnancy drop in the maternal arterial oxygen pressure to less than 90 mmHg may be noted in the supine position, presumably resulting from compression of inferior vena cava and subsequent decrease in cardiac output (6).

The airway mechanics during pregnancy generally remain unchanged. The forced vital capacity, forced expiratory volume in 1 s (FEV_1), peak expiratory flow rate (PEFR), and mean forced expiratory flow during the middle half of forced vital capacity (forced expiratory flow 25–75) remains unchanged (7). In general, all the measurements of

Table 1
Changes in Pulmonary Function Values During Pregnancy

Respiratory rate	Unchanged to slightly increased, but always less than 20
Total lung capacity	Unchanged to slightly low
Residual volume	Decreased by 15–20%
Tidal volume	Increased
Minute ventilation	Increased by 48%
Forced vital capacity (FVC)	Unchanged
Forced expiratory volume in 1s (FEV_1)	Unchanged
Peak expiratory flow rate	Unchanged
FEV_1/FVC	Unchanged
Maximum midexpiratory flow rate (forced expiratory flow 25–75)	Unchanged

Table 2
Arterial Blood Gas Values in Pregnant and Nonpregnant Women

	pH	PaO$_2$ mmHg	pCO$_2$ mmHg
Nonpregnant	7.4	91–95	36–39.4
Pregnant	7.43–7.46	102–106	29–30

pulmonary functions commonly used to make the diagnosis of airway obstruction do not change with pregnancy. In late pregnancy, diaphragmatic elevation caused by the enlarged uterus leads to the reduction in functional residual capacity and residual volume (Table 2).

CHANGES IN MATERNAL CARDIOVASCULAR PHYSIOLOGY AND FETAL OXYGENATION

Normal pregnancy is associated with a 20% increase in oxygen consumption and a 15% increase in the maternal metabolic rate. This extra demand is met by several compensatory mechanisms, such as increase in the minute ventilation and resting cardiac output by about 30% during early pregnancy (6). The arterial PO$_2$ of the fetus is only approx one-third to one-quarter of that of the maternal PO$_2$.

This probably results from the inefficient concurrent exchange system between the maternal and fetal circulation in the placenta. However, the fetus is capable of coping with this low-oxygen environment because of compensatory mechanisms involving high fetal cardiac output, high fetal hemoglobin concentration, and higher affinity of the fetal hemoglobin for the oxygen. This results in the leftward shift of oxygen dissociation curve. During maternal hypoxemia, the fetus has the ability to autoregulate the distribution of oxygenated blood to the heart, brain, and other vital organs (8,9). Prolonged maternal hypoxemia can, however, overwhelm the compensatory mechanisms and contribute to fetal complications, such as prematurity, low birth-weight, intrauterine growth retardation, and increased perinatal mortality. This is why aggressive control of asthma is so important during pregnancy.

INTERRELATIONSHIP BETWEEN ASTHMA AND PREGNANCY

Effect of Pregnancy on Asthma

The effect of pregnancy on asthma can best be described as variable. A review of more than 1000 pregnant patients with asthma in a combined series of studies by Gluck and Gluck *(10)* reported that asthma worsened in 23%, improved in 36%, and remained unchanged in 41% of the patients. Therefore, it is presumed to be a good generalization that during pregnancy, approximately one-third experience improvement in their asthma symptoms, one-third remain the same, and one-third get worse. Review of the data in this and other studies also suggests that women suffering from severe asthma are more prone to experience deterioration of their asthma during pregnancy. Worsening of asthma symptoms tends to occur more between 24 and 36 wk of gestation. In a study by Schatz et al. *(11)*, of 366 pregnant patients with asthma who were followed prospectively, 90% had no asthma symptoms during labor and delivery. Of those who experienced asthma symptoms half required no immediate treatment and only two patients required anything more than bronchodilator. Successive pregnancies tend to effect asthma severity similarly in an individual patient. Whatever the course of asthma during pregnancy, a majority of the patients tend to return to their prepregnancy status 3 mo after the delivery.

Potential mechanisms relating to the effects of pregnancy on asthma may include mechanical and hormonal factors, especially the bronchodilating effects of progesterone *(12)*.

Many women with asthma experience worsening of their symptoms because they stop their medications (especially inhaled corticosteroids [CSs]) because of their fear about the safety of medications during pregnancy.

The Effects of Asthma on the Mother and Fetus

A summary of the literature on the effects of asthma on pregnancy is presented in Table 3. Bronchial asthma during pregnancy can affect both the mother and the fetus. Several epidemiological studies have tried to determine the potential adverse effects of maternal asthma on pregnancy and the infant. One large study *(13)* showed a statistically significant increase in preterm birth and low birth-weight infants, decreased mean birth-weight, increased mortality, and increased neonatal hypoxia in the pregnancies of the women with asthma, compared with the control pregnancies. There was also an increased incidence of hyperemesis gravidarum, vaginal hemorrhage, and toxemia in the pregnant women with asthma as compared with the control pregnant women group. The other study *(14)* found a statistically significant increase in perinatal mortality in pregnant women with asthma vs pregnant women without asthma. Maternal chronic hypertensive disease was present in three out of eight of the fetal death cases. Subsequent control studies have reported an increase in low birth-weight, chronic hypertension, and preeclampsia in pregnant women with asthma, compared to pregnant women without asthma *(18,19,21,22)*. In a study by Schatz et al. *(16)*, lower maternal gestational FEV_1 during pregnancy was associated with intrauterine growth retardation. In another study by the same group *(20)*, patients treated by the asthma care specialist manifested a lower likelihood of the complications associated with asthma during the pregnancy. Therefore, it can be concluded indirectly that a better control of asthma during pregnancy would mean better perinatal outcomes.

Table 3

Effect of Asthma on Pregnancy: Summary of the Literature

Reference	Year of publication	Effects on pregnancy
14	1970	Increase in the perinatal mortality in pregnant women with asthma vs pregnant women without asthma. Neonatal mortality not reported.
13	1972	Increase in the preterm births, decreased mean birth-weight, increase in neonatal hypoxia, and neonatal mortality.
15	1986	Low-birth-weight infants in mothers admitted to hospital for the treatment asthma. Better outcome depended on good asthma control.
16	1990	Lower maternal mean FEV_1 during pregnancy was associated with lower birth-weight and asymmetric intrauterine growth retardation in infants of asthmatic women.
17	1991	Increased risk of transient tachypnea of the newborn in infants of mothers with asthma.
18	1992	Increased risk of preterm labor premature rupture of the membranes, preterm delivery, and increase in delivery by cesarean section in pregnant women with steroid and nonsteroid-dependent asthma. Increased frequency of both insulin-dependent and gestational diabetes mellitus in steroid-dependent pregnant asthmatics, compared to the control group.
19	1995	Increased risk of idiopathic preterm labor in pregnant women with asthma.
20	1995	Prospective, controlled, inception cohort study included 486 actively managed pregnant women with asthma. Not associated with increased incidence of preterm labor, preeclempsia, perinatal mortality, preterm or low-birth-weight infants, intrauterine growth retardation, or congenital malformations, compared with women without asthma with normal pulmonary function test results.
21	1998	Increased risk of preterm birth, low birth-weight, small for gestational age, and congenital anomalies. Increase in placenta previa, maternal hypertensive disorder, and cesarean delivery.
22	2000	Increased risk of preeclampsia, preterm birth, and low birth-weight. No evidence of increase in congenital malformation.

DIAGNOSIS OF ASTHMA IN PREGNANCY

Diagnosis of asthma in pregnant, as well as nonpregnant, women is based on history, physical examination, and spirometry. Clinical features may vary according to the severity of illness and underlying aggravating factors. Special consideration should be given to factors, such as emotional stress, gastroesophageal reflux, and an increase in viral and bacterial upper respiratory tract infections during pregnancy. Clinical impression should be confirmed by objective demonstration of reversible airway obstruction by spirometry (23). If a methacholine or histamine challenge test is required to confirm the diagnosis of asthma, it should be deferred until after the childbirth. Demonstration of a specific immunoglobulin E sensitization by skin testing carries a small risk of anaphylaxis; therefore, it should also be deferred until after the childbirth. During pregnancy, a radioallergosorbent (RAST) test is preferred instead of skin testing when specific allergen sensitization cannot be determined by careful history. RAST testing can provide adequate information while circumventing the possible risk of anaphylaxis.

Differential diagnosis of asthma should include the following (1,24,25):

1. Hyperventilation during early or late pregnancy, which may be associated with dyspnea, but no cough, wheezing, and chest tightness.
2. Peripartum cardiomyopathy.
3. Tocolytic therapy associated with pulmonary edema.
4. Amniotic fluid embolism.
5. Pulmonary embolism.

These may all be associated with acute dyspnea and occasional wheezing. Asthma can be ruled out by spirometry, which is normal in these patients.

MANAGEMENT OF ASTHMA IN PREGNANCY

For effective management of asthma during pregnancy, the National Asthma Education Program Working Group on Asthma and Pregnancy (1) recommends the following four integral components of an asthma management program:

1. Objective measures for accessing and monitoring of maternal lung functions and fetal well-being.
2. Environmental control.
3. Pharmacological treatment.
4. Patient education.

Goals of therapy for pregnant women should include the following:

1. Optimal therapy to maintain good control of asthma symptoms.
2. Maintaining normal or near-normal pulmonary function.
3. Maintaining normal activity level, including appropriate exercise.
4. Preventing acute exacerbation.
5. Avoiding adverse effects of asthma medication.
6. Delivering a healthy infant.

OBJECTIVE MEASURES FOR ASSESSMENT AND MONITORING

Maternal Monitoring

Pulmonary function tests are essential for estimating the severity of airway obstruction and can be achieved by simple spirometry in the physician's office. FEV_1 is considered the single best measure of pulmonary function for assessing the severity of airway obstruction. Therefore, it is recommended that office spirometry be conducted in the initial assessment of all pregnant patients being evaluated for asthma. Office spirometry should be repeated periodically during follow-up visits in the physician's office. Peak expiratory flow rate (PEFR), which can be measured by a simple, inexpensive, portable peak flow meter, correlates well with FEV_1. The patient can use this device at home to objectively assess the severity of airflow obstruction and follow the recommended treatment plan by her physician. Use of peak flow meter can further help in the maintenance of normal or near-normal pulmonary function (FEV_1 and PEFR) and provide an indirect measure of normal fetal oxygenation.

Fetal Monitoring

Early sonography, between weeks 12 and 20 of gestation, is recommended to determine the gestational age of the fetus as accurately as possible and to provide a benchmark against which future fetal growth can be measured. In addition, fetal growth during the second and third trimesters can also be determined by careful and serial measurements of fundal heights. Daily maternal recording of fetal activity, or kick counts, should also be encouraged. If the patient is admitted with acute asthma exacerbation or with hypoxemia, continuous electronic fetal monitoring is necessary and is continued until maternal status is stable. Careful fetal monitoring is also essential when women with asthma are admitted in labor.

Control of Environmental Triggers

Identification and avoidance of potential triggers is the integral part of asthma management. Environment control measures are especially helpful in pregnancy because they may improve the patient's well-being and, at the same time, may reduce the need for excessive medications. Patients should be instructed to avoid exposure to known specific irritants, including smoke, chemical sprays, fumes, and dust. If the patient herself smokes, she should be strongly encouraged to quit smoking and be referred to an appropriate smoking cessation program. If a house dust mite allergy is suspected or confirmed by RAST testing, appropriate measures should be taken to reduce the exposure to the house dust mite. Allergy-causing pets should be kept out of the house (1,23,26).

Immunotherapy

Immunotherapy reduces asthma-related symptoms triggered by allergens, such as the house dust mite, grass pollen, and cat dander. Abortion associated with systemic allergic reaction after grass pollen immunotherapy has been reported (27). In general, immunotherapy during pregnancy is considered safe. Metzger et al. (28) reported a retrospective study of 121 mothers with atopic pregnancies who had received immunotherapy during pregnancy, compared with a group of 147 untreated atopic gravidas. In the group of treated women, the incidence of prematurity, toxemia, abortion, neonatal death, and congenital malformation was no greater than in the untreated group. The incidence of atopic disease in the infants was the same in both groups. Based on this information, it is recommended that if a patient is on a maintenance dose of allergen immunotherapy, the dose should be reduced by one-half until delivery. The general recommendation is that the immunotherapy be discontinued in pregnant mothers who would require further significant increase in the dosage to achieve maximum therapeutic benefit (28,29).

PHARMACOLOGICAL THERAPY

General Considerations

Pharmacological therapy of asthma in pregnant women is not substantially different from the treatment of asthma in general. The prime goal of pharmacological therapy is to achieve a stable, asymptomatic state, using whatever medications necessary to achieve the best possible pulmonary functions. Because there are no randomized prospective human studies of asthma pharmacological therapy during pregnancy, recommendations for the treatment of asthma in pregnancy are based on published safety and efficacy data. There is no clear documentation of teratogenic effects of medications used in the treatment of asthma. The Working Group (1) recommends a step-wise (step up or step down) approach based on ongoing home PEFR monitoring. Twice-a-day PEFR monitoring will promote early detection of changes in air flow and enhance timely intervention.

Medications recommended for the outpatient management of mild, moderate, and severe persistent asthma and their Food and Drug Administration categories are shown in Tables 4 and 5. A step-care approach to the treatment of persistent asthma in pregnancy is the same as in nonpregnant women with asthma (see Table 6).

Short-Acting β₂-Agonist

Short-acting inhaled β_2-agonists used alone are usually sufficient for the treatment of mild intermittent asthma. This group of drugs may be administered by inhalation or given orally. Because of the minimal side effects, inhalation therapy is the preferred mode of administration of β_2-agonists bronchodilators (31,32).

Long-Acting β₂-Agonist

Two long-acting inhaled β_2-agonists (LABA), salmeterol and formoterol, are now marketed for the treatment of asthma. Their use is recommended as an adjunct to the anti-inflammatory therapy in moderate to severe persistent asthma. LABA should not be used for the relief of acute asthma symptoms.

Anti-Inflammatory Agents

Cromolyn sodium by inhalation is essentially devoid of any side effects and is an effective nonsteroidal anti-inflammatory drug available for use in mild persistent asthma. Its efficacy, however, is less predictable than the inhaled CSs. It requires 4–6 wk of trial before its efficacy can be determined. Nedocromil sodium has properties similar to cromolyn, but no significant data are available regarding clinical experience in pregnancy. Both cromolyn and nedocromil are less effective and more expensive than inhaled CSs.

Inhaled CSs are available for administration by inhalation, oral, or parenteral route. Steroids are by far the most effective anti-inflammatory agents available for the treatment of asthma. Only a minimal amount of inhaled CSs is systemically absorbed. Six studies regarding the gestational use of inhaled CSs have been published. In one large study from the Swedish Medical Birth Registry, 2968 mothers who reported use of inhaled budesonide for asthma in early pregnancy gave birth to infants of normal gestation age, weight, and length, with no increase in the rate of still births or multiple births (34). There is no evidence that in the recommended doses, any other inhaled CSs have adverse effects on pregnancy. Triamcinolone (33) and Beclomethasone (15) are also effective and have no significant adverse effects or teratogenic risks when used during pregnancy for the treatment of asthma.

Systemic steroid (prednisone, prednisolone) therapy should be used when other forms of therapy are maximized and asthma symptoms are still not well controlled. Some data (30) suggest that systemic CSs could increase the risk of preeclampsia and decrease intrauterine growth or infant prematurity. Severe asthma, however, can itself

Table 4
Food and Drug Administration Pregnancy
Risk Categories of the Pharmacological Agents
Used in Asthma and Rhinitis

Drugs	FDA category
• Bronchodilators	
Epinephrine (systemic)	C
Albuterol (inhaled or oral)	C
Levalbuterol	C
Metaproterenol (inhaled or oral)	C
Pirbuterol (inhaled)	C
Salmeterol (inhaled)	C
Formoterol	C
Ipratropium bromide (inhaled)	B
Theophylline (oral)	C
• Anti-inflammatory drugs	
Cromolyn sodium (inhaled)	B
Nedocromil sodium (inhaled)	B
• Inhaled corticosteroids	
Beclomethasone	B
Budesonide	B
Fluticasone	C
Flunisolide	C
Triamcinolone	C
• Oral corticosteroids	
Prednisone	C
Prednisolone	
• Leukotriene modifiers	
Montelukast	B
Zafirlukast	B
• Antihistamines	
Cetirizine	B
Chlorpheniramine	B
Diphenhydramine	B
Fexofenadine	C
Hydroxyzine	C
Loratadine	B

be associated with increased maternal and fetal morbidity. Thus, risk–benefit consider-ations still favor using systemic steroids when indicated for the management of severe and poorly controlled asthma during pregnancy.

Leukotriene Modifiers

Although there is no gestational human data for the zafirlukast and montelukast, ani-mal studies and postmarket surveillance data are reassuring. Their use could be consid-ered in patients with recalcitrant asthma who have shown favorable response before becoming pregnant (1).

Table 5
Food and Drug Administration Categories of Fetal Risks

Category	Risk
A	Controlled studies in the pregnant women. No risk to fetus demonstrated.
B	Animal studies have not demonstrated any fetal risk, but no controlled studies in the pregnant OR animal studies have shown an adverse effect that has no confirmed in women in the first trimester.
C	Animal studies have shown adverse effects on the fetus, and there are no controlled studies in pregnant women OR studies in women and animals are not available. Drug should be administered if potential benefit outweighs the risk to the fetus.
D	Positive evidence of fetal risk exists. Benefits from use in the pregnant women may make the drug acceptable.
X	Animal and human studies have demonstrated fetal abnormalities. Risk of the drug in the pregnant women clearly outweighs any potential benefits. These drugs are contraindicated in women who are or may become pregnant.

Theophylline

Various theophylline preparations have been used in the treatment of asthma for more than 50 yr. They are primarily used for their bronchodilator effect. With a better understanding of the pathophysiology of asthma and the advent of newer pharmacological agents, use of theophyllines has remarkably decreased. Sustained-release theophylline may be used for controlling nocturnal asthma symptoms. There is no evidence of adverse effects on pregnancy or increased risk of stillbirth *(35)*. Decrease in theophylline clearance during the third trimester of pregnancy has been reported, and, therefore, monitoring theophylline levels during pregnancy is essential, generally aiming for the levels of 8–12 mg/mL *(36)*.

Nebulized Ipratropium

Ipratropium bromide is a quaternary derivative of atropine and produces bronchial dilation by decreasing airway vagal tone. Use of inhaled ipratropium is not contraindicated in pregnancy but is seldom needed for long-term control of asthma.

Omalizumab

Omalizumab (Xolair®) is recombinant, humanized anti-immunoglobulin E monoclonal antibody that has demonstrated effectiveness in moderate to severe allergic asthma. Its use in pregnancy has not been studied and should be reserved for nonpregnant women with asthma only.

MANAGEMENT OF ACUTE EXACERBATION
OF ASTHMA IN PREGNANCY

The goal of treatment of chronic (persistent) asthma in pregnant women should be to keep the patient as free from symptoms as possible. However, acute or subacute

Table 6
Asthma Severity Classification and Step Therapy of Chronic Asthma During Pregnancy

	Symptoms	Nocturnal symptoms	Pulmonary functions	Treatment — Controller medications	Treatment — Reliever medications
Severe persistent asthma Step 4 care	Continued symptoms. Limited physical activity. Frequent exacerbation.	Frequent	Forced expiratory volume in 1 s (FEV_1) or peak expiratory flow rate (PEFR) 60% predicted variability.	High-dose inhaled steroids. Long-acting β_2-agonists (inhaled) and/or sustained-release theophylline. Consider oral steroids.	Inhaled short-acting β_2-agonist.
Moderate persistent asthma Step 3 care	Daily symptoms. Daily use of reliever medications. Exacerbation >2/wk, effects activity and lasts for days.	1/wk	FEV_1 or PEFR >60 and <80% predicted. PEFR variability 20–30%.	Medium-dose inhaled steroids OR low-medium-dose inhaled steroids and long-acting β_2-agonists and/or Sustained-release theophylline.	Inhaled short-acting β_2-agonist.
Mild persistent asthma Step 2 care	Symptoms >2/wk, but less than 1/d. Exacerbation may affect activity.	>2/mo	FEV_1 or PEFR >80% predicted. PEFR variability 20–30%.	Low-dose inhaled corticosteroid or Cromolyn sodium.	Inhaled short-acting β_2-agonist.
Mild intermittent asthma Step 1 care	Symptoms ≤2/wk. Asymptomatic between symptoms. Exacerbation brief.	≤2/mo	FEV_1 or PEFR ≥80% predicted. PEFR variability ≤20%.	No daily medications needed.	Inhaled short-acting β_2-agonist. (albuterol)

Adapted and modified from refs. 1 and 23.

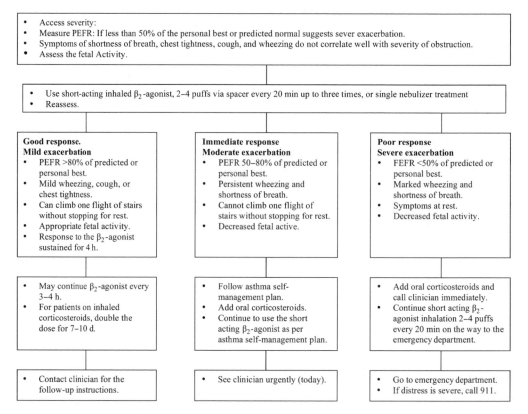

Fig. 1. Home management of acute exacerbation of asthma during pregnancy.

exacerbation of asthma symptoms cannot always be avoided and should be treated promptly. According to the report of the Working Group *(1)*, the following elements are essential in the treatment and prevention of the deterioration caused by exacerbation of asthma.

1. Recognition of early warning symptoms and worsening of objective measures, i.e., PEFR at home or FEV_1 in the physician's office.
2. Written action plan based on the deterioration of symptoms or objective parameters, i.e., PEFR or FEV_1.
3. Prompt communication between the patient and her physician.
4. Appropriate intensification of antiasthma therapy and administration of systemic CSs, if necessary.
5. Recognition and removal of any triggers from the patient's environment.
6. Patients with a history of potential fatal asthma should be followed closely.
7. For patients with moderate or severe asthma, regular visits (monthly or more often, if indicated), with monitoring of objective parameters and subjective status is essential.

For the treatment of acute exacerbation of asthma at home, emergency department, and hospital, refer to the accompanying Fig. 1 and Tables 7 and 8.

When evaluating these patients in the emergency department or in hospital, one must remember that blood gas analysis in healthy pregnant women routinely reveal lower PCO_2 and higher PO_2. PCO_2 of 35 mmHg or higher and PO_2 of 70 mmHg or lower

Table 7
Potential Neonatal Adverse Effects of Asthma/Antiallergy Drugs During Lactation

Medication	Maternal dose effect on infant
• **Inhaled**	
Bronchodilators	Very low serum levels in the mother, and will not result in significant
Cromolyn Na	dose to the infant through the breast milk.
Nedocromil	Considered compatible with breast-feeding.
Corticosteroids	
• **Oral**	
Bronchodilators	Not contraindicated during lactation.
β_2-agonist	May cause neonatal tachycardia, tremors, and hypoglycemia.
	Regularly scheduled use of oral β_2-agonists should be discouraged.
	Asthma control should be achieved by regular use of inhaled
	anti-inflammatory drugs.
• Theophylline	Less than 1% appears in breast milk. This is considered not clinically
	significant, but because of increased sensitivity in some infants,
	it may cause irritability, vomiting, jitteriness, and cardiac arrhythmia.
• Prednisone	Low concentration passes through the breast milk; 50 mg given orally
	to the mother will result in the infant receiving less than 20% of its
	normal daily physiological requirement.
	Considered compatible with breastfeeding.
• Antihistamine	Considered compatible with breastfeeding.
	Because of their anticholinergic properties, may have inhibitory
	effect on lactation.
• Decongestants	Considered compatible with breastfeeding.

From refs. *1* and *44–46*.

during acute exacerbation of asthma may represent a more severe respiratory compromise during pregnancy than the similar arterial blood gas in a nonpregnant patient. Therefore, it is essential that in a pregnant patient presenting with acute exacerbation of asthma in the emergency room, an O_2 saturation of more than 95% should be maintained by supplemental oxygen. If chest X-ray is needed, it must not be withheld because the patient is pregnant. Ionizing radiation from the chest X-ray is 0.2 rad, and it can be further minimized by abdominal shielding. Intravenous hydration is also important. Antibiotic therapy should be instituted when necessary. Tetracyclines, quinolones, and sulfonamides should be avoided in late pregnancy.

MANAGEMENT OF ASTHMA DURING LABOR AND DELIVERY

Acute asthma exacerbation, although uncommon during labor and delivery, may cause substantial distress to the gravidas and the infant. The Working Group *(1)* recommends that the patients should be continued on regularly scheduled asthma medications. Patients experiencing symptoms of acute asthma exacerbation during labor should be treated promptly. For the patients on chronic systemic steroids or who are treated with several short courses of systemic steroids during pregnancy, supplemental systemic CSs for the stress of labor and delivery are recommended. A dose of 100 mg of hydrocortisone intravenously on admission and 100 mg every 8 h until 24 h postpartum should be

Table 8
Hospital Management of Acute Exacerbation of Asthma During Pregnancy

Acute asthma exacerbation during pregnancy has the potential of causing serious conse-quences for the fetus. Therefore, asthma exacerbation during pregnancy should be managed aggressively. While managing acute exacerbation of asthma in a pregnant patient, the following points should be carefully observed:

Monitoring and assessment
- Careful ongoing assessment of mother and fetal monitoring (consult specialist).
- Patient with severe exacerbation should be hospitalized in the intensive care unit.

Treatment
- Supplemental oxygen to maintain oxygen saturation of 95% or better.
- Administer inhaled short acting β_2-agonist hourly or continuously.
- May add ipratropium bromide nebulizer solution.
- Systemic corticosteroids (methylprednisone, prednisone, or prednisolone): Doses of 120–180 mg/d in three or four divided doses for 48 h, then 60–80 mg orally daily until PEFR or FEV_1 is greater than 70% baseline. Taper over 7–14 d.

Outcome and follow-up
- Patient improved: minimal or no wheezing, good activity tolerance, PEFR or FEV_1 greater than 70% baseline, adequate oxygen saturation on room air, and no fetal distress. Consider discharge on inhaled β_2-agonist, inhaled and oral corticosteroid (to be tapered in 7–14 d) and long-acting β_2-agonist, if indicated.
- Patient education: appropriate use of controller vs rescue asthma medications, PEFR monitor-ing, written asthma action plan, environmental control measures, and follow-up plan. Close follow-up with asthma care specialist is highly recommended.

PEFR, peak expiratory flow rate; FEV_1, forced expiratory volume in 1 s.

administered. Intensive fetal monitoring of gravidas who enter labor with uncontrolled or severe asthma is recommended.

OBSTETRICAL MANAGEMENT

Detailed obstetric management of a pregnant woman with asthma is not possible in this chapter. However, the following points should be remembered. For induction of labor, oxytocin is preferred over various prostaglandin (PG) preparations. PGE1 and PGE2 are considered bronchodilators; however, intravenous administration of PGE2 has been reported to cause bronchoconstriction. PGF2α is a bronchoconstrictor, and should be avoided *(37,38)*. Intravaginal or intracervical PGE2 gel has not been reported to cause bronchospasm *(39)*.

Lumbar epidural analgesia reduces oxygen consumption and minute ventilation during the first and the second stages of labor and may considerably advantageous to patients with asthma *(40)*. Epidural analgesia has been reported to enhance the response to bronchodilator as well. If general anesthesia is needed, pretreatment with atropine and glycopyrrolate may provide a bronchodilating effect. Ketamine is the agent of choice for anesthesia induction *(1)*.

Oxytocin is also the drug of choice for postpartum hemorrhage. If tocolytic therapy is needed for preterm labor, care must be taken to avoid the use of more than one kind of β_2-agonist. Magnesium sulfate *(41)* or nifedipine may be used safely. Nonsteroidal anti-inflammatory drug, such as indomethacin, may exacerbate asthma and should be avoided in the treatment of preterm labor.

PATIENT EDUCATION

The patient plays a key role in the treatment of all asthma. Open communication and active participation by clinicians of all disciplines with the patient will not only improve the patient's understanding of the disease process but also enhance the total outcome. Building a partnership with the patient and the family must be done by the clinicians (obstetrician, asthma specialist, and primary care physician). The physician must inform the patient that although no medications for asthma, allergy, or, for that matter, any condition can be considered absolutely safe during pregnancy, relatively few medications have been proven harmful. It should be emphasized that potential direct and indirect consequences for the mother and for the baby of inadequately controlled asthma are worse than side effects of any of the medications used in the treatment of asthma. Patient education should be conducted in a relaxed atmosphere by the asthma care coordinator. Control of environmental triggers is important and should be emphasized. Appropriate use of peak flow meter metered-dose inhalers and dry powder inhalers should also be discussed and demonstrated. Written materials should be provided and telephone numbers should be given for easy accessibility to the care provider *(1,42–44)*.

Breast-Feeding

Almost all medications enter breast milk by diffusion from plasma. Milk concentrations are usually low, and it is uncommon for infants to receive a medication dosage in breast milk sufficient to produce toxic effect (*see* Table 7).

CONCLUSION

The goals of asthma management during pregnancy are essentially the same as the treatment of asthma in nonpregnant patients. However, the seriousness with which goals must be achieved is augmented because ineffective treatment and poor control of asthma will have adverse effects on not only the patient herself but also the fetus. It must be understood that harm to the fetus is more likely to come from the consequences of poorly controlled asthma than from medications for the treatment of asthma, including inhaled and systemic steroids. It is essential that clinicians caring for the pregnant patient with asthma work as a team and encourage the patient to actively participate in her care.

Currently, a registry study *(47)* that began in early 1998 under the Organization of Teratology Information Services is underway to prospectively evaluate pregnancy outcomes in relation to exposure to inhaled CSs. Information is also being collected for all other medications, including system steroids and leukotriene modifiers. It is hoped that the future will bring answers to the more complex questions of asthma management during pregnancy.

REFERENCES

1. Asthma and Pregnancy Update 2004. NAEP Working group Report on Managing Asthma during Pregnancy: Recommendations for Pharmacologic Treatment update 2004. NIH publication 05-3279. Bethesda, MD: US Department of Health and Human Services; National Institute of Health; National Heart, Lung, and Blood Institute, 2004.
2. Prouwe CM, Gaensler EA. Respiratory and acid–base changes during pregnancy. *Anesthesiology* 1965; 26: 381–392.
3. Weinberger SE, Weis ST, Cohn WR, et al. State of the art pregnancy and the lung. *Am Dev Respir Dis* 1980; 121: 559.

4. Libratoue SM, Pistelli R, Patalono F, et al. Respiratory function during pregnancy. *Respiration* 1984; 46: 145.

5. Templeton A, Kelman Gr. Maternal blood gases (PAO2-PaO2), physiologic shunt, VD/VT in normal pregnancy. *BP J Anaesth* 1976; 48: 100–104.

6. Aldrich CJ, O'Antona D, Spencer JAD, et al. The effect of maternal posture on fetal cerebral oxygenation during labor. *Obstet Gynecol* 1995; 102: 14–19.

7. Baldwin GR, Moorthisn DS, Whelton JA, et al. New lung functions and pregnancy. *Am J Obstet Gynecol* 1977; 127: 235.

8. Clark SL, Cotton DB, Lee W, et al. Central hemodynamic assessment of normal term pregnancy. *Am J Obstet Gynecol* 1989; 161: 1439–1442.

9. Peeters LLH, Sheldon RE, Jones MD, et al. Blood flow of fetal organs as a function of arterial oxygen content. *Am J Obstet Gynecol* 1979; 135: 637.

10. Gluck JC, Gluck PA. The effects of pregnancy on asthma: a prospective study. *Ann Allergy* 1976; 37: 165–168.

11. Schatz M, Hasoden K, Forsythe L, et al. The course of asthma during pregnancy, post partum and with successive pregnancies: a prospective analysis. *J Allergy Clin Immunol* 1988; 81: 509–517.

12. Juniper EF, Daniel EE, Roberts RS, et al. Effects of pregnancy on airway responsiveness and asthma severity. Relationship to serum progesterone. *Am Rev Respir Dis* 1991; 143: 578.

13. Bahna SL, Bjerbedal T. The course and outcome of pregnancy in women with bronchia asthma. *Acta Allergol* 1972; 27: 397–406.

14. Gordon M, Niswander KR, Berendes H, Kantos AG. Fetal morbidity following potentially atoxigenic obstetric condition: 7. Bronchial asthma. *Am J Obstet Gynecol* 1970; 106: 421–429.

15. Fitzsimons R, Greenberger PA, Patterson R. Outcome of pregnancy in women requiring corticosteroids for severe asthma. *J All Clin Immunol* 1986; 78: 349–353.

16. Schatz M, Zeiger RS, Hoffman CP. Intrauterine growth is related to gestational pulmonary function in pregnant asthmatic women. Kaiser Permanente Asthma and Pregnancy Study Group. *Chest* 1990; 98: 267.

17. Schatz M, Zeiger RS, Hoffman EP, et al. Increased transient tachypnea of the newborn in infants of asthmatic mothers. *Am J Dis Child* 1991; 145: 156–158.

18. Perlow JH, Montgomery D, Morgan MSA, Towers CV, Poto M. Severity of asthma and perinatal outcome. *Am J Obstet Gynecol* 1992; 967: 963–967.

19. Kramer MS, Coates AL, Michoud MC, et al. Maternal asthma and idiopathic preterm labor. *Am J Epidermiol* 1995; 142: 1078–1088.

20. Schatz M, Zeiger RS, Hoffman CP, et al. Perinatal outcomes in pregnancies of asthma women: a prospective controlled analysis. *Am J Respir Crit Case Med* 1995; 151: 1170–1174.

21. Demissie K, Breckenridge MB, Rhoades GG. Infants and maternal outcomes in the pregnancies of asthmatic women. *Am J Respir Crit Case Med* 1998; 158: 1091–1095.

22. Kare B, Rydhstroem H, Aberg A. Asthma during Pregnancy—A population-based study. *Eur J Epidemiol* 2000; 16: 167–171.

23. National Heart, Lung and Blood Institute National Asthma Education and Prevention Program. *Guidelines for the Diagnosis and Management of Asthma.* Expert Panel Report 2. NIH Publication 1997; No. 97-4051.

24. Hollingsworth HM, Irwin RS. Acute respiratory failure in pregnancy. *Clin Chest* Med 13; 4: 723–740.

25. Rizk NW, Kalassian KG, Gilligan T, Druzin MI, Daniel DL. Obstetric complications in pulmonary and critical medicine. *Chest* 1996; 110: 791–809.

26. Schatz M, Zeiger RS. Asthma and allergy in pregnancy. *Clinics Perinatol* 1997; 24: 407–432.

27. Francis N. Abortion after grass pollen injection. *J Allergy* 1971; 12: 559.

28. Metzger WJ, Turner E, Patterson R. The safety of immunotherapy during pregnancy. *J Allergy Clin Immunol* 1978; 61: 268–272.

29. Metzger WJ. Indications for allergen immunotherapy during pregnancy. *Comp Ther* 1990; 16: 17–26.

30. Schatz, M, Zeiger RS, Harden K, et al. Safety of asthma and allergy medications during pregnancy. *J Allergy Clin Immunol* 1997; 100: 301–306.

31. Schatz M, Zeiger RS, Harden KAA, et al. The safety of inhaled B-agonist bronchodilators during pregnancy. *J Allergy Clin Immunol* 1989; 92: 686–695.

32. Rayburn WF, Ateleinson BD, Gilbert K, et al. Short term effects of inhaled albuterol on maternal and fetal circulations. *Am J Obstet Gynecol* 1994; 171: 770–773.

33. Dombeowski MP, Brown CL, Berry SM. Preliminary experience with triamcinolone acetamide during pregnancy. *J Mat Fet Med* 1996; 5: 310–313.

34. Norjavaara E, Gerhardsson de Verdier M. Normal Pregnancy outcomes in a population-based study including 2968 pregnant women exposed to budesonide. *J Allergy Clin Immunol* 2003; 111: 736–742.

35. Neff RK, Leviton A. Maternal theophylline consumption and risk of stillbirth. *Chest* 1990; 11: 266–267.

36. Caster BL, Driscoll CE, Smith GD. Theophylline clearance during pregnancy. *Obstet Gynecol* 1986; 68: 555–559.

37. Karin SMM. Appearance of prostaglandin F2OC in lumen blood during labor. *Br Med J* 1968; 1: 618–621.

38. Shaw JO, Moser KM. The current status of prostaglandins and the lungs. *Chest* 1975; 68: 75–80.

39. Rayburn WF. Prostaglandin E2 gel for cervical ripening and induction of labor: a critical analysis. *Am J Obstet Gynecol* 1989; 160: 529.

40. Hagesdal M, Morgan CW, Sumner AE, Gertsche BB. Minute ventilation and oxygen consumption during labor and epidural analgesia. *Anesthesiology* 1983; 59: 425–427.

41. McLean RM. Magnesium and its therapeutic uses: a review. *Am J Med* 1994; 96: 63–96.

42. Patterson R, Greenberger PA, Frederick MC. Asthma and pregnancy: responsibility of physicians and patients. *Ann Allergy* 1990; 65: 469–472.

43. Gross G, Burdon JG. Patient education. Asthma and pregnancy. *Aust Fam Physician* 1991; 20: 1140.

44. Lipkowitz MA, Schatz M, Cook TJ, et al. When allergies and asthma complicate pregnancy. *Ann Allergy Asthma Immunol* 1998; 81: 30–34.

45. American Academy of Pediatrics Committee on Drugs. Transfer of drugs and other chemicals into human milk. *Pediatrics* 1989; 84: 924–936.

46. Bennett DN. *Drugs and Human Lactation*. New York: Elsevier; 1988.

47. Scialli AR. The Organization of Teratology Information Services (OTIS) Registry study. *J Allergy Clin Immunol* 1999; 103: S373–S376.

10 Infectious and Environmental Triggers of Asthma

Laurel J. Gershwin, DVM, PhD

CONTENTS

KEY POINTS

- Development of asthma can be enhanced by infection with respiratory viruses.
- Exposure to environmental tobacco smoke enhances development of Th2 response and subsequent sensitization to inhaled allergen.
- Ozone and allergen exposure during development can enhance airway remodeling, allergic sensitization, and airway hyperresponsiveness.
- Environment and genetics of the host contribute to the development of the allergic asthmatic phenotype.

INTRODUCTION

The incidence of asthma has been increasing during the past several decades, especially in industrialized nations. Although nobody knows the reasons for this increase,

From: *Current Clinical Practice: Bronchial Asthma:*
A Guide for Practical Understanding and Treatment, 5th ed.
Edited by: M. E. Gershwin and T. E. Albertson © Humana Press Inc., Totowa, NJ

there have been many theories proposed. Increased pollution in the form of tobacco smoke, ozone, and diesel fumes, as well as alteration in life styles, have been implicated *(1)*. The link between infection with certain respiratory viruses early in life and the development of chronic allergic asthma in adulthood has been strengthened in recent years by studies performed in laboratory animal models. Also, studies using animal models have demonstrated that environmental tobacco smoke (ETS), ozone, and diesel exhaust particulates can increase allergic sensitization to inhaled allergens, while data linking infection with respiratory viruses, particularly respiratory syncytial virus (RSV), have been further substantiated.

Complex genetic factors that govern both immunoglobulin (Ig)E responsiveness and the development of airway hyperreactivity are recognized as important to the etiology of asthma. It is widely known than individuals with one or more parents who are asthmatic/atopic are more likely to develop asthma than those individuals with a non-asthmatic/nonatopic family history. In recent years, progress has been made in the detection of gene polymorphisms associated with atopy and asthma. Using both candidate gene studies and genome-wide screens, several potential genetic factors for susceptibility to asthma have been identified *(2)*. Among the genes that are believed to be involved are: the cytokine gene cluster on chromosome 5 (coding for interleukins [ILs]-3, 4, 5, 9, and 13), the gene coding for the β chain of the IgE high-affinity receptor on chromosome 11, the gene coding for the IL-4 receptor on chromosome 16, and signal transducer and activator of transcription (STAT)6 on chromosome 12 *(3)*.

More recent data on IL-4 and IL-4 receptor gene polymorphisms were obtained from a study on Korean children. Polymorphisms in these genes were identified, and associations with eosinophilia and bronchial hyperresponsiveness were examined. It was concluded that the IL-4Rα Arg551 gene may play a role in susceptibility to atopic asthma *(4)*. The importance of STAT6 in signal transduction and transcriptional activation in T-helper (Th)2 cell differentiation has made polymorphisms in this gene a target for investigation. Polymorphisms in the STAT6 gene were examined in a cohort of white adults. A haplotype was identified that was associated with high levels of total IgE *(5)*.

In individuals with the appropriate genotype, the development of asthma is influenced by contact during infancy or early childhood with appropriate pathogens and/or indoor and outdoor sources of air pollution. It is highly likely that the increase in exposure to these adverse external conditions is an important factor influencing the increase in the incidence of asthma in the human population. According to the "hygiene hypothesis," exposure to bacterial products during childhood has a protective effect. However, the importance of the genetic background on which such stimuli have their effect should not be understated.

MODULATION OF THE ALLERGIC RESPONSE
BY INFECTIOUS DISEASES

There are two separate and opposite effects of infectious disease agents on asthma: those that promote the asthmatic phenotype and those that inhibit it. A basic feature of the immune response is the cooperation that occurs between T- and B-lymphocytes after exposure to antigen. In 1989, Mossman and Coffman described different patterns of cytokine secretion that leads to different patterns of immune responsiveness *(6)*. It is well recognized that CD4+ T-cells have two different profiles of cytokine production: Th1 and Th2. Cell-mediated immunity is stimulated by the Th1 cytokines, whereas humoral immunity is stimulated by Th2 cytokines. Th1 and Th2 responses are balanced in a normal immune system. Th1 cytokines (interferon (IFN)-γ, IL-2, and IL-12) can downregulate Th2 cytokine (IL-4, IL-5, IL-10, and IL-13) production. A strong Th2 response facilitates IgE production and the consequent development of allergy. The balance of Th1 and Th2 cytokines is maintained and determined by the specific dose of antigen, the genetic background of the host, and the local tissue environment (including co-stimulatory factors). Recently, the important role of the dendritic cells that act as professional antigen-presenting cells has been elucidated. Thus, disease agents that promote a Th1-type response are believed to have a protective role, whereas those associated with a Th2 response are associated with promotion of the asthmatic phenotype. The abundance of case studies and research data has created a paradox. The hygiene hypothesis, which has received wide attention, was originally based on epidemiological data. Children raised in rural farming communities have a lower incidence of asthma, presumably because there is a preferential stimulation of the Th1 cytokine response by exposure to bacteria and their products, such as endotoxin (7–9). The corollary is that lack of infection with bacteria containing endotoxin or simply a lack of natural aerosol exposure to such organisms causes the development of allergy. However, endotoxin inhalation promotes the clinical symptoms of asthma. Studies on cotton workers have documented the cause of "Monday Asthma" to be the inhalation of endotoxin present in the cotton dust (reviewed in ref. [10]). Yet, several recent studies have shown an association between less asthma in children raised with animals, despite the documentation of increased endotoxin levels in animal-containing homes (11).

Decreased microbial infection resulting from increased vaccination has been proposed as an explanation for the increased incidence of asthma. This was addressed in relation to both natural measles infection and vaccination in a 1998 study of British children (12). In this study of more than 6000, children with both measles infection and vaccination were associated with a reduced risk of hay fever. More recently, Roost et al. accumulated data from 1537 Swiss schoolchildren (13). They evaluated the effect of both natural infection and measles, mumps, and rubella (MMR) vaccination on incidence of sensitization to allergens and development of asthma (14). The study concluded that neither MMR vaccinations nor natural MMR infections are associated with an increase in atopic disease in the population examined. Other studies have had similar conclusions (15,16). In contrast, the IgE-promoting effects of *Bordetella pertussis* are well known (14–19), and it has been suggested that vaccination for whooping cough may stimulate development of allergy. However, Bjorksten and coworkers performed a large prospective study on the subject and have essentially concluded that *B. pertussis* vaccination is not a likely cause of increases in the incidence of allergy in the human population (20). Moreover, in a mouse model, whole cell pertussis vaccine played a protective role rather than a stimulatory role in the development of allergic asthma (21).

A recent study examined the relationship between occurrence of tonsillitis in children between the ages of 3 and 14 yr with and without asthma. The data revealed that children with recurrent tonsillitis were less likely to have asthma. It was believed that the tonsillar hyperplasia was indicative of a Th1 response (22). Such observations are consistent with the hygiene hypothesis.

A recent idea stimulated by the hygiene hypothesis suggests that the allergic phenotype might be prevented by infection with an organism capable of inducing an opposing type of immune response. The hallmark study that appeared to define the relationship between shifting the immune response toward a Th1 response by introduction of a Th1-inducing micro-organism and protection from asthma was performed by Shirakawa *(21)*. In this study of Japanese schoolchildren who received immunization against tuberculosis with the Bacille Calmette Guerin (BCG) vaccine results indicated that there was a strong inverse association between delayed-type hypersensitivity to *Mycobacterium tuberculosis* and the presence of type I immediate hypersensitivity. Thus, students who had positive tuberculin skin tests had lower serum IgE and a lower incidence of allergy. Moreover, the cytokine profile of these children showed a bias toward Th1 cytokines. It is well recognized that mycobacterial antigens stimulate a strong Th1 response, causing production of cytokines, such as IFN-γ. These Th1 cytokines downregulate the Th2 response and, thus, diminish the allergic response. The recognition that the BCG-vaccinated children had significantly less allergy than non-BCG-vaccinated children demonstrated that immune regulation during early life is likely an important factor influencing development of allergic respiratory disease in future years.

A more recent study was performed on infants and newborns from Thailand, Argentina, and Turkey (countries that routinely administer BCG vaccines). Children underwent both purified protein derivative (PPD) and allergen testing at 2 yr of age. There was a significant correlation between a negative PPD response vs a positive PPD response and having an allergic history at 2 yr of age for subjects in Thailand and Turkey but not in Argentina *(24)*.

Another study on the effect of BCG vaccination on the development of allergy was performed in Sweden *(25)*. In this study, 216 children with an atopic family history were vaccinated with BCG when they were less than 6 mo old. Another 358 age-matched children were not vaccinated with BCG. The family risk factors for developing allergy were similar in both groups. Results of the study showed that 36% of the BCG group and 41% of the control group developed clinical signs of atopy. Neither results of serum levels of allergen-specific IgE nor skin-prick tests were significantly different. The conclusion reached in this study was that in children with a family history of atopy, early vaccination with BCG did not affect the development of atopic disease in early childhood.

These studies have stimulated others to explore the potential of using BCG vaccination for modulation of the immune response in patients with asthma. Thus, in a recent study by Vargas et al., BCG- and placebo-immunized schoolchildren with asthma were tested for serum IgE, IL-4, and IFN-γ production by peripheral blood mononuclear cells. In the placebo group, the parameters of a Th2 response increased (IL-4 and IgE), whereas the Th1 cytokine IL-1 decreased. Th2 parameters did not change in BCG-treated patients. However, the severity and frequency of asthma did not change significantly and was the same in both groups *(26)*. Thus, although BCG treatment may alter the immune response, this study did not show a translation into clinical improvement. Animal models have been used to determine the validity of these observations on effects of BCG vaccination on development of allergic asthma. In one study by Herz et al., Balb/c mice were sensitized with BCG, ovalbumin (OA), or both *(27)*. Mice that were sensitized with OA developed the expected Th2 cytokine response, IgE production, airway hyperresponsiveness, and eosinophilia, whereas those mice that received BCG before OA immunization showed decreased IgE production and normalized cytokine production and lacked airway hyperresponsiveness and eosinophilia. In a study by Tukenmez et al., newborn mice were immunized with either *Mycobacterium bovis* and *Mycobacterium vaccae* or phosphate-buffered saline solution or were not injected *(28)*. At adulthood, mice were immunized with a series of intraperitoneal injections of OA followed by an aerosol challenge. Mice immunized with *M. bovis* and *M. vaccae* had significantly lower IgE levels than those mice in the phosphate-buffered saline solution groups. The effect of a potent Th1 stimulus (*M. vaccae*) on an already-primed animal was examined in another study, which used mice that were previously sensitized to OA. Wang et al., found that a single injection of *M. vaccae* caused a decrease in serum IgE and two injections inhibited IL-5 production as well *(27)*. Based on all of these findings, the potential for using a Th1 modulator, such as *M. vaccae*, for treatment of atopy has been suggested.

The importance of microflora in the intestinal tract for modulating development of the immune response is reviewed by Bjorksten *(28)*. The immune responses to microbes and food proteins presented by the oral route differ such that tolerance is the expected response to foods while active antibody production accompanies immune stimulation with microbial pathogens. Studies on infants in Estonia and in Sweden have demonstrated differences in intestinal microflora of atopic and nonatopic children. Postnatal colonization with lactobacilli was greater in the Estonian infants *(29)*. Shida et al. demonstrated that *Lactobacillus casei* inhibits antigen-induced IgE secretion through cytokine release, probably IL-12 *(30)*. Thus lack of the appropriate Lactobacilli may facilitate a further Th2 cell response in the infant.

VIRAL INFECTIONS AND ASTHMA

Recurrent wheezing in infants and young children has recently been reviewed by Hopp *(33)*. The large number of terms used to describe the infant with recurrent wheezing are described: "reactive airway disease," "recurrent bronchiolitis," "chronic bronchiolitis," "wheezy bronchitis," "chronic bronchitis," and "asthmatic bronchitis." Some of the children in all of these categories are truly asthmatic. An infection with RSV that causes bronchiolitis is often followed by episodes of recurrent wheezing. Hopp describes three types of episodic wheezing in young children: transient early wheezers, late wheezers, and persistent wheezers. The determination that episodes of wheezing with subsequent viral infection are likely to evolve into clinical asthma is affected by factors, such as a family history of atopy, the presence of eosinophilia and high IgE, and exposure to tobacco smoke. Generally, wheezing after the age of 6 yr is caused by asthma. Before the age of 6 yr, frequent viral infections with agents such as influenza virus, RSV, and rhinovirus (RV) are important causes of wheezing episodes.

Several viruses (RSV, RV, and parainfluenza) are implicated as triggers of acute exacerbation of clinical symptoms of asthma in both children and adults. Recently, the human meta pneumovirus (new variant) has been associated with acute and severe exacerbation of asthma in a child *(34)*. A suggested trigger for these viruses is the recruitment of Th2-type cells into the lungs *(35)*.

An association between production of the pleiotropic cytokine IL-11 in the lung and induction of airway hyperresponsiveness has been shown by Einarsson et al. *(36)*. After infection with RSV, RV, and parainfluenza virus, production of IL-11 by stromal cells was increased in the lung. In this same study, IL-11 production was also documented in nasal aspirates of virus-infected children with wheezing. This same group has found that viruses implicated as inducers of wheezing (RSV, RV, and parainfluenza virus) are all inducers of IL-11, whereas those pathogens that fail to induce wheezing (cytomegalovirus, herpes simplex virus, pyogenic bacteria) do not induce IL-11 production.

RESPIRATORY SYNCYTIAL VIRUS

Multiple viruses, as discussed, can trigger asthma in the infected patient. RSV has an even more significant role in asthma. RSV has been recognized as an important cause of bronchiolitis in infants and young children since 1957. The majority of all children are infected by 2 yr old. Subsequent reinfection occurs during childhood, but reinfection often consists of simply upper respiratory symptoms described as a "cold," except in some children that continue to wheeze.

There is increasing evidence that not only can RSV trigger asthma, but also early life infection can program an infant to become asthmatic. Evidence for this comes from both human case studies and animal experiments. Holtzman described this effect as a "hit-and-run" phenomenon in which the asthmatic phenotype was activated by viral infection in susceptible genotypes long after clearance of the virus *(37)*.

Welliver et al. *(38)* studied infants and children infected with RSV and grouped them into those with only upper respiratory tract disease, those with lower respiratory tract disease, and those with lower respiratory tract disease who showed evidence of wheezing. Interestingly, they reportedly found that RSV-specific IgE and nasal levels of histamine were increased in the group that wheezed.

Validation of the role for RSV-specific IgE in disease pathogenesis has come from several animal studies. Using a bovine model of RSV (cattle have a similar virus, bovine RSV, that causes natural infection of calves), Gershwin et al. found that there was a strong correlation between severity of disease and bovine RSV-specific IgE detected in serum *(39)*.

The role of RSV-specific IgE was also demonstrated in a mouse model. In that study, RSV-specific IgE was associated with airways hyperresponsiveness to methacholine; more importantly the presence of the high-affinity IgE receptor on mast cells was required for this effect to occur *(40)*. These studies suggest that the development of a virus-specific IgE response contributes to pathogenesis of airway hyperresponsiveness.

One study evaluated children who had RSV before age 3 yr. These children were followed for development of wheezing and atopy until the age of 13 yr. Results from this study showed that RSV lower respiratory tract illnesses were associated with an increase risk of wheeze by age 6 yr. The risk decreased as the children got older. There was no association with atopy. It was concluded that RSV infection early in life can influence subsequent wheezing up until age 11 yr, but this wheezing was not associated with increased sensitization to allergen *(41)*.

Another school of thought involving the role of RSV in asthma induction is that infection facilitates sensitization to inhaled allergens. The limitations of epidemiological data have led to performance of in vitro assays using specimens from human patients, as well as the establishment of several animal models, for examination of the potential augmentation of sensitization to inhaled allergens that appears to occur during or as a sequel to RSV infection. In one study by Noma et al., the relationship between the onset of recurrent wheezing and antigen-specific IL-2 responsiveness was analyzed *(42)*. IL-2 is the cytokine responsible for proliferation of antigen-specific T-lymphocytes. The data indicated that RSV infection of infants induced responsiveness to the respiratory allergen, *D. farinae* (house dust mite) and also to OA, a food antigen.

It has now been well established that RSV infection causes development of and often persistence of a Th2 cell response. This is accompanied by development of proinflammatory or immunoregulatory cytokines, such as IL-4, RANTES, CCL5, MIP-1α, IFN-γ, IL-2, IL-6, TNF-α, and MCP-1. Prostaglandin and leukotriene synthesis, activation of mast cells, and eosinophils have all been reported and implicated in pathogenesis of infection (reviewed in ref. *[43]*). It is easy to see that many of these same immune reactants are important constituents of the allergic response as well. In fact, transcriptional activation of genes important for inflammatory responses that occur in asthma pathogenesis is triggered by replication of RSV in respiratory epithelium.

Mouse models have been used to show that infection with RSV can enhance sensitization to inhaled allergen. One mechanism that has been examined involves the production of certain chemokines by RSV-infected epithelial cells. CCL5/RANTES is produced during infection *(44)*. This chemokine is also important in allergic asthma, causing the recruitment of inflammatory cells to the airways. The receptor for CCL5 is CCR1 and is important in RSV-induced exaggeration of allergic airway disease. CCR$^{-/-}$ mice showed a reduced response to aerosolized allergen after RSV infection compared with wild-type mice *(45)*.

OTHER RESPIRATORY VIRUSES AFFECTING ASTHMA

Viruses, such as influenza, RV, and parainfluenza, have also been studied for their asthma-enhancing effects. The incidence of respiratory tract infection in adults requiring hospitalization for asthma has been examined. The most common viral agents in these adult patients were influenza A and RV, although studies in children show that RV and RSV are the major respiratory infections associated with wheezing. Most observations support the hypothesis that wheezing with viral infections is of greatest significance to the under 6-yr-old population.

Several animal models have been developed to study the complex interaction of respiratory tract infections with viruses and the development of allergic sensitization and asthma. Several of these models have been reviewed by Hegele *(46)*. In one study, infection of Balb/c mice with influenza A caused development of an IgE response to flu antigen when it was injected intradermally *(47)*. In another study, Balb/c mice were infected with influenza A and then were sensitized to inhaled OA during the acute or convalescent phase of the infection. Those mice sensitized to the OA during the acute phase developed an IgE response, but not those sensitized during the recovery phase *(48)*. These results suggest that, at least in the mouse model, like RSV, influenza virus infection enhances allergic sensitization and airway hyperresponsiveness.

T-eosinophil, a hallmark of allergic airway disease, is often associated with viral-induced asthma exacerbation. Stimulation of eosinophil accumulation in airway interstitium is an anticipated result of secretion of proinflammatory mediators, cytokines/chemokines. Recruitment of eosinophils to airway nerves has been reported as a mechanism for inhibition of the muscarinic receptors on airway parasympathetic nerves *(49)*.

Multiple mechanisms, including but not limited to those cited, have been suggested for enhancement of asthma by respiratory viruses *(49)*. Effects of virus infection on the infant or child who is atopic may be primarily to promote sensitization to allergen and development of the allergic phenotype. The imprinting process may involve alterations to parasympathetic nerve fibers, programming the immune response toward a Th2 phenotype, or facilitating allergic sensitization through dendritic cell recruitment or stimulation. Recruitment of dendritic cells, important for antigen presentation, into the airway epithelium during the inflammatory response to virus and bacterial pathogens has been implicated as a factor favoring allergic sensitization *(50)*. In studies on rats challenged with live virus and/or bacterial pathogens, lungs were analyzed for cell recruitment. A variety of C-C chemokines were implicated in recruitment of the dendritic cells to the inflammation site.

Neuropeptides are expressed by the nonadrenergic, noncholinergic autonomic nervous system. These neurotransmitters include vasoactive intestinal peptide, which relaxes bronchial smooth muscle, and substance P, which contracts bronchial smooth muscle. These mediators and others in the class are undoubtedly important in asthma pathogenesis *(51)*. Alteration in expression of sensory neuropeptides occurs after RSV infection. Balb/c mice infected with RSV showed increased airway resistance to inhaled methacholine, and substance P expression was increased in airway tissue. Use of a neurokinin-1 receptor antagonist inhibited the development of this airway hyperresponsiveness *(39)*.

NONVIRAL INFECTIOUS AGENTS AND ASTHMA

Mycoplasma pneumoniae, often referred to as atypical bacterial pneumonia, has been associated with exacerbation of asthma in adults and children. Recent studies have implicated *M. pneumoniae* in the pathogenesis of chronic asthma. The increased presence of *M. pneumoniae* in the airways of patients with chronic asthma lends support to the hypothesis that the infection may have a role in chronic asthma.

More recently, the cytokines stimulated by *M. pneumoniae* infection were examined. One study focused on children with acute mycoplasma infection and wheeze. In this study, there was a significant increase in serum levels of IL-5, but not IL-4, IFN-γ, or IL-2 *(52)*. In an in vitro study using both human nasal epithelial cells from patients with and without asthma and peripheral blood mononuclear cells infected with *M. pneumonia*, it was found that there was no change in RANTES or IL-8 from nasal epithelial cells. The peripheral blood mononuclear cells from normal volunteers infected in vitro with *M. pneumoniae* showed increases in IL-2, IL-6, and tumor necrosis factor (TNF)-α. The conclusion was made that cytokine production was probably more important from mononuclear cells present at the airway surface than from the airway epithelial cells *(53)*. This is in contrast to a virus, such as RSV.

Another nonviral agent that has recently been associated with asthma is *Chlamydia pneumoniae*. Hahn examined the association between acute *C. pneumoniae* infection and asthmatic bronchitis in adults *(54)*. In this prospective study, serology, bacteriology, and clinical assessment were evaluated in 365 patients with signs of respiratory disease with and without serological titers positive for *C. pneumoniae*. Forty-seven percent of patients who had acute *C. pneumoniae* infection developed bronchospasm. Of these patients, 96% failed to show evidence of coinfection with any other respiratory pathogens. There was a significant association between antibody titer (after but not before infection) to *C. pneumoniae* and development of asthmatic bronchitis. The study concluded that repeated or prolonged exposure to *C. pneumoniae* may be a cause of wheezing, asthmatic bronchitis, and adult-onset asthma. A subsequent study by the same group attempted to further investigate the association of *C. pneumoniae* infection with adult reactive airway disease. In this study, serology and pharyngeal cultures were used to determine infection status, and lung function was also monitored by peak flow measurements in patients with wheezing and dyspnea. The conclusion was that seroreactivity to *C. pneumoniae* was indeed associated with both chronic asthma and acute asthmatic bronchitis. It is notable that 15 of 18 controlled epidemiological studies reviewed showed a significant association between *C. pneumoniae* infection and asthma. The disappearance of asthma symptoms after long-term antibiotic therapy was noted in several studies.

Childhood asthma has also been associated with *C. pneumoniae* infection. Both *C. pneumoniae* and *M. pneumoniae* have been detected in children with asthma, although RV and RSV were the most frequently detected pathogens. One UK study of 108 children aged 9–11 yr with asthma examined both *C. pneumoniae* and *M. pneumoniae* as potential compounding factors. The data suggested that chronic *C. pneumoniae* infection stimulates an immune response that interacts with the allergic inflammatory response and enhances asthma symptoms. This was not true for *M. pneumoniae (55)*.

MODULATION OF THE IMMUNE RESPONSE BY CpG CONTAINING OLIGONUCLEOTIDES AS TREATMENT OR PROPHYLAXIS FOR ASTHMA

The hygiene theory gave rise to the hypothesis that treatment with oligonucleotides containing unmethylated CpG motifs (as they occur in bacteria) could downregulate the Th2 response and potentially prevent or even reverse the asthmatic phenotype and restore immunological balance *(56)*. Oligodeoxynucleotides containing CpG motifs mimic the ability of microbial DNA to activate the immune system.

This novel therapeutic approach has recently been evaluated in mouse, primate, and feline models of asthma. In a primate model of allergic asthma oligodeoxynucleotides-containing CpG, motifs or sham were administered to house dust mite-allergic rhesus monkeys for a 33-wk period, during which time monkeys also received aerosolized house dust mite allergen (HDMA). Both airway hyperreactivity, airway remodeling, and airway eosinophilia (all hallmarks of asthma) were diminished in CpG-treated monkeys as compared with sham-treated monkeys *(57)*. Similar results were seen by several different groups using mouse asthma models.

ETS AND ASTHMA

The "second-hand" or ETS that contaminates the smoker's environment and is inhaled by the nonsmoker inhabiting the same space is now a well-recognized health threat. People with asthma have known, for more years than any documentation in the literature suggests, that their symptoms of asthma are readily initiated by inhabitation of smoky environments. Yet we have only recently begun to realize that aside from the irritant effect ETS has on hyperirritable airways, there is a more subtle role for ETS in initiation of allergic lung sensitization, particularly in children. Prenatal and postnatal ETS exposure exert independent effects on a variety of health parameters, including, but not limited to, development of asthma in the child *(58)*.

Data compiled from epidemiological studies performed in several countries provide evidence that supports a link between early exposure to ETS and the development of allergic asthma. For example, a study performed on 11,534 children from 24 communities between 1988 and 1990 showed that children who were exposed in the home to ETS had relative odds for wheezing of 1.42, compared with 1.0 for children never exposed to ETS ($p < 0.01$) *(59)*. The relative odds increased to 1.70 ($p < 0.01$) when there were three smokers in the home, as compared with none. The compounding effect of ETS and respiratory infection was demonstrated by the relative odds of wheezing with colds of 1.65 for children currently exposed to smoke as compared with 1.0 for those never exposed to smoke ($p < 0.001$).

Effects of maternal smoking during pregnancy often compound the effect of ETS inhalation on development of asthma in children. In one study performed by Ehrlich et al., maternal smoking and current exposure to second-hand smoke were independent contributing factors to asthma and wheezing in young children (60). Survey questionnaires, urinary cotinine levels, and parental interviews were used to determine the relative influence of household smoke on asthma/wheeze in schoolchildren ages 7–9 yr. Household smoking and maternal smoking were important risk factors in many studies. The odds ratio for development of asthma in children of mothers who smoked 0.5 packs per day was 2.1, compared with 1.0 for children of nonsmokers. The odds ratio for development of asthma during the first year of life of these children was 2.6. These data further support the hypothesis that ETS exposure enhances development of asthma in the infant and young child.

The importance of the interaction of genetics with the environmental insults inflicted on a child has been recently underscored by a study in which exposure to ETS and potential risk for asthma were evaluated for gene–environment interactions. In this study, Colilla et al. showed that three regions of the genome, which had only nominal evidence for linkage to asthma, showed a significant association with asthma only when ETS exposure was considered. They concluded that linkage of genes to asthma can depend on an environmental factor (61). This type of study is exactly what is needed to generate the information required for analysis of risk in this multifactored disease.

In an effort to demonstrate an irrefutable link between enhancement of allergic sensitization and inhalation of ETS and to determine the mechanism by which this might occur, animal models have again been employed. Using a mouse model system and an ETS generation and exposure system, the author's group has shown that ETS exposure not only enhances IgE production but also increases IL-4 production by pulmonary T-cells, thereby proving that ETS enhances a Th2-type response (62). In one experiment to understand how inhalation of ETS affects the response of previously sensitized mice to an inhaled allergen, Balb/c mice were sensitized by the intraperitoneal route with OA precipitated in aluminum hydroxide. For the next 17 d, mice were housed in chambers that containing ETS, produced by a generator system, or were housed in similar chambers containing filtered ambient air (controls). On day 17 after the priming OA injection, mice were exposed to aerosolized OA for 60 min. Smoke- or control-chamber exposures continued until day 43. T-lymphocytes from homogenized lung were stimulated in vitro and supernatants from cultures were analyzed for cytokine content. IL-4 production was significantly greater from cells in the lung of the OA-sensitized mice exposed to ETS than in those exposed to filtered ambient air. IFN-γ production was below the level of detection. Initial experiments performed with adult mice were repeated with neonatal mice, and the enhancement effect of the ETS was even greater if exposure to ETS commenced during first few days of life (63).

In another study by the same group, it was shown that both airway hyperreactivity and eosinophilia were enhanced in *Aspergillus fumigatus* allergen-sensitized mice when compared with mice breathing ambient air (64). Thus, animal models support environmental evidence that inhalation of ETS increases both sensitization to allergen and elicitation of airway hyperreactivity after respiratory challenge with allergen.

OUTDOOR AIR POLLUTION AND ASTHMA

The external environment is increasingly contaminated with substances that result from industrialization. The effects of air pollutants on development of allergic immune responses in the respiratory tract have recently been reviewed (65). Diesel fuel exhaust particles (DEP) induce IgE responses and allergic airway hyperresponsiveness in animal models. Ozone concentrations in areas of the country that have high ambient levels of photochemical smog are excessive. During times of particularly high ambient air ozone concentrations, emergency rooms report that they have increased numbers of asthma patients presenting with severe attacks of dyspnea. Levels of nitrogen dioxide have also been linked to severe asthma. A recent "case-crossover" study was performed to examine the acute effects of pollutant exposure on asthma attacks requiring emergency room (ER) visits. In this study, no association was shown between ER visits and levels of SO_2 or NO_2, but there was a statistically significant association between ER visits and ozone levels (66). Epidemiological observations have helped to prove associations between levels of pollutants and the increased incidence of asthmatic episodes among the population.

More recently, the effect of ozone exposure on airway responses to inhaled allergen was examined in subjects with asthma. Although the sample size was small (14 subjects), the protocol required subjects to inhale either 0.2 ppm ozone or filtered air (on alternate days) followed by exercise and HDMA challenge. This low level of ozone did not enhance inflammatory responses in the lung. However, the results suggested increased sensitivity to aeroallergens after ozone exposure (67).

Epidemiological studies have been substantiated by studies using animal models. These types of experiments allow researchers to delve into the mechanisms that are responsible for the pathogenic synergy involved in the multifactorial causation of asthma. For example, the data provided by Chen et al. cited above (67) are supportive of previously reported experimental studies using a mouse model in which ozone exposure enhanced allergic sensitization to aerosolized OA. In that study, the ozone concentration was 0.5 and 0.8 ppm (68,69).

A rhesus monkey model of allergic asthma has been used to evaluate the combined effects of episodic ozone exposure and allergen aerosolization on several parameters of asthma. Infant monkeys were exposed to 11 episodes of filtered air, HDMA, 0.5 ppm ozone, or HDMA and ozone. Each 5 d of exposure was followed by 9 d of filtered-air exposure. Monkeys that received allergen were exposed to the aerosolized HDMA for 2 h/d on days of exposure. This protocol resulted in increased levels of specific IgE in the ozone/HDMA group, increased plasma histamine, increased airway resistance, and increased eosinophils in the bronchoalveolar lavage. Lung pathology revealed increased volume of mucous cells in airway and bronchioles. In addition, the exposure of infant monkeys to HDMA and ozone caused an alteration in the normal development of the neural innervation of the epithelial compartment (70). These findings underscore the important role of air pollutants in enhancing the development of atopic asthma (71). Further work with this model showed that the remodeling of the tracheal basement membrane zone that occurred in infant monkeys exposed to both HDMA and ozone was not reversed during a recovery period that lacked ozone exposure but provided for occasional stimulation with allergen. The depletion of the perlecan from the basement membrane zone and the atypical collagen in this same region was resolved after the ozone exposure ended. These studies highlight that ozone and allergen together can have a lasting effect on asthmatic remodeling of the infant lung (72).

DIESEL EXHAUST PARTICLES AND RESPIRATORY ALLERGY

Exposure to DEP enhances allergic sensitization in humans and animal models (reviewed in ref. *73*). Studies on the effects of DEP on respiratory allergy in humans demonstrate that aerosolized DEPs increase local production of IgE in the upper respiratory tract, particularly in association with allergen. Studies using the mouse model have also demonstrated that DEPs produce an adjuvant effect on IgE production. Studies in humans and mice have shown that the cytokine profile elicited is that of the Th2 type, which promotes allergic responses. It seems clear that in both species, DEPs can enhance allergic sensitization. Most of the immune response effects are caused by the carbon core of the DEP. However, the polyaromatic polycarbons that constitute the major portion of the chemical part of the exhaust increase IgE production.

MECHANISMS OF ENHANCEMENT OF AIRWAY HYPERREACTIVITY

Constriction of bronchial smooth muscle with resultant wheezing and dyspnea can be stimulated by more than one mechanism. The variety of external triggers of asthma discussed (virus, ozone, ETS, DEP) undoubtedly share some, but not all, of these mechanisms (reviewed in ref. *74*). The increased sensitization with subsequent reactivity of IgE with mast cells and mediator liberation, influx of eosinophils, and synthesis of late-phase reactants, such as leukotrienes, is involved in mediation of the bronchoconstriction that occurs in allergic asthma. However, some environmental agents that cause exacerbation of asthma act via neurological pathways and modulation of the cytokine environment. The autonomic nervous system regulates smooth muscle tone and secretion of mucous glands, permeability, and blood flow in the bronchial circulation. The β-adrenergic receptors that are present on smooth muscle in bronchi are activated by catecholamines and are responsible for smooth muscle relaxation. A decrease in this β-adrenergic response can cause airway hyperreactivity. In contrast, the cholinergic nervous system controls constriction; stimulation of parasympathetic nerves causes constriction of airway smooth muscle. The cholinergic and adrenergic nervous systems act together to regulate homeostasis in the airways. A third nervous system is the "nonadrenergic noncholinergic" autonomic nervous system; it functions with neuropeptides as transmitters. Nerve fibers containing the neuropeptide vasoactive intestinal peptide, a substance that causes relaxation of smooth muscle, have been found in airway smooth muscle *(75)*. Because the airway epithelium is directly in contact with inhaled irritants, such as pollutants, and is the target of infection for some viruses (RSV), theories have been proposed suggesting that excitation of afferent receptors in the epithelium initiates reflexes that mediate constriction of bronchial smooth muscle. It is well established that there are intraepithelial nerves in human bronchi. Stimulation of sensory nerves in the respiratory tract can cause "neurogenic inflammation" as a result of the release of neuropeptides, such as substance P. The resultant increased capillary permeability, vasodilation, and smooth muscle contraction resembles the physiological effects of mediators, such as histamine. Activation of C-fibers causing neurogenic inflammation has been proposed as one mechanism for development of airway inflammation in asthma. It is possible that environmental pollutants and viral infection might act through this pathway to augment the inflammatory response in asthma *(75)*.

SUMMARY

There seems to be little doubt that oxidant air pollutants, DEP, ETS, and certain infections early in life can contribute to the development of allergic/atopic asthma. The mechanisms by which this occurs are gradually becoming evident. The development of the IgE response to inhaled allergen is enhanced by RSV infection, ETS, DEP, and ozone exposure. Cytokines are modulated by these asthma triggers. Viruses interact with bronchial epithelial cells to increase potent chemotactic chemokines that are important in asthma. Potentially, these alterations affect the antigen-presenting cells in the lung. Finally, innervation of the small airways is modified by exposure to these ozone and potentially other environmental influences early in life. Many of these observations were posed as questions in the previous edition of this book. Although there are still multiple questions to be resolved regarding the complex interactions between the atopic genotype and infectious and environmental insults, it is rewarding that the research performed during the past 5 yr has greatly increased our knowledge in this area.

REFERENCES

1. Kaiser HB. Risk factors in allergy/asthma. *Allergy Asthma Proc* 2004; 25: 7–10.
2. Howard TD, Wiesch DG, Koppelman GH, et al. Genetics of allergy and bronchial hyperresponsiveness. *Clin Exp Allergy* 1999; 29 Suppl: 86–89.
3. Borish L. Genetics of allergy and asthma. *Ann Allergy Asthma Immunol* 1999; 82: 413–424.
4. Lee SG, Kim BS, Kim JH, et al. Gene-gene interaction between interleukin-4 and interleukin-4 receptor alpha in Korean children with asthma. *Clin Exp Allergy* 2004; 34: 1202–1208.
5. Weidinger S, Klopp N, Wagenpfeil S, et al. Association of a STAT 6 haplotype with elevated serum IgE levels in a population based cohort of white adults. *J Med Genet* 2004; 41: 658–663.
6. Mossman TR, Coffman RL. Different patterns of cytokine secretion lead to different functional properties. *Ann Rev Immunol* 1989; 11: 245–268.
7. Elliott L, Yeatts K, Loomis D. Ecological associations between asthma prevalence and potential exposure to farming. *Eur Respir J* 2004; 24: 938–941.
8. Holt P, Sly P, Bjorksten B. Atopic versus infectious disease in childhood: a question of balance? *Pediatr Allergy Immunol* 1997; 8: 1–5.
9. Riedler J, Braun-Fahrlander C, Eder W, et al. Exposure to farming in early life and development of asthma and allergy: a cross-sectional survey. *Lancet* 2001; 358: 1129–1133.
10. Liu AH. Something old, something new: indoor endotoxin, allergens, and asthma. *Paediatr Resp Rev* 2004; 5(suppl A): S65–S71.
11. Hesselmar B, Aberg N, Aberg B, Eriksson B, Bjorksten B. Does early exposure to cat or dog protect against later allergy development? *Clin Exp Allergy* 1999; 29: 611–617.
12. Lewis SA, Britton JR. Measles infection, measles vaccination and the effect of birth order in the aetiology of hay fever. *Clin Exp Allergy* 1998; 28: 1493–1500.
13. Roost HP, Gassner M, Grize L, et al. Influence of MMR-vaccinations and diseases on atopic sensitization and allergic symptoms in Swiss schoolchildren. *Pediatr Allergy Immunol* 2004; 15: 401–407.
14. McKeever TM, Lewis SA, Smith C, Hubbard R. Vaccination and allergic disease: a birth cohort study. *Am J Public Health* 2004; 94: 985–989.
15. Da Cunha SS. No epidemiological evidence for infant vaccinations to cause allergic disease. *Vaccine* 2004; 22: 3375–3385.
16. Benke G, Abramson M, Raven J, Thein FC, Walters EH. Asthma and vaccination history in a young adult cohort. *Aust NZJ Public Health* 2004; 28: 336–338.
17. Dong W, Selgrade MK, Gilmour MI. Systemic administration of *Bordella pertussis* enhances pulmonary sensitization to house dust mite in juvenile rats. *Toxicol Sci* 2003; 72: 113–121.
18. Hirano T, Kawasaki N, Miyataka H, Satoh T. Wistar strain rats as the model for IgE antibody experiments. *Biol Pharm Bull* 2001; 24: 962,963.
19. Ryan M, McCarthy L, Rappuoli R, Mahon BP, Mills KH. Pertussis toxin potentiates Th1 and Th2 responses to co-injected antigen: adjuvant action is associated with enhanced regulatory cytokine production and expression of the co-stimulatory molecules B7-1, B7-2 and CD28. *Int Immunol* 1998; 10: 651–662.

20. Nilsson L, Kjellman NI, Bjorksten B. A randomized controlled trial of the effect of pertussis vaccines on atopic disease. *Arch Pediatr Adolesc Med* 1998; 152: 734–738.

21. Ennis DP, Cassidy, JP, Mahon BP. Whole-cell pertussis vaccine protects against Bordetella pertussis exacerbation of allergic asthma. *Immunol Lett* 2005; 97: 91–100.

22. Ceran O, Aka S, Oztemel D, Uyanik B, Ozkozaci T. The relationship of tonsillar hyperplasia and asthma in a group of asthmatic children. *Int J Pediatr Otorhinolaryngol* 2004; 68: 775–778.

23. Shirakawa T, Enomoto T, Shimazu S, Hopkin JM. The inverse association between tuberculin responses and atopic disorder. *Science* 1997; 275(5296): 77–79.

24. Townley RG, Barlan IB, Patino C, et al. The effect of BCG vaccine at birth on the development of atopy or allergic disease in young children. *Ann Allergy Asthma Immunol* 2004; 92: 350–355.

25. Alm JS, Lilja G, Pershagen G, Scheynius A. Early BCG vaccination and development of atopy. *Lancet* 1997; 350: 400–403.

26. Vargas MH, Bernal-Alcantara DA, Vaca MA, Franco-Marina F, Lascurain R. Effect of BCG vaccination in asthmatic schoolchildren. *Pediatr Allergy Immunol* 2004; 15: 415–420.

27. Herz U, Gerhold K, Gruber C, et al. BCG infection suppresses allergic sensitization and development of increased airway reactivity in an animal model. *J Allergy Clin Immunol* 1998; 102: 867–874.

28. Tukenmez F, Bahceciler NN, Barlan IB, Basaran MM. Effect of pre-immunization by killed *Mycobacterium bovis* and *vaccae* on immunoglobulin E response in ovalbumin-sensitized newborn mice. *Pediatr Allergy Immunol* 1999; 10: 107–111.

29. Wang CC, Rook GA. Inhibition of an established allergic response to ovalbumin in BALB/c mice by killed *Mycobacterium vaccae*. *Immunology* 1998; 93: 307–313.

30. Bjorksten B. The intrauterine and postnatal environments. *Curr Allergy Clin Immunol* 1999; 104: 1119–1127.

31. Bjorksten B, Naaber P, Sepp E, Mikelnar M. The intestinal microflora in allergic Estonian and Swedish 2year old children. *Clin Exp Allergy* 1999; 29: 342–346.

32. Shida K, Makino K, Morishita A, et al. Lactobacillus casei inhibits antigen-induced IgE secretion through regulation of cytokine production in murine splenocyte cultures. *Int Arch Allergy Immunol* 1998; 115: 278–287.

33. Hopp RJ. Recurrent wheezing in infants and young children: a perspective. *J Asthma* 1999; 36: 547–553.

34. Schildgen O, Geikowski T, Glatzel T, et al. New variant of the human metapneumovirus (HMPV) associated with an acute and severe exacerbation of asthma bronchiale. *J Clin Virol* 2004; 31: 283–288.

35. Tan WC. Viruses in asthma exacerbations. *Curr Opin Pulm Med* 2005; 11: 21–26.

36. Einarsson O, Geba GP, Zhu Z, Landry M, Elias JA. Interleukin-11: stimulation in vivo and in vitro by respiratory viruses and induction of airways hyperresponsiveness. *J Clin Invest* 1996; 97: 915–924.

37. Holtzman MJ, Shornick LP, Grayson MH, et al. "Hit-and-run" effects of paramyxoviruses as a basis for chronic respiratory disease. *Pediatr Infect Dis J* 2004; 23(11 Suppl): S235–S245.

38. Welliver RC, Wong DT, Sun M, Middleton E Jr, Vaughan RS, Ogra PL. The development of respiratory syncytial virus-specific IgE and the release of histamine in nasopharyngeal secretions after infection. *N Engl J Med* 1981; 305: 841–846.

39. Gershwin LJ, Gunther RA, Anderson ML, et al. Bovine respiratory syncytial virus-specific IgE is associated with interleukin-2 and -4, and interferon-gamma expression in pulmonary lymph of experimentally infected calves. *Am J Vet Res* 2000; 61: 291–298.

40. Dakhama A, Park JW, Taube C, et al. Alteration of airway sensory neuropeptide expression and development of airway hyperresponsiveness following respiratory syncytial virus infection. *Am J Physiol Lung Cell Mol Physiol* 2004; 288: L761–L770.

41. Stein RT, Sherrill D, Morgan WJ, et al. Respiratory syncytial virus in early life and risk of wheeze and allergy by age 13 years. *Lancet* 1999; 354: 541–545.

42. Noma T, Mori A, Yoshizawa I. Induction of allergen-specific IL-2 responsiveness of lymphocytes after respiratory syncytial virus infection and prediction of onset of recurrent wheezing and bronchial asthma. *J Allergy Clin Immunol* 1996; 98: 816–826.

43. Ogra PL. Respiratory syncytial virus: the virus, the disease and the immune response. *Paediatr Respir Rev* 2004; 5 Suppl A: S119–S126.

44. Miller AL, Bowlin TL, Lukacs NW. Respiratory syncytial virus-induced chemokine production: linking viral replication to chemokine production in vitro and in vivo. *J Infect Dis* 2004; 189: 1419–1430.

45. John AE, Gerard CJ, Schaller M, et al. Respiratory syncytial virus-induced exaggeration of allergic airway disease is dependent upon CCR1-associated immune responses. *Eur J Immunol* 2005; 35: 108–116.

46. Hegele RG. Role of viruses in the onset of asthma and allergy: lessons from animal models. *Clin Exp Allergy* 1999; 29 Suppl 2: 78–81.
47. Grunewald SM, Hahn C, Wohlleben G, et al. Infection with influenza a virus leads to flu antigen-induced cutaneous anaphylaxis in mice. *J Invest Dermatol* 2002; 118: 645–651.
48. Yamamoto N, Suzuki S, Suzuki Y, et al. Immune response induced by airway sensitization after influenza A virus infection depends on timing of antigen exposure in mice. *Virology* 2001; 75: 499–505.
49. Jacoby DB. Virus-induced asthma attacks. *J Aerosol Med* 2004; 17: 169–173.
50. McWilliam AS, Napoli S, Marsh AM, et al. Dendritic cells are recruited into the airway epithelium during the inflammatory response to a broad spectrum of stimuli. *J Exp Med* 1996; 184: 2429–2432.
51. Underner M, Millet C, Charriere V, et al. [Neuropeptides and respiratory diseases: prospects in the treatment of asthma.] *Rev Pneumol Clin* 1989; 45: 144–151.
52. Esposito S, Droghetti R, Bosis S, et al. Cytokine secretion in children with acute *Mycoplasma pneumoniae* infection and wheeze. *Pediatr Pulmonol* 2002; 34: 122–127.
53. Kazachkov MY, Hu PC, Carson JL, et al. Release of cytokines by human nasal epithelial cells and peripheral blood mononuclear cells infected with *Mycoplasma pneumoniae*. *Exp Biol Med* 2002; 227: 330–335.
54. Hahn DL, Dodge RW, Golubjatnikov R. Association of *Chlamydia pneumoniae* (strain TWAR) infection with wheezing, asthmatic bronchitis, and adult-onset asthma. *JAMA* 1991; 266: 225–230.
55. Freymuth F, Vabret A, Brouard J, et al. Detection of viral, *Chlamydia pneumoniae* and *Mycoplasma pneumoniae* infections in exacerbations of asthma in children. *J Clin Virol* 1999; 13: 131–139.
56. Hussain I, Kline JN. DNA, the immune system, and atopic disease. *J Invest Dermatol Symp Proc* 2004; 9: 23–28.
57. Fanucchi MV, Schelegle ES, Baker GL, et al. Immunostimulatory oligonucleotides attenuate airways remodeling in allergic monkeys. *Am J Respir Crit Care Med* 2004; 170: 1153–1157.
58. DiFranza JR, Aligne CA, Weitzman M. Prenatal and postnatal environmental tobacco smoke exposure and children's health. *Pediatrics* 2004; 113(4 Suppl): 1007–1015.
59. Cunningham J, O'Connor GT, Dockery DW, Speizer FE. Environmental tobacco smoke, wheezing, and asthma in children in 24 communities. *Am J Respir Crit Care Med* 1996; 153: 218–224.
60. Ehrlich RI, Du Toit D, Jordaan E, et al. Risk factors for childhood asthma and wheezing. Importance of maternal and household smoking. *Am J Respir Crit Care Med* 1996; 154(3): 681–688.
61. Colilla S, Nicolae D, Pluzhnikov A, et al. Evidence for gene-environment interactions in a linkage study of asthma and smoking exposure. *J Allergy Clin Immunol* 2003; 111: 840–846.
62. Seymour BW, Pinkerton KE, Friebertshauser KE, Coffman RL, Gershwin LJ. Second-hand smoke is an adjuvant for T helper-2 responses in a murine model of allergy. *J Immunol* 1997; 159: 6169–6175.
63. Seymour BW, Friebertshauser KE, Peake JL, et al. Gender differences in the allergic response of mice neonatally exposed to environmental tobacco smoke. *Dev Immunol* 2002; 9: 47–54.
64. Seymour BW, Schelegle ES, Pinkerton KE, et al. Second-hand smoke increases bronchial hyperreactivity and eosinophilia in a murine model of allergic aspergillosis. *Clin Dev Immunol* 2003; 10: 35–W42.
65. Gershwin LJ. Effects of air pollutants on development of allergic immune responses in the respiratory tract. *Clin Dev Immunol* 2003; 10: 119–126.
66. Boutin-Forzano S, Adel N, Gratecos L, et al. Visits to the emergency room for asthma attacks and short-term variations in air pollution. A case-crossover study. *Respiration* 2004; 71: 134–137.
67. Chen LL, Tager IB, Peden DB, et al. Effect of ozone exposure on airway responses to inhaled allergen in asthmatic subjects. *Chest* 2004; 125: 2328–2335.
68. Gershwin LJ, Osebold JW, Zee YC. Immunoglobulin E-containing cells in mouse lung following allergen inhalation and ozone exposure. *Int Arch Allergy Appl Immunol* 1981; 65: 266–277.
69. Osebold JW, Gershwin LJ, Zee YC. Studies on the enhancement of allergic lung sensitization by inhalation of ozone and sulfuric acid aerosol. *J Environ Pathol Toxicol* 1980; 3: 221–234.
70. Larson SD, Schelegle ES, Walby WF, et al. Postnatal remodeling of the neural components of the epithelial-mesenchymal trophic unit in the proximal airways of infant rhesus monkeys exposed to ozone and allergen. *Toxicol Appl Pharmacol* 2004; 194: 211–220.
71. Schelegle ES, Miller LA, Gershwin LJ, et al. Repeated episodes of ozone inhalation amplifies the effects of allergen sensitization and inhalation on airway immune and structural development in Rhesus monkeys. *Toxicol Appl Pharmacol* 2003; 191: 74–85.

72. Evans MJ, Fanucchi MV, Baker GL, et al. Atypical development of the tracheal basement membrane zone of infant rhesus monkeys exposed to ozone and allergen. *Am J Physiol Lung Cell Mol Physiol* 2003; 285: L931–L927.

73. Polosa R, Salvi S, Di Maria GU. Allergic susceptibility associated with diesel exhaust particle exposure: clear as mud. *Arch Environ Health* 2002; 57: 188–193.

74. Wardlaw AJ. The role of air pollution in asthma. *Clin Exp Allergy* 1993; 23: 81–96.

75. Nadel JA. Decreased neutral endopeptidases: possible role in inflammatory diseases of airways. *Lung* 1990; 168(Suppl): 123–127.

11 Exercise-Induced Asthma

Sports and Athletes

Rahmat Afrasiabi, MD

CONTENTS

KEY POINTS

- Exercise-induced asthma (EIA) occurs in 90% of individuals with asthma.
- The prevalence of EIA among athletes ranges between 3 and 11%.
- EIA is characterized by transient airway obstruction occurring after strenuous exertion.
- Pathophysiological mechanisms that could possibly explain the phenomenon of EIA include respiratory, heat or water loss (or both), hyperventilation leading to the release of bronchospastic chemical mediators, or rebound rewarming of the blood in the airway tissues.
- Coughing, wheezing, shortness of breath, chest tightness, fatigue, or stomach ache in children are common symptoms of EIA during or immediately in postexercise period. The symptoms usually peak 8–15 min after exercise and resolve spontaneously in approx 60 min.
- EIA may occur at any age and is equally common in adults and children.
- EIA could be the only symptom in patients with mild asthma and indicates inadequate control of asthma.
- The severity of EIA cannot be predicted from the resting level of the lung function.
- EIA is one of the most common precipitating factors of acute asthma attacks in children.
- The diagnosis of EIA is established by demonstration of a drop of 13–15% in forced expiratory volume in 1 s or a drop of 15–20% in peak expiratory flow rate after exercise.
- Prevention is the main goal in the management of EIA.
- Early detection of EIA in school-aged children through screening would facilitate early treatment and could enhance exercise-related activities and decrease school absences.

From: *Current Clinical Practice: Bronchial Asthma:*
A Guide for Practical Understanding and Treatment, 5th ed.
Edited by: M. E. Gershwin and T. E. Albertson © Humana Press Inc., Totowa, NJ

Table 1
Clinical Features of Exercised-Induced Asthma

1. A common phenomenon in patients with asthma with prevalence of up to 90%.
2. 12–15% of the general population suffers from exercised-induced asthma (EIA).
3. Coughing, wheezing, chest tightness, shortness of breath, fatigue, and stomachache in children are common symptoms.
4. The symptoms of EIA peak in 8–15 min after exercise cessation.
5. Symptoms of EIA resolve spontaneously in 60 min, and there is a refractory period of up to 3 h.
6. There is a late asthmatic phase to EIA that is seen in 30–89% of patients and is seen 3–8 h after EIA.

- Proper pharmacological management would allow athletes with EIA to participate and compete at any level of exercise.
- Aerobic fitness and adequate and good control of preexisting bronchial reactivity could help to diminish the effect and intensity of EIA.
- Inhaled β-agonists are medications of choice in the prevention of EIA.
- Inhaled sodium cromoglycate (Intal) or nedocromil (Tilade) may also be used in the treatment of EIA.

INTRODUCTION

Exercise as a common cause of bronchospasm in patients with asthma was first reported in 1962 by Jones and coworkers. Exercise-induced asthma (EIA) occurs in up to 90% of patients with asthma and in 40% of patients with allergic rhinitis (1–3). The prevalence of EIA varies depending on the populations studied. The general prevalence among athletes ranges between 3 and 11%. It is estimated that EIA affects from 12 to 15% of the general population (3), and 2.8–14% of the world-class athletes manifest EIA (4).

EIA may occur at any age and is equally common in adults and children. The common symptoms of EIA include coughing, wheezing, shortness of breath, chest tightness, fatigue, or stomach ache in children (3) (see Table 1).

EIA is defined as a transient increase in airway resistance usually occurring several minutes after strenuous exercise with a pace sufficient to raise an approximate heart rate of 170 beats per minute (bpm) (5,6). EIA symptoms reflecting bronchospasm usually peak 8–15 min after cessation of exercise and spontaneously resolve in approx 60 min, and a refractory period of up to 3 h has been observed. EIA could be the only manifestation of patients presenting with mild asthma and could indicate inadequate control of their asthma (8).

EIA is one of the most common precipitating factors of acute asthma attacks in children (10). The laboratory definition of EIA is a drop of 10% in forced expiratory volume in 1 s FEV_1 or same drop in peak expiratory flow rate (PEFR) after strenuous exercise capable of increasing heart rate to 170–180 bpm, with an increase of oxygen uptake of 65–85% (5,7). The most significant drop in spirometric parameters is seen between 2 and 10 min after exercise (10).

Early detection of EIA in school-aged children through screening could lead to earlier treatment, which could eventually enhance the exercise-related activities and decrease school absences (11).

Table 2
Pathophysiological Mechanisms Explaining the Phenomenon
of Exercise-Induced Bronchospasm

1. Airway cooling, dehydration, and hyperosmolality of airway epithelium.
2. Histamine and leukotrienes release from mast cells triggered by physical changes, including cooling, dehydration, and hyperosmolality.
3. Neutrophil chemotactic factor, such as LTB4, which could lead to appearance of CR1, the C3b receptor on neutrophils.
4. An increase in the number of CD25-positive T-cells or T-helper (Th) type-2 cells in peripheral blood.
5. An increase in the number of CD23-positive B-cells in peripheral blood, which could lead to more IgE synthesis.
6. An increase in the number of Th2 cells leads to the release of proallergy and proinflammatory mediators, including interleukin (IL)-3, IL-4, IL-5, and granulocyte macrophage colony-stimulating factor.

EIA could cause athletes to suffer needlessly; however, through appropriate instruction, conditioning, and treatment, these athletes could control their symptoms and possibly even win Olympic gold medals. EIA should not prohibit athletes from competing at the world level.

An International Olympic Committee-approved program comprising 67 athletes (11% of the US Olympic team) who had asthma or EIA provided coordinated medical care and appropriate use of medications and enabled 41 of the 67 athletes to win medals.

Prevention is the main goal in the management of EIA. A warm-up period of 15 min before exercise and avoiding exercising in cold air and outdoors in the peak of allergy season for patients with history of allergy could be helpful in ameliorating or eliminating EIA. Inhaled β_2-agonists are the medications of choice for preventing EIA.

- EIA is a common occurrence in patients with asthma.
- The presence of EIA should alert the practitioner that he or she may be dealing with a patient who has inadequate control of his or her asthma.
- With proper prophylaxis, mainly short-acting β_2-agonist, and with adequate control of asthma, EIA should not be a prohibitive factor to regular physical and athletic activity.

PATHOPHYSIOLOGY

There has been tremendous progress in understanding the underlying mechanism of EIA in the last three decades (see Table 2). The debate regarding the exact factor or factors leading to EIA continues. There is no simple answer to explain the pathophysiology of EIA. There are several physiological changes that occur with increasing minute ventilation of greatly increased volumes of inhaled air during exercise, which in turn, results in cooling of the air and dehydration of the respiratory mucosa. Dehydration leads to increase in osmolality of epithelial lining fluid, which could trigger the release of bronchoconstricting mediators in the airway tissues, which could ultimately manifest as an increase in airway resistance and a drop in FEV_1.

The role for histamine and bronchoconstrictor leukotrienes, including the cysteinyl leukotriene (LTS), C4, D4, and E4, in enhancement of airway resistance in EIA have been documented in several studies (13–16). In some, but not all, patients with EIA, increase in arterial or venous plasma histamine after exercise has been shown on a molar basis. Leukotriene (LT)C4 and LTD4 are 200 times more potent in affecting bronchoconstriction than histamine. Leukotrienes increase vascular permeability, which could lead to airway edema, as well as increase in mucous production. Further support to the role of leukotrienes in the pathophysiology of EIA comes from the effectiveness of leukotriene antagonist in amelioration of EIA. In an elaborate study using a 5-lipoxygenase inhibitor, Israel and his colleagues showed that zileuton significantly inhibited cold air-induced bronchoconstriction supportive of the effect and role of leukotrienes in the phenomenon of exercise induced bronchoconstriction *(17)*. These authors showed a 47% increase in the amount of cold dry air required to reduce FEV_1 by 10% in patients given zileuton compared with the group receiving placebo. Hyperpnea-induced bronchoconstriction in guinea pigs is an animal model of EIA. Using this animal model, recent studies have been conducted to study the role of other causatory factors, including neuropeptides in the pathogens of EIA.

It has been reported that hyperpnea-induced bronchoconstriction in guinea pigs is mediated through tachykinin release from airway sensory nerve *(18)*; depletion of tachykinin through pretreatment of guinea pigs with capsaicin attenuates the hyperpnea-induced bronchoconstriction *(18)*. Calcitonin gene-related peptide (CGRP) is a 37 amino acid peptide that is made by sensory C fibers throughout the respiratory tree *(19)*. Using a guinea pig model, CGRP attenuated the hypercapnia-induced bronchoconstriction *(19)*. Pretreatment with CGRP attenuates the LTD4-induced bronchoconstriction, suggesting that CGRP may modulate LTD4-mediated responses.

Dimarzo and coworkers have shown that CGRP inhibits the release of leukotrienes, including LTC4 and LTD4, from platelet-activating factor-stimulated rat lungs and ionophores-stimulated guinea pig lungs *(20)*. CGRP can also cause vasodilation, which could in turn, effect heat and water transfer through the bronchial mucosa.

In guinea pigs, Gerland and coworkers have shown that hyperpnea-induced bronchoconstriction was reduced by 50–90% by either LTD4 receptor antagonist or 5-lipoxygenase inhibitor *(21)*. There is cumulating evidence that there are also cellular changes in peripheral blood early in exercise-induced bronchospasm (EIB). These changes include appearance of CR 1, the C3b receptor on neutrophils, which could be the result of neutrophil chemotactic factors, such as LTB4 released through mast cell activation *(22,23)*. There is additional evidence documenting an increase in the number of CD25-positive T-cells (T-helper [Th] type-2 cells), as well as a similar increase in CD23-positive B-cells in the peripheral blood during EIB *(24)*. These changes have meaningful implication in supporting the concept of expansion of inflammatory components in airway in patients with EIB.

Hallstrand and colleagues' studies indicate that there is an increase in Th2 activity in peripheral blood of patients with atopic asthma, as well as an increase in number of CD23-positive B-cells *(24)*. The number of these T- and B-cells increases in EIB. In turn, these activated Th2 cells release a specific set of cytokines, including interleukin (IL)-3, IL-4, IL-5 and granulocyte macrophage colony-stimulating factor. IL-4 is an important cytokine in switching B-cells to active immunoglobulin (Ig)E-producing cells. Further production of specific IgE on exposure to specific allergens leads to mast cell activation and release of several chemical mediators of allergic inflammation, which contribute to clinical symptoms of asthma. IL-5 is also important in eosinophil activation and recruitment. The eosinophils are important cells that are actively involved in the expanding airway inflammation through the release of a variety of chemicals, including major basic protein, which can cause damage to the epithelial airway cells.

There is mounting evidence that manifestations of Th2 activity can be seen in peripheral blood in both children and adults with stable atopic asthma, and these changes are augmented in EIB *(24)*.

Th2 activity is translated into upregulation of B-cells producing IgE, which in turn, could lead to activation of mast cells. The release of chemical mediators by mast cells leads to bronchospasm manifested by wheezing, as seen in EIB.

- Airway cooling, dehydration, and hyperosmolality are major factors in initiating a series of reactions leading to bronchoconstriction.
- Leukotrienes play a pivotal role in mediating bronchoconstriction in EIA.
- Amelioration of EIA by leukotriene antagonists supports the contention that leukotrienes are major mediators of bronchoconstriction in EIA.
- Recent evidence suggests that Th2 cell activity and number is increased in the peripheral blood of patients with EIA.
- Th2 cells release a specific set of cytokines, including IL-2, IL-3, IL-4, IL-5, and granulocyte macrophage colony-stimulating factor, which lend to upregulation and enhanced synthesis of IgE and recruitment and enhanced survival of eosinophils, the key cells in allergic inflammation.

ATHLETES AND ASTHMA

EIA does not preclude athletes from extensive training programs. Anywhere from 2.8 to 14% of world-class athletes manifest EIA *(4)*.

US athletes with history of EIA or asthma won 41 medals at the 1984 Olympic Summer Games in Los Angeles *(1–3)*. Of 667 US athletes in the 1998 Olympic Summer Games in Seoul, South Korea, 52 had confirmed EIA. In those games, the same percentage of athletes who had and did not have EIA won medals; the athletes with a history of asthma have been able to even win medals in Olympic events requiring high ventilatory efforts, such as bicycling, swimming, and cross-country skiing. Through long-term training, these athletes develop certain adaptive mechanisms in their airways, enabling them to do well in sports demanding such high performance levels. Of 699 athletes who participated in the 1996 Summer Olympic Games in Atlanta and completed the US Olympic Committee Medical History Questionnaire, 107 (15.3%) had a previous diagnosis of asthma and 97 (13%) had a of history using asthma medications *(32)*.

Athletes with the highest prevalence of asthma were athletes participating in cycling and mountain biking. Frequency of active asthma varied from 45 of cyclists and mountain bikers to none of the divers and weight lifters.

The frequency of EIA varies with different sports (*see* Tables 3 and 4). The requirement for prophylactic medication depends on the type of exercise.

Exercising in a warm humid environment, such as swimming, is probably least likely to be associated with EIA and may not require prophylactic medications. Other exercises, including badminton, tennis, and football, in which there are short periods of exertions followed by short periods of rest, are also less likely to be associated with EIA and may not require prophylaxis. On the other hand, exercises (such as figure skating) that expose the athlete to cold air are more likely to be associated with EIA. The incidence of EIA in figure skaters is as high 30–35% *(33)*.

Table 3
Sports Most Commonly Associated
With Exercise-Induced Asthma

1. Running
2. Cycling
3. Figure skating
4. Mountain biking

Table 4
Sports That Are Less Commonly Associated
With Exercise-Induced Asthma

1. Swimming
2. Walking
3. Badminton
4. Tennis
5. Football
6. Volleyball

Several simple and practical measures can help reduce the frequency of EIA. Breathing slowly through the nose, which helps to humidify the air and reduce minute ventilations, could possibly help to control EIA.

Improving humidity through swimming in a heated pool and wearing a mask or scarf in cold weather can lower the frequency of EIA.

Exercising in spurts of less than 5 min, with each spurt less than 40 min apart, is less likely to be associated with EIA and may be necessary in some patients with asthma.

CLINICAL FEATURES AND DIFFERENTIAL DIAGNOSIS

Clinically, the classical symptoms of EIA occur within 10–15 min after exercise cessation. The typical symptoms include coughing, wheezing, chest tightness, shortness of breath, fatigue, and stomachache in children (*see* Table 5).

A dual response, which includes a late-phase asthmatic response, within 3–8 h after exercise has been reported in 30–89% of patients *(26–28)*.

There is ongoing debate regarding the mere existence and genuine nature of the late asthmatic response. A recent study by Sunil et al. *(28)* shows that late-phase asthmatic response in EIA is a true phenomenon. In this study, there was no obvious or physiological predictor of the late-phase response after an EIA attack. There is a refractory period of 30–90 min, during which there is little or no bronchoconstriction.

McFadden and Zawadski reported vocal cord dysfunction masquerading as EIA in a group of seven elite athletes *(29)*. These athletes with psychogenic vocal cord dysfunction present with acute dyspnea and wheezing during competitions (*see* Table 3).

The critical clinical features that could help differentiate vocal cord dysfunction from true EIA included lack of consistency in the development of symptoms when these athletes were exposed to identical stimuli, the onset of breathing difficulties occurred during exercise, and they had poor therapeutic response to a prophylactic anti-EIA treatment program *(29)*.

Table 5
Clinical Features of Disorders Simulating Exercise-Induced Asthma

1. Vocal cord dysfunction presents with symptoms such as choking, wheezing, stridor, cough, and dyspnea during exercise.
2. There is a strong psychological component with extreme vulnerability to internal and external pressure not to fail.
3. Vocal cord dysfunction is usually seen in elite athletes with success-oriented background in whom the fear of failure is strong.
4. Clinical features, including absence of nighttime symptoms, history of choking, and lack of response to usual exercised-induced asthma (EIA) treatments, are main differentiating features.
5. Exertional gastroesophageal reflux (GER) is seen up to 91% of patients with documented acid reflux disease and could present with symptoms simulating EIA.
6. Exertional GER is worse with sports like running and weight training, which require greater body movement.

Exercise-induced laryngeal prolapse (EILP) is an important differential diagnosis that mimics EIA and exercise-induced vocal cord dysfunction. Patients with EILP present with dyspnea and chest tightness during exercise. The symptoms of EILP result from mucosal edema prolapsing from aryepiglottic folds into the endolarynx. EILP should be suspected especially in patients with refractory EIA on maximal asthma therapy, including inhaled bronchodilators, inhaled corticosteroid, and leukotriene antagonists. Spirometry after exercise shows a typical pattern of extrathoracic obstruction. This condition can be diagnosed by fiberoptic laryngoscopy during maximal exertion coinciding with the onset of severe respiratory distress. Bjornsdottir and colleagues described six elite athletes referred to their center for evaluation of refractory EIA, despite maximal asthma therapy. The researchers documented EILP on fiberoptic laryngoscopy during maximal exertion, coinciding with symptoms of extreme dyspnea and audible stridor. The prolapsed edematous tissue partially obscured vision of vocal cords and resulted in glottic obstruction; four of these athletes underwent surgical correction using laser laryngoplasty and could compete again at gold-medal levels in their respective sports (43). Exercise-induced stridor owing to abnormal movement of the arytenoid area was recently reported in four patients who developed severe symptomatic stridor during maximal cardiopulmonary exercise testing. The baseline nasal fiberoptic laryngoscopy showed normal findings. Nasal fiberoptic laryngoscopy after maximal exercise testing showed normal vocal cord motion during exercise, but developed abnormal anterior motion of the arytenoid and aryepiglottic folds only at peak exercise leading to partial airway obstruction and severe stridor (44).

It has been questioned whether the gastroesophageal reflux (GER) is a factor in EIA, especially in the light of recent reports of exertional gastroesophageal acid reflux. Wright and Sagatelian studied 10 athletes with EIA for occurrence of GER during exercise. Continuous monitoring of intraesophageal pH and motility were conducted. Although 60% showed some degree of GER, only three individuals demonstrated a pathological degree of GER. In the two individuals who were tested postprandially, the change in FEV_1 was not different in one and improved in the other, despite worsening of GER in both. The authors of this study concluded that there was no correlation between GER and EIA (30).

Table 6
Diagnosis of Exercise-Induced Asthma: Summary of Diagnostic Features and Methods Used to Diagnose Exercise-Induced Asthma

1. Exercised-induced asthma (EIA) is defined as a 10% drop in forced expiratory volume in 1 s (FEV_1) from pre-exercise level.
2. The gold standard test to diagnose EIA is treadmill test.
3. A standard treadmill test is 3–8 min of exercise capable of maintaining a heart rate at 80% of maximal predicted value.
4. Peak expiratory flow rate (PEFR) or FEV_1 is measured every 5 min during the first 15–30 min after exercise cessation.
5. In a standard treadmill test, a drop in FEV_1 of more than 15% of baseline is considered diagnostic.
6. Free running for 1 mile in an outdoor environment with measuring of PEFR before running and 5, 15, and 30 min after cessation is an alternative test to standard treadmill.
7. A free running test is more practical and can be used in large scale screening for EIA.

It is clinically relevant and important not only to diagnose and prevent EIB but also to be able to predict the severity of EIB. In doing so, clinical strategies to prevent and treat EIB in asthmatic patients will be created. Otoni and colleagues studied 23 patients with asthma to determine the predictors of EIB. The methacholine provocation test, eosinophils in induced sputum, and vascular permeability index, which is defined as the ratio of albumin in induced sputum and serum, were the parameters used to predict the severity of EIB in this patient population. By using stepwise multiple regression analysis, the researchers showed a significant correlation between these parameters and EIB after exercise testing on all 23 patients. There was no significant correlation between baseline FEV_1 and the severity of EIB *(45)*.

The most classical and common clinical presentation of EIA occurs in the postexercise period usually in the first 10–15 min after exercise cessation.

A late asthmatic response, which occurs within 3–8 h after exercise, is a true and genuine phenomenon in EIA.

DIAGNOSIS

EIA is defined in laboratory as exercise that reduces the PEFR or the FEV_1 by at least 10% when compared with preexercise levels *(5)*. A typical test to diagnose EIA is a standard treadmill test, which consists of 3–8 min of exercising at a level to maintain heart rate at 80% of maximal predicted value. The PEFR or FEV_1 is measured every 5 min during the first 15–30 min after exercise cessation *(7)*. A significant drop more than 15% of baseline is considered diagnostic of EIA *(see* Table 6).

Free running for 1 mile in an outdoor environment with monitoring of PEFR before running and then 5, 15, and 30 min thereafter has been considered another alternative to standard treadmill test, which may not be practical in a large population study *(10)*. EIB is defined as a decrease of 15% of PEFR at any point after exercise. Using this method, Kukafka and colleagues found a substantial number of unrecognized EIB among varsity athletes. These authors, by looking at stepwise regression analysis of their data, noted that history of wheezing and residence in a poverty-stricken area were most closely associated with EIB. Therefore, they suggested that active screening for EIB, especially for students residing in poverty-stricken areas, may be indicated to identify individuals who are at risk for EIB and asthma *(31)*.

Eucapnic voluntary hyperventilation (EVH) is able to identify airway hyperrespon-siveness (AHR) in elite cold-weather athletes. In a recent study by Rundell and col-leagues, EVH was compared with exercise in the field. EVH setting protocol in laboratory was defined that athletes inhaled dry air at 19°C, containing 5% carbon dioxide for 6 min at a target ventilation equivalent to 30 times baseline FEV_1. The exercise included cross-country skiing, ice skating, or running for 6–8 min. AHR consistent with EIB was defined as a fall in FEV_1 by 10% or more. A total of 19 out of 38 athletes had AHR; 58% were identified by exercise and 89% were identified by EVH. The authors concluded that EVH in laboratory for 6 min had a greater chance of identifying AHR in these athletes compared with 6–8 min of field exercise in cold weather *(46)*.

TREATMENT

The short-acting β_2-agonist albuterol is most commonly used as prophylaxis and is effective prophylaxis for EIA.

Cromolyn sodium and nedocromil are equally effective in controlling EIA.

In addition to conditioning and modified training techniques, there are several medica-tions that have been used to prevent or treat EIA (*see* Table 7). These include short- and long-acting β_2-adrenergics, cromolyn sodium, nedocromil, leukotriene antagonists, inhaled furosemide, inhaled indomethacin, theophylline, glucocorticoids, antihistamines, and anticholinergics. The β_2-adrenergic agents provide protection from EIA in 80–95% and have few side effects.

The inhalant form of the β_2-adrenergic agent commonly used is albuterol, which has a rapid onset of action and induces bronchodilation for 4–6 h. The usual dosage is two puffs 15 min before exercise initiation. Another common and widely prescribed medicine that is used as prophylaxis is cromolyn sodium, which is effective in preventing EIA in 70–87% of patients and has minimal side effects. Cromolyn should be given 10–20 min before exer-cise to prevent the onset of EIA. The long-acting β_2-adrenergic agent salmeterol has been used as a single dose in prevention of EIA. In a placebo-controlled crossover study by Green and Price using 50 µg dose of salmeterol aerosol in children prevented EIA at 1, 5, and 9 h after dosing. The mean maximum fall in FEV_1 in salmeterol-treated children was 3.4% after 9 h of exercise challenge compared with 26.6% fall in FEV_1 with placebo *(34)*.

Occasionally it appears more practical for children with EIA to receive salmeterol before leaving for school in view of the difficulty they may face in the school setting using prn medication or some other barrier, including some children forgetting to take asthma medication before exercise.

Cromolyn sodium at a 10-mg dose and 4 mg nedocromil in the form of metered-dose inhalers are equally effective in controlling EIA in children, and their protective effect lasts less than 2 h in most patients *(38)*. The EIA inhibitory effect of cromolyn sodium in a nebulized form increases with escalating concentration of the drug from 2 to 40 mg *(36)*. A similar dose–response effect was shown with a pressurized aerosol at doses from 2 to 20 mg *(37)*. On the other hand, the inhibitory effect of nedocromil on EIA has not been shown to be dose dependent when the dose range of 0.5–20 mg through metered-dose inhalers was used. The practical message from these studies is that the 2-mg dose of cromolyn, which is used in some countries, is suboptimal and should be changed to at least 10 mg.

Part of our understanding of the role of leukotrienes in the pathogenesis of EIA has come from studies showing the effectiveness of leukotriene antagonist in attenuating EIA.

Table 7
Prophylactic Pharmacological Management of Exercise-Induced Asthma

Type and class of medication	Mechanism of action	Dosing and administration (min before exercise)	Duration of action (h)
β₂-Adrenergic:	Relaxation of smooth muscles of airway		
Albuterol MDI		2 puffs, 15	4–6
Metaproterenol			
Sulfate MDI		2 puffs, 10	2–4
Terbutaline sulfate MDI		2 puffs, 15	3–6
Salmetrol discus		50 μg, 30–60	12
Cromolyn sodium MDI	Stabilizing mast cell membrane inhibiting histamine release	2 puffs, 10–20	4–6
Nedocromil MDI	Similar to cromolyn-	2 puffs, 10–20	4–6
Theophyline, oral	blocking phosphodiesterase enzyme and, hence, increasing intracellular cAMP, leading to smooth muscle relation and anti-inflammatory property	Serum levels at 6 mg/L, 30–60	4–12 24
Anticholinergics Ipratrapium bromide MDI	Blocking cholinergic pathway	2 puffs, 60	Unknown
Leukotriene receptor Antagonists, oral	Blocking the effect of leukotrienes, leading to smooth muscle relaxation of airways, decreased mucus production, and decreased airway inflammation	5–10 mg For montelukast	Up to 20–24 h After dose

MDI, metered-dose inhaler.

When zafirlukast, which is a selective LTD4-recepter antagonist at a single dose ranging from 5 to 40 mg, was used as prophylaxis against EIA in a group of children, the maximum mean fall of FEV_1 after exercise was 8.7–11%, compared with 16.3–17.1% after placebo, confirming the effectiveness of this agent in reducing bronchoconstriction in EIA *(39)*. The result of this latter study *(39)* show that the drug was effective for most patients at the time of challenge, which was 4 h after administration. The long duration of this medication offers a practical advantage over other prophylactic medications, the majority of which are shorter lived.

Leff and colleagues evaluated another recently approved leukotriene receptor antagonist, montelukast, in a 12-wk placebo-controlled study using 10 mg of montelukast once daily. The montelukast therapy offered significantly greater protection against EIB than placebo therapy. There was no evidence of tolerance to medication in this 3-mo study; neither was there evidence of residual rebound 2 wk after treatment cessation *(40)*.

Another study evaluated the effectiveness of 400 µg daily beclomethasone for a 3-mo period compared with placebo in a group of children ranging in age from 7 to 9 yr, with EIB. The result of this study showed significant improvement of asthma control at 1 and 2 mo (41).

One of the clinical problems in the treatment and prevention of EIA is the development of tolerance. Tolerance develops after 1 wk of treatment with a short-acting inhaled β-agonist, albuterol, and similar tolerance develops 4 wk after salmeterol treatment. There was no tolerance observed in a 3-mo study with the leukotriene-receptor antagonist montelukast (40).

The oral theophylline given at least 1–2 h before exercise has a variable and dose-related bronchoprotective effect, a blood level of 15–20 ng/mL is required for maximum inhibition (44). However, for patients who are not accustomed to theophylline, these concentrations cause side effects, such as gastrointestinal complaints, headaches, and tachycardia. Therefore, the routine use of theophylline for prevention and treatment of EIA is not recommended unless the patient requires asthma medications continuously.

A recent study has reported that inhaled furosemide significantly inhibits bronchoconstriction caused by exercise (42). The exact mechanism through which furosemide works is not known. However, it appears that it resembles cromolyn sodium by acting on post-ganglionic cholinergic fibers in addition to its mast cell membranes' stabilizing properties (42). Furosemide at the dose of 20 mg/m^2 body area prevents EIA without increasing diuresis with efficacy comparable to cromolyn sodium (42). Another potential mechanism through which furosemide works is an increase in production of prostaglandin E2 in kidneys with similar effects in airways. Prostaglandin E2 has a significant bronchoprotective effective in patients with asthma and could attenuate EIA (42).

Tolerance is a common problem with the use of β$_2$-agonists.

Leukotriene antagonists are new effective treatment for EIA; they have the advantage of longer duration and less tendency to cause tolerance.

REFERENCES

1. Kawabori I, Pierson WE, ConQuest LL, et al. Incidence of exercise induced asthma in children. *J Allergy Clin Immunol* 1976; 58: 447–455.
2. McCarthy P. Wheezing and breezing through exercise-induced asthma. *Physician Sports Med* 1989; 17: 125–130.
3. Afrasiabi R, Specter SL. Exercise induced asthma. It need not sideline your patients. *Physician Sports Med* 1991; 19: 49–60.
4. Godfrey S. Symposium on special problems and management of allergic athletes: Part 2. *J Allergy Clin Immunol* 1984; 73: 630–633.
5. Anderson SD. Issues in exercise-induced asthma. *J Allergy Clin Immunol* 1985; 76: 763–772.
6. Exercise and asthma: a round up table. *Physician Sports Med* 1984; 12: 58–77.
7. Godfrey S, Silverman M, Anderson S. The use of treadmill for assessing EIA and the effect of varying the severity and duration of exercise. *Pediatrics* 1975; 56: 893–899.
8. Spector SL. Update on exercise induced asthma. *Ann Allergy* 1993; 71: 571–577.
9. Tar RA, Spector SL. Exercise-induced asthma. *Sports Med* 1998; 25: 1–6.
10. Garcia de la Rubia S, Pajaron-Fernandez MJ, Sanchez-Solis M, Martinez-Gonzalez MI, Perez-Plores D, Pajaron-Ahumada M. Exercise-induced asthma in children: a comparative study of free and treadmill running. *Ann Allergy Asthma Immunol* 1998; 80: 232–236.
11. The free running asthma screening test: an approach to screening for exercise-induced asthma in rural. *AL J School Health* 1997; 67: 83–88.
12. Anderson SD. Exercise-induced asthma: The state of the art. *Chest* 1985; 87(suppl 5): 1915–1925.

13. Barnes PJ, Brown NJ. Venous plasma histamine in exercise and hyperventilation-induced asthma in man. *Clin Sci* 1981; 36: 259–267.

14. MacGlashan DW, Schleimer RP, Peters SP, et al. Generation of leukotrienes by Purifield Human lung mast cells. *Jelin Invest* 1982; 70: 747–751.

15. Shaw RJ, Walsh GM, Cromwell O, Moqbel R, Spry CJF, Kay AB. Activated eosinophils generate SRS-A leukotrienes following IgG-dependent stimulation. *Nature* 1985; 316:150–152.

16. Dahlen SE, Hedqvist P, Hammarstrom S, Samuelsson B. Leukotrienes are potent constrictors of human bronchi. *Nature* 1980; 288: 484–486.

17. Israel E, Dermarkarian R, Rosenberg M, et al. The effects of a 5-Lipoxygenase inhibitor on asthma induced by cold, dry air. *N Engl J Med* 1990; 323: 1740–1744.

18. Ray DW, Hernandez C, Leff AR, Drazen JM, Solway J. Tachykinins mediate bronchoconstriction elicited by isocapnic hyperpnea in guinea pigs. *J Appl Physical* 1989; 63: 1108–1112.

19. Nagase T, Ohga E, Katayama H, et al. Roles of calcitonin gene-related peptide (CGRP) in hyperpnea-induced constriction in guinea pigs. *Am J Respir Crit Car Med* 1996; 154: 1551–1556.

20. DiMarzo VJR, Tippins, Morris HR. The effect of vasoactive intestinal peptide and calcitonin gene-related peptide on peptide leukotriene release from platelet activating factor stimulated rat lung and ionophore stimulated guinea pig lungs. *Biochem Int* 1986; 13: 933–942.

21. Gerland A, Jordan JE, Ray DW, et al. Role of eicosanoids in hyperpnea-induced airway responses in guinea pigs. *J Appl Physiol* 1993; 75: 2792–2804.

22. Arm JP, Walport MJ, Lee TH. Expression of complement receptor type I (CR 1) and type 3 (CR 3) on circulating granulocytes in experimentally provoked asthma. *J Allery Clin Immunol* 1989; 83: 649–655.

23. Venge P, Henriksen J, Dahl R, Hakanson L. Exercise-induced asthma and the generation of neutrophil chemotactic activity. *J Allerg Clin Immunol* 1990; 85: 498–504.

24. Teal S, Hallstrand MD, et al. Peripheral blood manifestations of TH2 lymphocyte activation in stable atopic asthma and during exercise induced bronchospasm. *Ann Allergy Asthma Immunol* 1998; 80: 424–432.

25. Lee TH, Nagakura T, Papageorgiou N, et al. Exercise-induced late asthmatic reaction with neutrophil chemotactic activity. *N Engl J Med* 1983; 308: 1502–1505.

26. Horn CR, Jones RM, Lee D, Brennan SR. Late response in exercise-induced asthma. *Clin Allergy* 1984; 14: 307–309.

27. Bierman CW, Spiro SG, Petheram I. Characteristics of late response in exercise-induced asthma. *J Allergy Clin Immunol* 1984; 74: 701–706.

28. Sunil K, Chhabra MD, Umesh Cojha DTCD. Late asthmatic response in exercise induced asthma. *Ann Allergy Asthma Immunol* 1998; 80: 323–327.

29. McFadden ER Jr, Zawadski DK. Vocal cord dysfunction masquerading as exercise-induced asthma. *Am J Respir Crit Care Med* 1996; 153: 942–947.

30. Wright RA, Sagatelian MA, Simons ME, McClan SA, Roy TM. Exercise-induced asthma: is gastroesophageal reflux a factor? *Digest Dis Sci* 1996; 41: 921–925.

31. Kukafka DS, Lang DM, Porter S, et al. Exercise-induced bronchospasm in high school athletes via a free running test. *Incidence Epidemiol Chest* 1998; 114: 1613–1622.

32. Weiler JM, Llayton T, Hunt M. Asthma in United States Olympic Athletes who participated in the 1996 Summer Games. *J Allergy Clin Immunol* 1998; 102: 722–726.

33. Mannix ET, Manfredi F, Farber MO. A comparison of two challenge tests for identifying exercise-induced bronchospasm in figure skaters. *Chest* 1999; 115: 651–653.

34. Green CP, Price JF. Prevention of exercise-induced asthma by inhaled Salmeterol xinafoate. *Arch Dis Child* 1992; 67: 1014–1017.

35. Fernando M, Benedicts DE, Tuteri G, et al. Cromolyn versus nedocromil: duration of action in exercise-induced asthma in children. *J Allergy Clin Immunol* 1995; 96: 510–514.

36. Patel KR, Berkin KE, Kerr JW. Dose response study of sodium cromoglycate in exercise induced asthma. *Thorax* 1982; 37: 663–666.

37. Tullett WM, Tan KM, Wall RT, Patel KR. Dose response effect of sodium cromoglycate pressurized aerosol in exercise-induced asthma. *Thorax* 1985; 40: 41–44.

38. DeBenedcits FM, Tuteri G, Bertotto A, Bruni L, Vaccaro R. Comparison of the protective effect of sodium cromoglycate and nedocromil sodium in exercise induced asthma in children. *J Allergy Clin Immunol* 1994; 94: 684–688.

39. Pearlman DS, Ostrom NK, Bronsky EA, Bonuccelli CM, Hanby LA. The leukotriene D4-receptor antagonist Zafirlukast attenuates exercise-induced bronchoconstriction in children. *J Pediatr* 1999; 134:273–279.

40. Leff JA, Busse WW, Pearlman D, et al. Montelukast, a leukotriene receptor antagonist, for the treatment of mild asthma and exercise-induced bronchoconstriction. *N Engl J Med* 1998; 339: 147–152.
41. Freezer NJ, Crousdell H, Dovll IJM, Holgate ST. Effect of regular inhaled beclomethasone on exercise and methacholine airway responses in school children with recurrent wheeze. *Eur Res PJ* 1995; 8: 1488–1493.
42. Bianco S, Vaghi A, Robuschi M, Pasargiklian M. Prevention of exercise-induced bronchoconstriction by inhaled Furosemide. *Lancet* 1988; 2: 252–255.
43. Bjornsdottir US. Exercise induced laryngeal prolapse in elite athletes—"curable asthma." *J Allergy Clin Immunol* 2004; 113: PS271.
44. Fahey JT, Bryant NJ, Karas D, et al. Exercise-induced stridor due to abnormal movement of arytenoid area: videoendoscopic diagnosis and characterization of the "at risk" group. *Pediatric Pulmonol* 2005; 39: ST-55.
45. Otani K, Kanazalva H, Fujiwara H, et al. Airway vascular hyperpermeability, eosinophlic inflammation and bronchial hyperreactivity are independent factors predicting the severity of EIB. *J Asthma* 2004; 41: 271–278.
46. Rundell KW, Andersen SD, Piering BA, Judelson DA. Field exercise vs. laboratory voluntary hyperventilation to identify airway hyperresponsiveness in elite cold weather athletes. *Chest* 2004; 125: 909–915.

12

How Can Foods, Additives, and Drugs Affect the Patient With Asthma?

Suzanne S. Teuber, MD

KEY POINTS

Foods

- Food-induced asthma is uncommon but especially worth considering in patients with atopic dermatitis and moderate to severe asthma.
- The key to diagnosing food-induced asthma is not the history but a double-blind, placebo-controlled challenge with spirometry pre- and postchallenge.
- An important condition in the differential diagnosis of isolated food-induced asthma is systemic food allergy with asthma as one part of the symptom complex. Epinephrine by self-injection is the preferred treatment in this case.

Additives

- Sulfites have been proven to cause bronchospasm or anaphylactic responses in some individuals with asthma. Asking patients about the presence of wheezing after ingestion of white wine is a relevant screening question.
- Aside from sulfites, no other food additive has been clearly associated with asthma in well-controlled studies, contrary to public perception.
- The key to diagnosing food additive-induced asthma is a double-blind, placebo-controlled challenge.

Nonsteroidal Anti-Inflammatory Drugs

- Aspirin and the other nonsteroidal anti-inflammatory drugs can cause worsening of asthma in approx 10–15% of patients with asthma, but many will not be aware of it.
- Desensitization can be helpful in reducing asthma and rhinitis symptoms.

From: *Current Clinical Practice: Bronchial Asthma:*
A Guide for Practical Understanding and Treatment, 5th ed.
Edited by: M. E. Gershwin and T. E. Albertson © Humana Press Inc., Totowa, NJ

INTRODUCTION

The individual roles of foods, additives, and medications, specifically aspirin and nonsteroidal anti-inflammatory drugs (NSAIDs), in asthma have been the focus of ongoing clinical research—and controversy in the case of food additives. There is still much to be defined, but this is certainly an area in which asthma caregivers can give patients practical information, particularly to counteract some common misperceptions. The influence of diet on asthma has long attracted attention. It must be remembered, however, that a significant proportion of a person's life is spent in the procurement, preparation, and enjoyment of food. It is to be expected, then, that many people have strong beliefs about how certain foods affect their sense of well-being, both physically and emotionally. Certain foods in different cultures are believed to be "good" for asthma and others as possibly causative. It is clear, however, that patients with asthma who have immunoglobulin (Ig)E-mediated food allergy (e.g., to shrimp, peanut, and hen's egg) are both at higher risk for life-threatening asthma in general in childhood, and at higher risk for more severe systemic reactions and death resulting from the food allergy than those with the food allergy but without underlying asthma (1,2). In addition, recent double-blind, placebo-controlled food challenge (DBPCFC) studies have established food-induced asthma as a rare but distinct clinical entity apart from a systemic allergic reaction to a food. Blinded challenges have also been critical in the study of additive reactions. NSAID hypersensitivity, especially in the setting of nasal polyposis and chronic rhinosinusitis, has been a particular challenge to some patients with asthma. In this chapter, each of the three topics is reviewed separately.

FOODS AND ASTHMA

Beneficial Effects of Food

Although there have been many hypotheses about the effect of diet on asthma, randomized controlled trials are generally difficult with whole foods; thus, the approaches have been to use supplemental extracts of foods or surveys of dietary habits. Supplements and vitamins are covered in more detail in Chapter 8. Supplementation with dietary fish oil, because of potential anti-inflammatory effects, has been studied most comprehensively in both adults and children with asthma and has been the subject of two Cochrane Database Systemic Reviews, most recently in 2002 (3). The reviewers found no consistent beneficial effect, but they point out that no adverse events were noted. The effects of preventive dietary supplementation have been further pursued in children who are at risk for asthma. The 3-yr outcomes of the Childhood Asthma Prevention Study in Australia are available. This randomized, controlled study enrolled 616 high-risk children antenatally and assigned them to dust mite reduction measures, n-3 fatty acid supplements, or placebo. There was no effect on wheezing at 3 yr by either active intervention, but there was a significant decrease in cough in children who were atopic on the active dietary supplement ($p = 0.003$, number needed to treat = 10) (4). The same group also studied a larger birth cohort to identify children with asthma and controls to use in a case-control study. A diet survey at age 8 was used to calculate the current n-6 to n-3 fatty acid ratio of the diet. A difference was found between the patients with asthma and controls ($p = 0.02$), suggesting that diets higher in n-3 fatty acids may be beneficial regarding a current diagnosis of asthma (5). It must be remembered, however, that after a diagnosis of asthma is made in a young child, families may be advised to delay introduction of fish and seafood because of concerns about the development of food allergy in a child who is atopic, which could bias surveys of this type. Interestingly, a group of 1601 young adults was extensively studied for associations of food with atopy or asthma. No association or protective effect was found with oily fish ingestion or the ratio of n-6 to n-3 fatty acids in the diet. Instead, whole milk, apples, and pears were protective against current asthma by logistic regression analysis, whereas soy beverages were associated with current asthma. By plasma fatty acid analysis, no protective effect was seen with the level of n-3 fatty acids, or n-6:n-3 fatty acid ratio, but dihomo γ-linolenic acid was positively associated with a current diagnosis of asthma (odds ratio [OR] = 1.34, 95% confidence interval [CI]: 1.13–1.60) (6,7). Obviously, further work is warranted in the area of primary prevention and dietary factors, as well as modification of established disease by diet or supplements.

Adverse Effects of Food

FOOD INTOLERANCE AND FOOD ALLERGY

Subtle psychological associations could be the source of some adverse reactions to foods. In fact, surveys from the 1980s and 1990s revealed that up to 25% of households in the US general population report at least one family member with a perceived food allergy (8,9). Chocolate and cow's milk were most frequently reported (9). In reality, cow's milk allergy (both IgE-mediated and non-IgE-mediated) affects approx 2.5% of infants, with 80% tolerant by age 5 (10), and proven clinical IgE-mediated allergy to processed chocolate (rather than peanut, tree nut, or cow's milk contaminants or occupational allergy to cacao bean dust) is actually not described in modern literature.

Food intolerance resulting from psychological or metabolic factors is far more common than an allergic, or immune-mediated, response to the food in question. Subjective symptoms are particularly prone to psychological factors. DBPCFCs in 24 patients with subjective symptoms (fatigue, bloating, migraines, nausea, itching, etc.) revealed only one patient with a positive food-induced reaction (soy-induced migraine) (11). There are some challenges in understanding the terms used to describe reactions to foods. The European Academy of Allergy and Clinical Immunology convened a committee to propose universal definitions, published in 1995, and updated in 2001; however, not all the changes have been adopted (12,13). In the United States, the umbrella term "adverse food reaction" describes any reaction to a food (14). Reproducible adverse food reactions can stem from "food intolerances," or to reactions mediated by the immune system called "food allergy" (14). Food intolerances may be caused by metabolic factors, such as lactase deficiency, that are specific to the individual. On the other hand, some adverse food reactions may result from toxic or pharmacological effects of foods that could affect anyone when given a large enough dose, for instance, solanine poisoning from the alkaloids in green potato skins, reactions to high levels of histamine in scombroid fish poisoning, or nervousness from too much caffeine or related compounds. Food intolerances owing to psychological factors are not reproducible when the food is given in a blinded challenge.

Table 1 shows the estimated prevalence of various food allergies (10,15–20). Random-digit dial telephone surveys were used to obtain the estimates that approx 1% of the adult population self-reported allergy to peanuts or tree nuts and 2% to fish or crustaceans (18,19).

Approximately 6% of children are believed to have definite food hypersensitivity (IgE-mediated or other immune mechanism) and perhaps up to 4% of adults. This is not

Table 1
Estimated Prevalence of Food Allergies

Food	Young children, %	Adults, %
Cow's milk	1.9–3.2	0.3
Peanut	0.8	0.6
Tree nut	0.2	0.5
Fish	0.1	0.4
Shellfish	0.1	2.0
Egg	1.6	0.2
Fruits/vegetables	Uncertain	Uncertain

including patients with pollen-induced allergic rhinitis who may have itching in the mouth and throat brought on by cross-reacting proteins present in pollen and fresh fruit or vegetables. Exact data on prevalence are lacking, but food hypersensitivity is more common in patients with a history of atopic dermatitis. It is this group of patients that is most likely to exhibit food-induced asthma and is also the group most likely to have systemic food allergy, which can progress to full-blown anaphylaxis. There is not enough room here for a full discussion of food allergy, but the interested reader is referred to recent reviews (10,14).

FOOD-INDUCED ASTHMA

Consider the diagnosis of food-induced asthma as a contributing factor to wheezing in all patients with a history of atopic dermatitis, especially those with onset of asthma early in life and those of any age with significant atopy whose asthma is poorly controlled. In particular, young children with atopic dermatitis may have cow's milk allergy contributing to both asthma and the atopic dermatitis.

Among patients with asthma, studies reveal that from 20 to 73% of patients believe that certain foods are a trigger, and up to 61% modify their diet in response, primarily by restriction (21). Double-blind food challenges in one study, however, showed only positive results (drop in forced expiratory volume in 1 s [FEV_1]) in approx 2.5% of a population that included both adult and pediatric patients with asthma (22). The prevalence of positive food challenges increased to 6–8% in studies examining only pediatric patients with asthma (23,24). Therefore, the actual prevalence of food-induced asthma in standard clinical practice is much lower than perceived by patients, but if diagnosed, the possibility for clinical improvement via eliminating exposure to the specific food in a chronic asthma patient is real. Interestingly, a DBPCFC study of patients with food-induced asthma showed that in a subset of patients, the food allergy could be contributing to the immunopathology of asthma, as evidenced by increases in bronchial hyperresponsiveness measured by methacholine challenge (25). A previous small study, however, failed to show such an association (26).

EVALUATION OF THE PATIENT

History

The historical information that is most helpful in evaluating the possibility of food-induced asthma follows:

1. The food believed to be associated with asthma.
2. The amount that needs to be ingested to develop symptoms.

Table 2
Inhalational Food Allergy Causing Asthma

Food	Exposure
Fish	Cooking vapors
Crustaceans	Cooking vapors
Hot dogs	Cooking vapors
Lentils	Cooking vapors
Chickpea	Cooking vapors
Peanut	Particulates in air when bags are popped open
Buckwheat	Cooking vapors and flour in buckwheat chaff-stuffed pillows

Table 3
Foods Associated With Occupational Asthma

Wheat, barley, rye flours
Dried cow's milk
Lupine seed flour
Soybean flour
Fish
Crustaceans
Clam
Dried fruits
Dried tea leaves
Green coffee beans
Cacao bean dust
Dried egg white

3. Whether symptoms have occurred with each exposure.
4. Whether other factors, such as exercise, are necessary in the development of symptoms.
5. The temporal association between ingestion of the food and onset of wheezing. Food-induced asthma usually is apparent within 1 h of food ingestion.
6. Presence of atopic dermatitis because this group is at greatest risk for food-induced asthma.
7. Whether symptoms are with food ingestion or food inhalation (e.g., steam from cooking crab, shrimp, fish, hot dogs, or lentils).
8. Presence of other symptoms that suggest a systemic reaction to a food on ingestion: nausea, vomiting, urticaria, angioedema, stridor, hoarseness, flushing, itching mouth/throat, nasal congestion/itching, watery/itchy eyes, lightheadedness, and fainting.
9. Whether symptoms occur after eating certain histamine-rich foods, such as red wine, aged cheeses, and fish.

Some patients with IgE-mediated food allergy will also experience bronchospasm on inhalation of the food particles or vapors, such as those emitted during boiling (see Table 2) (27–33). Exposures to aerosolized food allergens have also been reported to cause occupational asthma via an IgE mechanism, but it is not common in this setting to subsequently experience a reaction on eating the food (see Table 3) (34–41). The history should also focus on questions that relate to conditions that mimic food-induced asthma

Table 4
Differential Diagnosis of Food-Induced Asthma

- Systemic food allergy
    Can include any ONE of the following *with* bronchospasm or upper respiratory tract
    symptoms:
        Urticaria
        Angioedema
        Nausea/vomiting
        Diarrhea/abdominal pains
        Flushing
        Lightheadedness/fainting
- Food-induced asthma
    Isolated asthma
    Asthma and other upper respiratory tract symptoms:
        Laryngoedema (hoarseness of voice or frank stridor)
        Nasal congestion/rhinorrhea of acute onset
        Itchy/watery eyes of acute onset
- Inhalation of a food that may or may not cause a systemic reaction upon ingestion
    (e.g., boiling shrimp vapors)
- Gastroesophageal reflux
- Histamine intolerance

and are more common, such as gastroesophageal reflux *(42)*. In addition to dyspepsia and acid taste in the mouth, ask about chronic throat clearing at the level of the larynx because chronic reflux can result in subtle or overt laryngitis. Sensitivity to sulfites in some foods and beverages should also be considered; asking questions about wheezing in association with white wine (which often contains more sulfites than red) can be helpful (*see* Table 4).

Physical Examination

There are no distinct physical examination findings to suggest a diagnosis of food-induced asthma. However, because this entity is more common in patients with atopic dermatitis, careful attention to the skin examination is warranted.

Differential Diagnosis

Because true food-induced asthma is actually uncommon as proved by double-blind challenges, wheezing after eating is more likely to be related to other factors. Most important is the baseline variability in lung function. Such variability in patients with poorly or moderately controlled asthma can result in misleading historical information as it relates to foods or food additives. Other important conditions include gastroesophageal reflux, sulfite sensitivity, and systemic allergic reactions to foods with bronchospasm as one of several primary symptoms.

Rarely, histamine intolerance could account for some cases of food-induced asthma *(43)*. Scombroid fish poisoning is the classic example of histamine overdosage, resulting in flushing, sweating, nausea, vomiting, urticaria, palpitations, and headache as prominent symptoms when improperly stored fish is served. The fish may not taste spoiled, but may have a "peppery" taste and contains elevated levels of histamine caused by decarboxylation of histidine by bacteria *(44)*. Bronchospasm is not usually a feature in scombroid poisoning, except in severe cases. However, patients with asthma are more sensitive to elevated levels of plasma histamine and would be more likely to wheeze under such circumstances *(43)*. It has been proposed, but backed up by only a few reports, that some people are sensitive to endogenous histamine in foods, including the baseline levels of histamine in scombroid fish (tuna, mackerel, and bonito), other fish (including mahi mahi), some red wines, certain aged cheeses, and perhaps spinach and eggplant *(45–47)*. Sensitivity to histamine is also more likely in conjunction with antituberculous therapy with isoniazid, a potent inhibitor of diamine oxidase, one of key enzymes in the breakdown of dietary histamine *(48)*.

Diagnostic Tests

Skin-prick or -puncture testing with commercially prepared glycerinated extracts or with fresh foods (in the case of fruits and vegetables) is a good starting point to evaluate possible IgE-mediated food-induced asthma (believed to account for most food-associated asthma). A negative control (saline) and positive control (histamine) must be included. However, such testing should not performed unless the suspicion of a food-induced reaction is high and the physician is willing to follow-up positive results with food challenges (except in the case of severe reactions). Indiscriminate "food allergy panels" can give multiple false-positive results in an individual with atopy. Results are considered positive if the wheal is at least 3 mm greater than the wheal of the negative control *(49)*. Intradermal skin tests with foods are not recommended because of the increased risk of severe reactions *(10)*. Skin-prick testing has been demonstrated to possess high specificity, i.e., if the skin-prick test to a suspected food is negative, there is a greater than 95% probability that the food is not involved. However, positive results must be interpreted with caution because the positive predictive accuracy of a positive skin-prick test is only approx 50% *(10,14,50)*. It is not uncommon for individuals with atopy, particularly those with atopic dermatitis, to exhibit IgE against foods without *any* clinical symptoms or signs on ingestion—such foods do not need to be avoided. In adults, the most commonly implicated foods in IgE-mediated reactions are peanuts, tree nuts, shrimp, and fish. In young children, cow's milk, egg, soy, wheat, and peanut are the most common allergens. *See* Fig. 1 for a suggested algorithm to follow in the diagnosis of food-induced asthma.

If skin-prick testing is not available or if the patient has active atopic dermatitis involving the area to be tested or to screen for specific IgE in cases of life-threatening, sudden onset of wheezing in which the physician is concerned about a possible systemic reaction to the skin-prick test, in vitro quantitative specific IgE assays are an alternative. Recent studies have shown that it is possible to predict which children may outgrow their food allergy by assessing the level of specific IgE over time. If specific IgE to a food is below cut-off thresholds, then that child has a greater likelihood of now being tolerant to the food in question and a food challenge may be warranted *(10,14)*. Alternatively, certain high values have been determined to have a high likelihood of predicting that the individual is truly clinically allergic to the food assayed *(10)*. There is no role for specific IgG, IgG4, or food immune complex assays at this time in the diagnosis of food allergy because these procedures are considered unproven or experimental *(14)*.

If life-threatening asthma has resulted after exposures to the food in question and the skin-prick test or in vitro IgE assay is positive, it is reasonable to diagnose food-induced asthma and eliminate the food from the diet, both microscopic and macroscopic amounts.

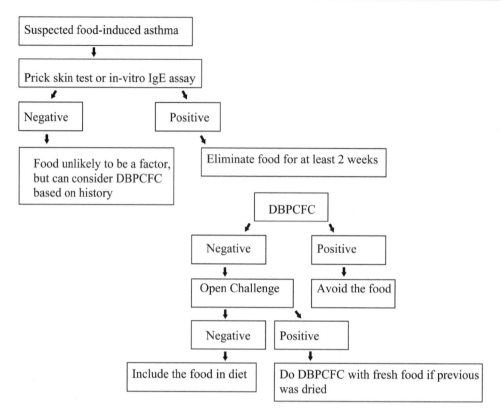

Fig. 1. Algorithm for diagnosis of food-induced asthma. DBPCFC, double-blind, placebo-controlled food challenge.

However, the history is not usually that compelling in cases of food-induced asthma, unlike acute systemic allergic reactions (anaphylaxis) to peanut, tree nuts, shrimp, or fish, where acute bronchospasm may be part of a multisystem reaction often easily linked to the food ingestion; symptoms in these cases have been known to start within 1 min of food ingestion. Instead, the next step is an elimination diet and food challenge. An elimination diet by itself cannot be used to screen for food-induced asthma because such individuals are usually atopic and multiple factors may contribute to peak flow variability, although, there are case reports of improvement in some patients after elimination of one suspect food *(51)*. Rather, the elimination of the food leads up to a food challenge, which can be performed in the office setting as long as the capability to treat severe asthma exists.

Food challenges should be double-blind and placebo-controlled. Guidelines for the performance of office-based food challenges have been published *(52)*. Single-blind challenges can be used initially if there are more than one or two foods suspected. Ideally, the patient should have avoided the suspect food for at least 2 wk, and asthma should be under good control. The latter point is critical, because if sequential spirometry on a non-challenge day shows variability of 10% or more, the results could be falsely skewed toward a positive challenge. Antihistamines should be held for several days before the challenge, but usual asthma controller medications continued. On the day of challenge, baseline spirometry should be performed. Challenge can usually begin with 25–200 mg of the suspected food in dried or freeze-dried form (most common foods are available in many grocery stores, natural food stores, and camping outlets) given in capsules or disguised in another food. For example, a fruit smoothie is a good way to disguise dried milk, wheat flour, soy, or egg powders. The dose is then doubled every 15–20 min (particularly when the suspect food or placebo is administered as a liquid in a patient with a history of rapid reactions) or up to 1 h, depending on the patient history. Spirometry should be repeated before the next dose is given. A drop of 15% in FEV_1 is considered a positive challenge. Alternatively, if other signs of a food allergic reaction develop, such as a morbilliform rash, urticaria, and lip/oral mucosa swelling, before a drop in FEV_1 is seen, the challenge can be stopped because these symptoms are consistent with food allergy and further incremental doses increase the risk for a severe reaction. If a total of 10 g (adding all increments given) of the suspected food has been tolerated, it is exceedingly unlikely that the food is a factor in the patient's asthma. Equal numbers of placebo and food challenges should be done. Ideally, it is recommended that two challenges and two placebos be given for each food suspected *(52)*. Such testing should occur on separate days and is obviously time-consuming for the patient but worth the effort, particularly if a pediatric patient has been on a restricted diet (e.g., milk and wheat restriction) because of positive skin-prick tests which are, statistically, most likely to be clinically irrelevant.

Anecdotally speaking, many adults choose to avoid the food in question rather than take the time to perform challenges, but it is *very* important to clarify the situation in children because children on restricted diets can face malnutrition and stigmatization by peers.

After a negative challenge, an open challenge with the food as the patient usually eats it should be scheduled because there are occasional instances of dried foods not provoking a reaction when the fresh food is indeed allergenic.

Treatment

Currently, the primary treatment for food-induced asthma, as with food allergy in general, is avoidance. Avoiding the food can be extremely difficult in some cases. Referral to a dietitian may be advisable if the food has been an important component of the diet, such as cow's milk in a young child. The patient and family must be educated on how to read food labels and the problems and pitfalls of cross-contamination in homes, bakeries, and restaurants. Although we are fortunate in the United States to have fairly stringent food labeling laws, cross-contamination of commercially prepared foods with undeclared allergens is a real concern as evidenced by numerous product recalls each year *(53)*. Table 5 is an example list of ingredients to avoid if a patient is allergic to cow's milk. However, starting on January 1, 2006, food labels in the United States will be required to use source ingredient labeling to inform food-allergic consumers of allergen presence as a result of passage of the Food Allergen and Consumer Protection Act (FALCPA) (included as Title II of Senate Bill 741, 2004). For example, instead of "casein" or "natural flavors," a label will also need to indicate "cow's milk." Patients may find additional assistance and information from local or national organizations dealing with food allergy, such as the Food Allergy and Anaphylaxis Network (www.foodallergy.org). There is currently no role for immunotherapy in foods, but a bright future for immune modulation in food allergy does exist *(54)*. There is also no role at this time for alternative therapies that are unproven, including acupuncture, homeopathy, provocation/neutralization, or "4-day rotary diets" *(14,55)*.

Another important point is that if there is evidence of systemic food allergy after accidental ingestion of the food, if an isolated lower respiratory reaction is severe, if

Table 5
Cow's Milk Avoidance Diet

Reading labels: less-obvious names for milk-containing ingredients
Artificial butter flavoring
Butter
Casein hydrolysates
Ghee
Lactose (it can be contaminated with the proteins)
Lactalbumin
Lactoglobulin
Rennet casein
Whey
Whey hydrolysate

Less-obvious products and ingredients that may contain milk proteins
Chocolate
Caramel coloring
High-protein flour
Margarine
Natural flavoring
Fat substitutes

laryngoedema is present, or if there is a history of a severe reaction to the food, the initial treatment should be with self-injected epinephrine rather than reliance on inhaled β_2-agonists or liquid/chewable antihistamines. All individuals with food-induced asthma should have self-injectable epinephrine available because the natural history of this condition is unknown. For instance, it is possible that an individual who normally experiences an episode of mild wheezing easily relieved by albuterol after accidental ingestion of peanut may go on to have status asthmaticus or a systemic reaction with cardiovascular collapse the next time the food is ingested. The same recommendations apply to those with asthma after inhaling cooking fumes from foods because the risk for laryngoedema or status asthmaticus is unknown.

The long-term natural history for food-induced asthma is similar to food allergy in general. If the reaction is to peanut, tree nuts, shrimp, or fish, then it is likely that the hypersensitivity is permanent; however, approx 20% of children with peanut allergy will lose their sensitivity over time *(56)*. If sensitivity to other antigens, such as cow's milk, egg, soy, or wheat, is present, there is a good chance that the patient will become tolerant of the food after several years of avoidance, especially if the onset of the allergy was in infancy or young childhood *(10)*.

ADDITIVES AND ASTHMA

Much maligned food and medication additives were targeted in the 1970s and 1980s as common precipitants of asthma. With the exception of sodium metabisulfite and the benzalkonium chloride that is now banned from use in some bronchodilator preparations *(57)*, double-blind, placebo-controlled trials or well-designed, single-blind trials have exonerated many of the additives in common use or suggested that sensitivity to such agents is actually exceedingly rare. In the case of monosodium glutamate (MSG), dyes, and other additives, earlier reports suggested that patients with aspirin-sensitive asthma (ASA) were most likely to react, whereas such reactions were rarely reported in patients with aspirin-tolerant asthma. Stevenson et al. and Weber et al. deserve much credit for pioneering the use of challenges in patients who are aspirin sensitive that showed that such patients have intrinsically unstable airways and, as a consequence, many of the trials implicating additives were likely falsely positive because of baseline instability of airway tone. This problem was most evident when bronchodilators were then withdrawn before challenges that involved populations with aspirin-induced asthma *(58–61)*.

Evaluation of the Patient Suspected of Having Adverse Reactions to Additives

HISTORY

Sulfite sensitivity can be screened for during the patient's history by asking questions related to asthma reactions after eating in restaurants in the early 1980s (before the regulations of use of sulfite on foods served as fresh in salad bars went into effect), after drinking white wine, wine in general, and problems with eating dried fruit with sulfites. White wine generally has higher levels of sulfites than red and is thus more commonly reported as a trigger. Regarding food additives, because sulfite sensitivity occurs with measurable prevalence in the population with asthma, questions should address this entity and patients can be asked to watch for any associations of asthma with sulfite exposure in follow-up appointments, because reactions can range from mild to severe. However, it may take a fairly high sulfite exposure to elicit asthma. For the other additives, patients can be queried about whether they modify their diet as a result of beliefs about other food or chemical sensitivities playing a role in their asthma.

PHYSICAL EXAMINATION

There are no identifying features on physical examination to suggest additive sensitivity.

DIFFERENTIAL DIAGNOSIS

If a patient believes that he or she has an additive allergy, the main concern in the differential diagnosis is coincidental lability of pulmonary function, which has been suggested to account for almost all cases of asthma possibly associated with additives besides sulfites. Food allergy, histamine intolerance, and reflux must be considered (*see* Tables 6 and 7).

DIAGNOSTIC TESTS

There are no in vitro diagnostic tests to aid in identifying individuals with sulfite sensitivity or adverse reactions to the other food additives. Challenge tests with sulfite preparations or with other additives are desirable if indicated.

TREATMENT

The treatment of sulfite-induced asthma is rapid institution of β-adrenergic agonist therapy; additional therapy will depend on the severity of the attack. Some patients with severe reactions will need self-injectable epinephrine immediately on recognition of a significant exposure, along with a call to activate the local emergency medical response system. Epinephrine is indicated even though the self-injectable epinephrine preparations are preserved with sulfites—fortunately, the beneficial effects outweigh the potential for harm. The best treatment, however, is prophylactic avoidance of the offending

Table 6
Food Additives Evaluated In Asthma

Additive	Found in	*Percentage of patients with asthma with positive challenges under double-blind, placebo-controlled conditions (with airway stability documented in patients who are aspirin-sensitive)*
Sulfites	Wines (especially white), juices, dried fruits, refrigerated commercial salsa, potatoes in restaurants, and shrimp	4–5%
Monosodium glutamate	Normal diet Packaged foods Asian restaurant cooking	0% of patients with asthma who are aspirin-sensitive; 0% of other patients with asthma
Tartrazine	Commercial foods and medications with yellow coloring added	0% of patients with asthma who are aspirin-sensitive; 0% of other asthmatics
Other dyes	Many commercial foods	Not studied in this manner
Benzoates	Soda pops, beverages	0–4%
Parabens	Rare in foods	Not studied in this manner
Butylated hydroxyanisole/ butylated hydroxytoluene	Packaged baked goods, mixes	Not studied in this manner

Table 7
Differential Diagnosis of Food Additive-Induced Asthma

- Inadequately controlled asthma
- Food allergy
    Systemic food allergy
    Food-induced asthma by ingestion
    Food-induced asthma by inhalation
- Histamine intolerance
    Increased intolerance secondary to enzyme inhibition by isoniazid
- Gastroesophageal reflux
- Additive sensitivity
    Sulfites
    Others

compounds, reviewed in the following section. It is unclear how often other additives truly elicit bronchospasm, but the primary treatment of avoidance remains the same.

Review of Individual Additives

SULFITES

Sulfite sensitivity is a potentially fatal clinical syndrome that is most commonly seen in patients with asthma, possibly secondary to the increased sensitivity of the asthma patient's airway to sulfur dioxide (SO_2) and bisulfite. It was first reported in 1973 in a child with asthma who, on several occasions, opened packages of SO_2-treated dried fruits, ate some, and developed shortness of breath and wheezing *(62)*. The term "sulfites" is a general term that refers to SO_2, sulfurous acid, and the inorganic salts: sodium and potassium metabisulfite, sodium and potassium bisulfite, and sodium and potassium sulfite. Sulfites can occur naturally in foods but are often added to inhibit nonenzymatic browning, enzymatic browning, or for antimicrobial preservative effects *(63)*.

Clinical Concerns

Approximately 4–5% of patients with asthma in challenge studies exhibit sulfite-sensitivity with decreases in FEV_1 of 20% or more on challenge *(64,65)*. However, approx 8% of patients with steroid-dependent asthma in one study were sensitive to sulfites *(65)*. Sensitivity most commonly presents as bronchospasm, sometimes with tingling, flushing, and loss of consciousness, but can include urticaria, rhinoconjunctivitis, angioedema, or anaphylaxis. There are a few reports of patients without asthma reacting to sulfites in foods with anaphylactic reactions and positive skin tests to sulfites *(66,67)*. For some patients with subsequently steroid-dependent asthma, their first wheezing episodes were in conjunction with reactions to ingested sulfites *(68)*.

Clinically, the reaction usually comes on within 1–5 min of ingestion of beverages or foods with substantial liquid content and in up to 30 min after eating solid foods that contain sulfites.

Public awareness of sulfite sensitivity became prominent in the early 1980s when there were fatalities and near-fatalities relating to acute asthma attacks after patients with asthma unknowingly ingested sulfite-treated produce in restaurants. It was common practice at that time to spray sulfite solutions on fresh fruits and vegetables, such as lettuce. Sulfite sensitivity also raised awareness about the role of the federal government in regulating potentially harmful additives. In 1985, the US Food and Drug Administration (FDA) issued a ruling that sulfite levels in shrimp (often dipped in sulfite solutions to prevent enzymatic darkening) should not exceed 100 ppm SO_2 *(69)*. The 1986 rulings prohibiting the use of sulfites on fruits and vegetables to be sold fresh (as in restaurant salad bars), with the sole exception of potatoes, and requiring the declaration of detectable sulfites (values >10 ppm) on the label were important steps *(70)*. The federal government also issued a regulation that SO_2 in wine should not exceed 350 ppm *(71)*. Manufacturers are required to use the minimum sufficient sulfite to achieve the desired effect, but missteps are reported. For instance, two patients in California developed status asthmaticus after eating small amounts of a refrigerated brand of salsa, which was labeled with the misleading term "fresh"—both patients were unconscious when emergency help arrived. The salsa in question had a mean SO_2 level of 1803 ppm, which is far in excess of reasonable amounts *(72)*. Despite such reports, since the FDA imposed regulations on the use and labeling of sulfites in foods went into effect, there has been a substantial decrease in adverse event reporting to the FDA. From 1980 to 1987, the FDA received an average of 111 reports per year of adverse reactions believed to result from sulfites, whereas from 1996 to 1999, an average of 10 reports per year were received *(73)*.

Patients with sulfite-sensitive asthma exhibit a threshold of tolerance to sulfites, above which they will experience a reaction, but below which the food is tolerated.

Characteristics of the food are important, too; sulfites in beverages or liquids elicit more responses, whereas low amounts within solid foods may be tolerated *(74)*. A recent study in Australia assessed sulfite sensitivity in 24 patients with asthma who gave excellent histories for wine-induced asthma (repeated episodes of worsening asthma within 30 min of wine consumption), 9 of whom had histories extremely suggestive of sulfite sensitivity (white wine and cheaper wines worse, or sulfited fruits or vegetables also causing symptoms). Interestingly, only 4 of the 9 with the stronger histories, and none of the other 15 patients, had positive single-blind challenges with 150 mL white wine containing 300 ppm sulfites (the maximum allowable level in Australian wines). It was suggested that other factors may also be important (e.g., pollen exposure, cigarette exposure, and baseline asthma control) in precipitating an asthmatic response away from the research laboratory. In subsequent double-blind, dose-response challenges, none of these four reacted to doses less than 300 ppm *(75)*.

Pathogenesis

Several mechanisms have been proposed, and more than one may be operative in any one patient:

1. Bronchospasm resulting from SO_2 inhalation.
2. IgE-mediated response.
3. Sulfite oxidase deficiency.

First, patients with asthma are extraordinarily sensitive to directly inhaled SO_2 and bisulfite. Less than 1 ppm of SO_2 can induce a fall in FEV_1 in patients with asthma *(76)*. Because the most severe reactions are with beverages, it has been proposed that inhalation of SO_2 given off from the liquid may be the etiology, but this does not explain why only a small subset of patients with asthma react to sulfites in food and drink. An interesting challenge study was performed in patients with sulfite-sensitive asthma using an acidic metabisulfite solution swished and swallowed vs instilled directly in the stomach via a nasogastric tube. The subjects reacted in the former situation, but not the latter *(77)*. The sensitivity to SO_2 in asthma may be mediated by cholinergic reflexes and perhaps also stem from increased levels of involved neuropeptide mediators in this pathway that could be of more prominence in patients with sulfite-sensitive asthma *(78,79)*.

Some individuals have immediate positive skin-prick or intradermal tests with metabisulfite solutions. Transfer of skin reactivity by passive transfer (and abolition of the effect by heating) have also been shown and are supportive of an IgE-mediated mechanism in some people *(66,67)*. IgE directed against sulfite compounds has not been shown, nor has the candidate haptenated protein been identified.

Simon described decreased sulfite oxidase activity in the cultured fibroblasts of six patients with sulfite sensitivity patients but no follow-up studies on these intriguing findings with larger numbers of patients and controls have been published *(80)*.

Diagnostic Sulfite Challenges

The clinical history does not correlate as well as would be expected with clinical challenges *(75)*. Unfortunately, there is variability in the challenges as well, depending on the type of solution used or if capsules are used. Such challenges are rarely performed. Acidic beverages are most likely to be associated with reactions, but virtually all patients with asthma are sensitive to inhaled SO_2, so if this is the main mechanism, it is possible that such challenges using acidic solutions may overestimate sensitivity to sulfites in foods. Taylor et al. recommend using potassium metabisulfite in capsules because this most closely mimics the exposures encountered in foods (*see* Table 8) *(74,81)*. If such a challenge is negative and the history is positive for reactions to wines or juices, for instance, a neutral- or acid-solution metabisulfite challenge could be done (*see* Table 9). As with other challenges, it is desirable that baseline stability in lung function be demonstrated. If the individual is aspirin-sensitive, bronchodilators should be continued. Sulfite challenges can induce severe reactions and should only be performed in a setting where such responses can be properly managed. In summary, challenges may be extremely complex and are only practical for individual patients who have a strong motivation to prove or disprove sensitivity. There is no role for skin-prick testing at the current time because the positive predictive value of a positive test is not defined and persons with near-fatal reactions have been skin-test negative.

Avoidance

Extremely sensitive patients must be counseled to read labels carefully. Some patients may specifically tolerate sulfites in solid foods, but as with all sulfite challenges, such determination should be made by food challenge in a place where the capability to treat a severe reaction exists *(74)*. Sensitive individuals must be advised to avoid not only SO_2 but also any term containing the word "sulfite" buried within it. Potatoes were exempted from the ban on sulfite use; thus, patients should avoid all potatoes in restaurants except baked potatoes served with the skins on, because sulfites would not be used on these *(63)*.

All medications should likewise be checked for sulfite content, because patients have reacted after aerosol (nebulizer) exposure and some after parenteral exposure. Alternatives exist, except the 1:1000 preparation of epinephrine for subcutaneous/intramuscular injection; but, as noted, when this is indicated, the beneficial effects outweigh any potential for negative side effects. If racemic epinephrine is needed for nebulization, such as postintubation, the intravenous preparations of epinephrine (1:10,000) without sulfites can be used *(57)*.

MONOSODIUM GLUTAMATE

A study published in 1987 stimulated great interest in whether ingestion of MSG from both natural and food additive sources could be contributory to the pathogenesis of asthma *(82)*. Natural sources of MSG actually dominate the average diet, approx 1 g/d is typical, with approx 0.5 g/d from prepared foods *(83)*. The original study reported that 14 out of 32 patients had 20% decreases in peak expiratory flow rate (PEFR) anywhere from 1 to 12 h after challenge with 2.5 g MSG *(82)*. It should be immediately apparent that bronchospasm at up to 12 h after a challenge is difficult to correlate with the challenge itself, especially when baseline stability of lung function has not been demonstrated. There were other criticisms of the study design as well, such as use of PEFR instead of spirometry and challenge of some subjects at night and others in the morning. All subsequent studies have failed to support this original report, including a recent rigorous trial of 100 subjects, 30 of whom had a history of asthma attacks after eating in an Oriental restaurant, and 70 with a history of ASA, a group originally believed to be at higher risk for MSG-triggered asthma *(84)*. A review of the clinical

Table 8
Capsule and Neutral-Solution Metabisulfite Challenge[a]

Preparing the patient and collecting preliminary data
- Withhold short-acting aerosol sympathomimetics and cromolyn/nedocromil sodium for 8 h and short-acting antihistamines for 24–48 h before pulmonary function testing.
- Measure pulmonary function: forced expiratory volume in 1 s (FEV_1) must be greater than or equal to 70% of predicted normal value and greater than or equal to 1.5 L in adults. (Test contraindicated in patients with an FEV_1 below those levels. Standards for children have not been defined.)

Performing the single-blind challenge
- Administer placebo (powdered sucrose) in capsule form. Measure FEV_1 at 30 min.
- Administer capsules containing 1, 5, 25, 50, 100, and 200 mg of potassium metabisulfite at 30-min intervals. Measure FEV_1 30 min after administering each dose and if the patient becomes symptomatic.
- If no response, administer 1, 10, and 25 mg of potassium metabisulfite in water-sucrose solution at 30-min intervals. Measure FEV_1 30 min after each dose and if symptoms occur. Positive response is indicated by a decrease in FEV_1 of 20% or more.

Performing the double-blind challenge
- Perform challenge and placebo procedures on separate days, in random order.
- Placebo day: Administer only sucrose in capsules and solution. Measure FEV_1 30 min after each dose and if patient becomes symptomatic.
- Challenge day: Same protocol as single-blind challenge day.

[a]Perform this test only where the capability to treat severe asthmatic reactions exists.
(Reprinted with permission from ref. *81*.)

Table 9
Acid-Solution Metabisulfite Challenge[a,b]

Preparing the patient and collecting preliminary data
- Withhold short-acting aerosol sympathomimetics and cromolyn/nedocromil sodium for 8 h and short-acting antihistamines or 24 to 48 h before pulmonary function testing.
- Measure pulmonary function: forced expiratory volume in 1 s (FEV_1) must be greater than or equal to 70% of predicted normal value and greater than or equal to 1.5 L in adults. (Test contraindicated in patients with an FEV_1 below those levels. Standards for children have not been defined.)

Performing the bisulfite challenge
- Dissolve 0.1 mg of potassium metabisulfite in 20 mL of a sulfite-free lemonade crystal solution. Have the patient swish the solution around for 10 to 15 s, then swallow.
- Measure FEV_1 10 min after the first dose. Then administer 0.5, 1, 5, 10, 15, 25, 50, and 75 and 100[c] mg per 20 mL of the solution at 10-min intervals. Measure FEV_1 10 min after each incremental increase in dose. Positive response is signified by a decrease in FEV_1 of 20% or more.

[a]Protocol investigated by the Bronchoprovocation Committee—American Academy of Allergy, Asthma and Immunology *(81)*.

[b]Perform this test only where the capability for managing severe asthmatic reactions exists.

[c]Doses in excess of 100 mg/20 mL may cause nonspecific bronchial reactions and are thus left off of this protocol *(81)*. (Adapted with permission from ref. *81*.)

Table 10
Monosodium Glutamate Food Additive Challenge

Suggested procedure for an outpatient challenge

Day 1	Day 2
Start time: 0800	Start time: 0800
Baseline spirometry	Baseline spirometry, if FEV_1 no more than 5% different than at start of Day 1, proceed[a]
Give 2.5 gm sucrose placebo, single-blind	Give 2.5 gm monosodium glutamate, single-blind
Hourly spirometry for 4–6 h[b]	Hourly spirometry for 4 to 6 h
If FEV_1 variability less than 10%, proceed	If a drop in FEV_1 of 20%, proceed to double-blind challenges

[a]Monosodium glutamate (MSG) and sucrose can be purchased from local grocery stores and 500 mg placed in gelatin capsules by the clinic or hospital pharmacy.

[b]If the patient believes reactions have always occurred within an hour of MSG exposure, then 4-h monitoring is enough. (Adapted with permission from ref. *84*.)

trials now shows that it is extremely unlikely that this entity exists and patients thus can be counseled *(85)*. It may be helpful to point out the preponderance of MSG that naturally occurs in the diet.

However, some patients who strongly believe that asthma is precipitated by exposure to MSG, e.g., after dining in a Chinese restaurant, and who currently go to great extremes to avoid MSG in the diet may be greatly benefited by undergoing a challenge. A negative challenge can go a long way in alleviating anxiety. Single-blind challenges with MSG are adequate for screening purposes and are easy and practical to perform in an outpatient primary care or specialty clinic, as in Table 10, but with the important caveat that baseline lung function must be stable. In the outpatient setting, this can be partially addressed by having the patient come in on the day before the single-blind challenges for a placebo challenge. If the FEV_1 that day varies by more than 10%, or if the FEV_1 on the day of challenge is more than 5% different from the placebo day, the results may be affected by the variability, and the test is best postponed *(84)*. Any positive results should be followed up by double-blind, placebo-controlled challenges, which, in this case, can also be easily performed in the outpatient clinic setting.

TARTRAZINE AND OTHER DYES

Until the last 20 yr, physicians were taught that patients with ASA should avoid all tartrazine in the diet. Tartrazine is a yellow food colorant, or dye, also referred to as Food Dye and Coloring Act (FD&C) yellow no. 5. It is an azo dye, meaning that it possesses an N::N bond, derived from coal tar. Of the coal tar-derived dyes still approved in the United States, the other commonly used azo dyes are FD&C red no. 4 (ponceau) and FD&C yellow no. 6 (sunset yellow). Approval of FD&C red no. 5 (amaranth) was pulled in 1975 after controversial claims linking this dye to carcinogenesis. The three best known nonazo dyes are FD&C blue no. 1 (brilliant blue), FD&C blue no. 2 (indigotin), and FD&C red no. 3 (erythrosine). Although it has now been generally accepted that a few patients experience urticaria after exposure to tartrazine, the mechanism is not related to cross-reactivity to aspirin, but may be IgE mediated. There is no cyclooxygenase (COX) inhibition by the azo dyes, and the chemical structure is not related to aspirin. In several careful studies, patients with aspirin-sensitive urticaria failed to show evidence of cross-reactivity, whereas a few patients with non-aspirin sensitive urticaria did react *(86,87)*.

In asthma, a series of studies in the 1960s and 1970s were published that attempted to link aspirin-sensitive asthma with tartrazine sensitivity. One of the largest was by Spector et al. in 1979; 11 of 44 (25%) patients with aspirin-sensitive asthma experienced a 20% decrease in FEV_1 on the tartrazine challenge day, whereas none of the 233 control patients with asthma had a decrease. However, bronchodilators were withheld for 6–12 h before beginning the challenges and 5 of the 11 reactors did not undergo placebo challenges *(88)*. In another study, 50% of patients who were aspirin sensitive were reported to react to tartrazine (12 of 24) based on falls in peak flow *(89)*. Because it is now known that patients with aspirin-sensitive asthma tend to have unstable airways, the chance of coincidental decreases in FEV_1 is quite likely after discontinuation of bronchodilators. Such patients will still react strongly to aspirin in blinded challenges with their usual bronchodilators administered beforehand, showing that bronchodilators do not mask a response. Because cross-reactivity with aspirin has been proposed, if such a mechanism existed, one would expect tartrazine to result in a reaction under similar circumstances to aspirin. In 1988, a European study of 156 patients who were aspirin sensitive showed that 4 patients reacted with a drop in FEV_1 of at least 25% on single-blind and subsequent double-blind challenges *(90)*. However, although the challenges were well controlled, baseline variability in lung function was not documented to be stable, so it is likely that the estimate of 2.6% sensitivity was an overestimate. Stevenson et al. performed two tightly controlled challenge studies in a total of 194 patients with aspirin-sensitive asthma. Six of 194 had at least a 20% decrease in FEV_1 on single-blind tartrazine challenge, but none reacted in subsequent double-blind challenges *(86,91)*. There are no convincing reports of asthma related to the other dyes in use, although there are case reports indicating systemic or gastrointestinal reactions to several dyes *(92,93)*. Overall, the risk of patients with ASA truly reacting to tartrazine or other dyes is extremely small. In the occasional situation where a challenge is desired, the protocol by Stevenson et al. could be adapted *(91)*.

BENZOATES

Sodium benzoate and benzoic acid are food preservatives that have been commonly employed in beverages, as well as in other products, for nearly 90 yr. Interestingly, many plants naturally contain benzoates, likely as part of the chemical defense repertoire against pathogens. Such plant sources include berries (cranberries and raspberries have high levels), prunes, cloves, and tea. Some case reports have indicated a possible role of benzoate sensitivity in some patients with asthma (and in some urticarial or anaphylactoid reactions), but larger clinical trials have failed to show convincing evidence because most of the studies did not demonstrate baseline stability of the FEV_1 or use placebos and double-blind challenges in those initially positive on single-blind challenge (reviewed in ref. *94*). Very few studies used changes in FEV_1 (as opposed to peak flow) and double-blind protocols. An abstract in 1976 reported that 1 out of 30 (3%) patients responded to sodium benzoate *(95)*. In another double-blind trial, 1 of 43 reacted (2%), but when rechallenged 2 yr later, the results were negative *(58)*. Tarlo and Broder reported one patient as sensitive to benzoates (3%), but an additive-free diet made no difference in his asthma control *(96)*.

PARABENS

The parabens are esters of *p*-hydroxybenzoic acid and have been in use in the United States since the 1930s (reviewed in ref. *94*). Methylparaben and propylparaben are approved for use in food. These preservatives are used in foods to a much lesser degree than the benzoates, but more commonly in medications and cosmetics, and in the latter preparations, contact dermatitis reactions have been well characterized. There are no adequate studies evaluating the role of these additives in populations of patients with asthma, but there is one case report of a patient who experienced bronchospasm and pruritus after intravenous administration of hydrocortisone solution preserved with methyl- and *n*-propylparaben. Skin tests were positive to the parabens, including by passive transfer, which was strongly suggestive of an IgE-mediated reaction *(97)*.

BUTYLATED HYDROXYANISOLE AND BUTYLATED HYDROXYTOLUENE

No evidence for asthma related to butylated hydroxyanisole and butylated hydroxytoluene ingestion has been published, although there may be rare patients with urticaria provoked by these agents *(98)*.

ADDITIVES IN BRONCHODILATOR SOLUTIONS

Preservative compounds, particularly benzalkonium chloride (BAC), have been added to nonsterile unit-dose bronchodilator solutions used for nebulizers in high enough concentrations to cause clinically relevant paradoxical bronchospasm (reviewed in ref. *57*). BAC-induced bronchospasm is potentially clinically relevant in countries where such solutions may still be available *(99)*. Nonsterile unit-dose solutions have been phased out in the United States.

In countries that allow nonsterile unit-dose medications, consider an adverse reaction to additives in nebulized bronchodilator solutions in the emergency department patient or intensive care unit patient who is not responding well to standard nebulized bronchodilator therapy, particularly if paradoxical bronchospasm results.

Such adverse reactions are more likely if repeated, continuous doses are administered. BAC was the preservative of choice in the nonsterile albuterol preparations in the United States. Inhalation challenge studies with BAC demonstrate a dose-dependent and, interestingly, cumulative effect of BAC on the decrease in FEV_1 in a majority of studied patients *(100)*. Thus, if a patient received repetitive doses or continuous nebulization of albuterol containing sufficient quantities of BAC, particularly unit-dose vials containing 300 µg BAC/vial, the potential for paradoxical bronchospasm or poor response to the bronchodilator was real *(57)*. Sterile, preservative-free, unit-dose vials are now the only option for single-use purchase in the United States, which bypasses this potential adverse reaction.

Ethylenediamine tetraacetic acid (EDTA) is added to some solutions to prevent color changes. This agent too has been associated with bronchospasm in a study using a small number of patients, but the doses required were high *(100)*. In another randomized, controlled, cross-over study comparing responses to BAC, EDTA, or placebo, there was no difference between EDTA and placebo. Routine use of products containing small amounts of EDTA is unlikely to be associated with paradoxical bronchospasm or poor bronchodilator responsiveness *(57)*.

DRUGS AND ASTHMA

Aspirin and NSAIDS

Of drugs that have significant effects on asthma, if not speaking of therapeutic agents, it is aspirin and NSAIDs that are implicated. Although most patients tolerate aspirin and NSAIDs well, a subset of patients with asthma experience clinical symptoms to aspirin or NSAIDs in a dose-responsive manner, ranging from mild nasoocular reactions (rhinorrhea, nasal congestion, and periorbital angioedema) to severe, life-threatening bronchospasm. These patients are said to have aspirin-exacerbated respiratory tract disease, or aspirin-induced asthma (AIA).

PREVALENCE

Based on three recently performed population-based surveys in Finland, Poland, and Australia, AIA affects from 4.3 to 11% of patients with diagnosed asthma, but this is believed to be an underestimate because up to 15% of challenge-positive patients in another study were unaware of their condition *(101–104)*. Recent studies on the natural history of the disorder show that it is extremely unusual in children—the average age of onset is 30–34 yr *(104,105)*. AIA usually starts with persistent rhinitis, often following what is reported to be a typical viral upper respiratory infection; this is followed by chronic sinusitis, asthma, aspirin sensitivity, and nasal polyposis. Approximately one-third of patients are atopic—in this subgroup, the rhinitis and asthma appeared earlier. The asthma is often moderate to severe; 50% required chronic oral corticosteroids (CSs) at a mean dose of 8 mg/d *(104)*.

Pathogenesis

The mechanism of aspirin-exacerbated respiratory tract disease is not fully elucidated at this time, but the advent of 5-lipoxygenase inhibitors, leukotriene (LT) receptor blockers, and cyclooxygenase (COX)-2 inhibitors have facilitated study (reviewed in ref. *106*). The original hypothesis that AIA patients were overly sensitive to blockade of COX by aspirin and NSAIDs, thus shunting arachidonic acid metabolism toward products of the lipoxygenase pathway, has been greatly refined with the discovery of different COX enzymes. Picado et al. that suggested abnormally low COX-2 activity may be part of the AIA pathogenesis, because the COX-2 pathway produces beneficial prostaglandin $(PG)_{E2}$ *(107)*. They studied nasal polyp tissue from patients with aspirin-tolerant asthma and patients with AIA for COX-2 mRNA expression; expression in the aspirin-sensitive group was sevenfold lower ($p < 0.0001$). There were no differences in COX-1 mRNA expression. Another study, using immunostaining of cells from bronchial biopsies, found fivefold higher counts of cells expressing LTC_4 synthase in cells from patients with AIA than patients with aspirin-tolerant asthma ($p = 0.0006$). The authors suggested that aspirin may result in a removal of PG_{E2}-mediated suppression of overabundant LTC_4 synthase, with subsequent high production of cysteinyl leukotrienes *(108)*. Significantly lower PG_{E2} production from bronchial fibroblasts obtained from patients with AIA has also been found *(109)*. A striking finding in support of these hypotheses is that COX-2 inhibitors are tolerated in AIA with only a few case reports otherwise *(110,111)*. PG_{E2} normally functions as an important immunomodulator—lack of which can result in an increase in synthesis of the cysteinyl leukotrienes and PGD_2 release by inflammatory cells. A recent human genetic study of polymorphisms in genes associated with the arachidonic acid metabolic cascade found a significant association of multiple single nucleotide polymorphisms (SNPs) in the PG_{E2} receptor subtype 2 with AIA. Examined further, SNPs in the promoter region of this gene, especially a SNP in the regulatory region of the gene, were significantly associated with AIA. If this SNP affects the function of the gene in further studies, it is further support for the hypothesis that a reduction in PG_{E2} immunomodulatory activity is key in the pathogenesis of this disorder (112).

The oversynthesis of cysteinyl leukotrienes is a prominent feature of AIA. In fact, even at baseline, patients with asthma with AIA have elevated urinary LTE_4 concentrations, but this is not a diagnostic test (113). With oral challenges, urinary levels of LTE_4 rise significantly higher, and the increase correlates with the onset of respiratory symptoms, typically 1–4 h later. Patients with asthma without AIA do not show increases in urinary LTE_4 with aspirin challenges (114). Moreover, not only are the levels of LTE_4 in urine higher, but patients with asthma with AIA in one study had a greater decrease in FEV_1 after challenge with inhaled LTE_4 than patients who do not have AIA, suggesting that patients with AIA synthesize more LTE_4 and are also more sensitive to its bronchoconstrictive effects (115). Immunochemical staining of leukocytes from patients with AIA has demonstrated increased expression of Cys-LT1 receptors (these receptors bind LTC_4, LTD_4, and LTE_4), which could explain the greater sensitivity of patients with AIA (116).

EVALUATION OF THE PATIENT

AIA is underdiagnosed among patients with asthma, so physicians are urged to think of the diagnosis in patients with persistent rhinitis and asthma. Many patients have not had aspirin or NSAIDs in sufficient dose to provoke symptoms or may not have associated flares of asthma with aspirin/NSAID ingestion resulting from the delay in nasoocular or asthma symptoms of up to 4 h.

History

- Ask about recent use of aspirin or NSAIDs and nasoocular or asthma symptoms occurring within 4 h.
- Ask about history of anosmia, polyps, and acute and chronic sinusitis.
- Ask about a family history of aspirin/NSAID sensitivity.
- Many patients who are aspirin sensitive are CS-dependent or have otherwise difficult-to-control asthma.

Physical Examination

The presence of nasal polyps and chronic sinusitis on physical examination or screening sinus computed tomography scan should raise the suspicion of AIA.

Diagnostic Tests

For now, the key to *definitive* diagnosis of AIA is an oral challenge test, but this is not routinely performed unless there is a specific need to determine tolerance to aspirin in a patient with an unclear history. Biochemical markers sensitive or specific for AIA have not been described. There is the potential for a severe asthmatic response with oral challenges, so such testing should be performed in a place where the ability to treat a severe reaction exists, such as in a hospital setting with an intensive care unit nearby. Three-day oral challenges can be combined with desensitization (106,117) (*see* Table 11).

Table 11
Single-Blind 3-d Aspirin Diagnostic Challenge[a]

Time	Day 1	Day 2	Day 3
0800	Placebo	Aspirin, 30 mg	Aspirin, 150 mg
1100	Placebo	Aspirin, 60 mg	Aspirin, 325 mg
1400	Placebo	Aspirin, 100 mg	Aspirin, 650 mg

[a]Only perform where the capability to treat a severe reaction exists. Measure forces expiratory volume in 1 s (FEV_1) hourly after each dose. Challenge should be stopped after any sign of reaction: decrease of 20% in FEV_1, rhinorrhea, ocular injection, periorbital edema, or, rarely, stridor, flushing, abdominal cramps, diarrhea, or urticaria. (Adapted with permission from ref. *117*.)

However, provocation testing with inhaled Lysine-ASA has been developed that does not provoke such severe respiratory reactions, the fall in FEV_1 occurs within 20–45 min (faster), and is reversible with β_2-agonists. Overall the test is believed to be safer *(118)*.

Treatment

There is no cure for AIA, but there are some options for ongoing management.

- Strict avoidance of aspirin/NSAIDs.
- Leukotriene receptor antagonist therapy.
- Desensitization to aspirin (this induces tolerance to other NSAIDs also) with subsequent daily aspirin/NSAID therapy.

Strict Avoidance of Aspirin/NSAIDs

Multiple products contain aspirin or NSAIDS, so the patients with ASA must be well educated to scrutinize all over-the-counter products carefully and make sure a pharmacist has reviewed prescription products. For example, patients who are aspirin-sensitive have been administered ketorolac eyedrops for allergic conjunctivitis, and in a scenario repeated all too often, have received intramuscular ketorolac as a pain medication postoperatively. Table 12 shows medications that are generally safe in AIA. Some patients with aspirin-sensitive asthma may react to weak inhibitors of COX-1 if adequately high doses are given. Stevenson et al. studied 10 patients with AIA and found two who reacted to 2 g salsalate. When the patients were desensitized to aspirin, they no longer reacted to salsalate either *(119)*. Settipane and Stevenson studied three patients with AIA by double-blind, placebo-controlled challenges and two had a fall in FEV_1 more than 20%, with 1000 mg acetaminophen, a weak inhibitor of COX-1 at higher doses *(120)*. Two were desensitized to aspirin and were subsequently able to tolerate 1000 mg of acetaminophen without bronchospasm. Another study now suggests that up to 30% of patients with aspirin-sensitive asthma may react to acetaminophen, but only in large doses of 1000–1500 mg, and the bronchospasm seen has only been mild or moderate *(121)*. Thus, patients do not need to avoid acetaminophen in the standard dose range. Meloxicam and nimesulide (not in the United States) have mixed COX-1 and COX-2 inhibitory activity but are relatively COX-2 specific. These have induced asthma in AIA, but may be tolerated by most patients at lower doses *(122)*.

No cross-reactivity with tartrazine has been seen in properly controlled studies. Naturally occurring salicylates in foods have not been shown to cross-react with aspirin.

Table 12
Usually Tolerated in Patients With Asthma Who Are Aspirin-Sensitive

Salicylates
Sodium salicylate
Salicylamide
Salsalate
Diflunisal
Choline magnesium trisalicylate
COX-3 inhibitor (very weak COX-1 inhibitor), used at 650 mg or less
Acetaminophen
Selective COX-2 inhibitors
Rofecoxib
Celecoxib
NSAIDs with COX-2 inhibition more than COX-1 inhibition, used at lower doses
Nimesulide
Meloxicam

NSAIDs, nonsteroidal anti-inflammatory drugs; COX, cyclooxygenase.

Leukotriene Receptor Antagonist Therapy

There exists only one randomized, double-blind, placebo-controlled trial of the currently available $CysLT_1$ receptor blocker, montelukast, in the treatment of AIA, which is often moderate to severe in grade. Montelukast competitively antagonizes binding of LTC_4, LTD_4, and LTE_4 to its receptor. The trial studied 80 patients with challenge-proven AIA. After 4 wk of 10 mg of montelukast or placebo added nightly to their usual asthma therapy (glucocorticoids in 85–90% or theophylline), the montelukast group showed significant improvement in FEV_1 (10.2% increase, $p < 0.001$) and morning and evening PEFR ($p < 0.001$). There were also improvements in asthma-specific quality of life ($p < 0.05$) *(123)*. Previously, zileuton, a 5-lipoxygenase inhibitor, had also shown benefit in AIA management, but it is no longer marketed *(124)*.

Neither montelukast nor zileuton was able to provide adequate or consistent protection against provoked upper respiratory symptoms on oral aspirin challenge, however, so while taking such medication may be indicated for control of asthma, such therapy does not allow for use of NSAIDs in these patients *(106)*.

Aspirin Desensitization

If aspirin or standard NSAIDs are needed, or if the patient desires to better control severe asthma or hyperplastic sinus disease, desensitization can be performed. In this procedure, the patient is challenged with aspirin as in Table 11, but after a positive challenge has been obtained, the patient is then challenged the following day with the same dose that caused a reaction, and doses are continued upward until a reaction is obtained. The placebo day can be skipped if it is already demonstrated that the patient is aspirin sensitive. If a reaction is seen before 650 mg, the challenges are again stopped until the next day. The following day, challenges again start with the last dose to incite a reaction. When 650 mg is reached without a reaction, a refractory state results in which further doses of aspirin, or any other NSAID, will not induce a reaction *(106)*. This state persists for 2–5 d, then full sensitivity to aspirin returns. The mechanisms underlying this phenomenon are not clear. The patient is then instructed to take 650 mg of aspirin twice per day, but unfortunately, many desensitized patients experience gastritis and stop the medication *(125)*. Desensitization can be maintained by doses as low as 81–325 mg/d, but low doses have not been studied over the long term for beneficial effects on asthma or nasal polyposis. The beneficial clinical effects of desensitization, in 172 patients followed for 1–5 yr on 650 mg aspirin bid, included decreased nasal symptoms, decreased dosages of oral CSs (or taper off), fewer hospitalizations for asthma, and a lower frequency of sinus surgeries *(125)*. The same group also reported significantly improved asthma, nasal, and olfactory symptom scores in the first month of desensitization ($p < 0.0001$) *(126)*.

REFERENCES

1. Roberts G, Patel N, Levi-Schaffer F, Habibi P, Lack G. Food allergy as a risk factor for life-threatening asthma in childhood: a case-controlled study. *J Allergy Clin Immunol* 2003; 112: 168–174.
2. Bock SA, Munoz-Furlong A, Sampson HA. Fatalities due to anaphylactic reactions to foods. *J Allergy Clin Immunol* 2001; 107: 191–193.
3. Woods RK, Thien FC, Abramson MJ. Dietary marine fatty acids (fish oil) for asthma in adults and children. *Cochrane Database Systemic Rev* 2002; 3: CD001283.
4. Peat JK, Mihrshahi S, Kemp AS, et al. Three-year outcomes of dietary fatty acid modification and house dust mite reduction in the Childhood Asthma Prevention Study. *J Allergy Clin Immunol* 2004; 114: 807–813.
5. Oddy WH, de Klerk NH, Kendall GE, Mihrshahi S, Peat JK. Ratio of omega-6 to omega-3 fatty acids and childhood asthma. *J Asthma* 2004; 41: 319–326.
6. Woods RK, Raven JM, Walters EH, Abramson MJ, Thien FC. Fatty acid levels and risk of asthma in young adults. *Thorax* 2004; 59: 105–110.
7. Woods RK, Walters EH, Raven JM, et al. Food and nutrient intakes and asthma risk in young adults. *Am J Clin Nutr* 2003; 78: 414–421.
8. Sloan AE, Powers ME. A perspective on popular perceptions of adverse reactions to foods. *J Allergy Clin Immunol* 1986; 78: 127–133.
9. Altman DR, Chiaramone LT. Public perception of food allergy. *J Allergy Clin Immunol* 1996; 97: 1247–1251.
10. Sampson HA. Update on food allergy. *J Allergy Clin Immunol* 2004; 113: 805–819.
11. Parker SL, Leznoff A, Sussman GL, et al. Characteristics of patients with food-related complaints. *J Allergy Clin Immunol* 1990; 86: 503–511.
12. Bruijnzeel-Koomen C, Ortolani C, Aas K, et al. Adverse reactions to food. *Allergy* 1995; 50: 623–635.
13. Johansson S, Hourihane JO'B, Bousquet J, et al. A revised nomenclature for allergy. An EAACI position statement from the EAACI nomenclature task force. *Allergy* 2001; 56: 813–824.
14. Sicherer SH, Teuber SS, and the Adverse Reactions to Foods Committee. Current approach to the diagnosis and management of adverse reactions to foods. *J Allergy Clin Immunol* 2004; 114: 1146–1150.
15. Jakobsson I, Lindberg T. A prospective study of cow's milk protein intolerance in Swedish infants. *Acta Pediatr Scand* 1979; 68: 853–859.
16. Host A, Halken S. A prospective study of cow milk allergy in Danish infants during the first 3 years of life. *Allergy* 1990; 45: 587–596.
17. Schrander JJP, van den Bogart JPH, Forget PP, et al. Cow's milk protein intolerance in infants under 1 year of age: a prospective epidemiological study. *Eur J Pediatr* 1993; 152: 640–644.
18. Sicherer SH, Munoz-Furlong A, Sampson HA. Prevalence of peanut and tree nut allergy in the United States determined by means of a random digit dial telephone survey: a 5-year follow-up study. *J Allergy Clin Immunol* 2003; 112: 1203–1207.
19. Sicherer SH, Munoz-Furlong A, Sampson HA. Prevalence of seafood allergy in the United States determined by a random telephone survey. *J Allergy Clin Immunol* 2004; 114: 159–165.
20. Eggesbo M, Botten G, Halvorsen R, Magnus P. The prevalence of allergy to egg: a population-based study in young children. *Allergy* 2001; 56: 403–411.
21. Woods RK, Weiner J, Abramson M, Thein F, Walters EH. Patients' perceptions of food-induced asthma. *Austr N Z J Med* 1996; 26: 504–512.

22. Onorato J, Merland N, Terral C, et al. Placebo-controlled double-blind food challenge in asthma. *J Allergy Clin Immunol* 1986; 78: 1139–1146.

23. Novembre E, de Martino M, Vierucci A. Foods and respiratory allergy. *J Allergy Clin Immunol* 1988; 81: 1059–1065.

24. Oehling A, Cagnani CEB. Food allergy and child asthma. *Allergol Immunopathol* 1980; 8: 7–14.

25. James JM, Eigenmann PA, Eggleston PA, Sampson HA. Airway reactivity changes in asthmatic patients undergoing blinded food challenges. *Am J Respir Crit Care Med* 1996; 153: 597–603.

26. Zwetchkenbaum JF, Skufca R, Nelson HS. An examination of food hypersensitivity as a cause of increased bronchial responsiveness to inhaled methacholine. *J Allergy Clin Immunol* 1991; 88: 360–364.

27. Martin JA, Compaired JA, de la Hoz B, et al. Bronchial asthma induced by chick pea and lentil. *Allergy* 1992; 47: 185–187.

28. Roberts G, Golder N, Lack G. Bronchial challenges with aerosolized food in asthmatic food-allergic children. *Allergy* 2002; 57: 713–717.

29. Polasani R, Melgar L, Reisman RE, Ballow M. Hot dog vapor-induced status asthmaticus. *Ann Allergy Asthma Immunol* 1997; 78: 35–36.

30. Goetz DW, Whisman BA. Occupational asthma in a seafood restaurant worker: cross-reactivity of shrimp and scallops. *Ann Allergy Asthma Immunol* 2000; 85: 431–433.

31. Sicherer SH, Furlong TJ, DeSimone J, Sampson HA. Self-reported allergic reactions to peanut on commercial airliners. *J Allergy Clin Immunol* 1999; 104: 186–189.

32. Lee SY, Lee KS, Hong CH, Lee KY. Three cases of childhood nocturnal asthma due to buckwheat allergy. *Allergy* 2001; 56: 763–766.

33. Pascual CY, Crespo JF, Dominguez-Noche C, et al. IgE-binding proteins in fish and fish steam. *Monogr Allergy* 1996; 32: 174–180.

34. Houba R, Doekes G, Heederik D. Occupational respiratory allergy in bakery workers: a review of the literature. *Am J Ind Med* 1998; 34: 529–546.

35. Bernaola G, Echechipia S, Urrutia I, et al. Occupational asthma and rhinoconjunctivitis from inhalation of dried cow's mild caused by sensitization to alpha-lactalbumin. *Allergy* 1994; 49: 189–191.

36. Jeebhay MF, Robins TG, Lehrer SB, Lopata AL. Occupational seafood allergy: a review. *Occup Environ Med* 2001; 58: 553–562.

37. Crespo JF, Rodriguez J, Vives R, et al. Occupational IgE-mediated allergy after exposure to lupine seed flour. *J Allergy Clin Immunol* 2001; 108: 295–297.

38. Zuskin E, Kanceljak B, Schachter EN, Mustajbegovic J. Respiratory function and immunologic status in workers processing dried fruits and teas. *Ann Allergy Asthma Immunol* 1996; 77: 317–322.

39. Zuskin E, Kanceljak B, Schachter EN, et al. Respiratory function and immunologic status in cocoa and flour processing workers. *Am J Ind Med* 1998; 33: 24–32.

40. Smith AB, Bernstein DI, London MA, et al. Evaluation of occupational asthma from airborne egg protein exposure in multiple settings. *Chest* 1990; 98: 398–404.

41. Larese F, Fiorito A, Casasola F, et al. Sensitization to green coffee beans and work-related allergic symptoms in coffee workers. *Am J Ind Med* 1998; 34: 623–627.

42. Harding SM. Gastroesophageal reflux and asthma: insight into the association. *J Allergy Clin Immunol* 1999; 104: 251–259.

43. Simon RA, Stevenson DD, Arrygave CM, Tan EM. The relationship of plasma histamine to the activity of bronchial asthma. *J Allergy Clin Immunol* 1977; 60: 312–316.

44. Morrow JD, Margolies GR, Rowland BS, Roberts LJ. Evidence that histamine is the causative toxin of scombroid-fish poisoning. *N Engl J Med* 1991; 324: 716–720.

45. Feldman JM. Histaminuria from histamine rich foods. *Arch Intern Med* 1983; 143: 2099–2102.

46. Wantke F, Hemmer W, Haglmuller T, Gotz M, Jarisch R. Histamine in wine. Bronchoconstriction after a double-blind placebo-controlled red wine provocation test. *Int Arch Allergy Immunol* 1996; 110: 397–400.

47. Wohrl S, Hemmer W, Focke M, Rappersberger K, Jarisch R. Histamine intolerance-like symptoms in healthy volunteers after oral provocation with liquid histamine. *Allergy Asthma Proc* 2004; 25: 305–311.

48. Uragoda CG, Kottegoda SR. Adverse reactions to isoniazid on ingestion of fish with a high histamine content. *Tubercle* 1977; 58: 83–89.

49. Bock S, Buckley J, Holst A, et al. Proper use of skin tests with food extracts in diagnosis of food hypersensitivity. *Clin Allergy* 1978; 8: 559–564.

50. Sampson HA, Albergo R. Comparison of results of skin tests, RAST, and double-blind placebo-controlled food challenges in children with atopic dermatitis. *J Allergy Clin Immunol* 1984; 74: 26–33.

51. Bousquet J, Chanez P, Michel F. The respiratory tract and food hypersensitivity. In: *Food Allergy: Adverse Reactions to Foods and Food Additives.* Metcalfe D, Sampson H, Simon R (eds.). Blackwell Scientific Publications, Boston, 1991, pp. 139–149.

52. Bock SA, Sampson HA, Atkins FM, et al. Double-blind, placebo-controlled food challenge as an office procedure: a manual. *J Allergy Clin Immunol* 1988; 82: 986.

53. Vierk K, Falci K, Wolniak C, Klontz KC. Recalls of foods containing undeclared allergens reported to the US Food and Drug Administration, fiscal year 1999. *J Allergy Clin Immunol* 2002; 109: 1022–1026.

54. Burks W, Lehrer SB, Bannon GA. New approaches for treatment of peanut allergy: chances for a cure. *Clin Rev Allergy Immunol* 2004; 27: 191–196.

55. Teuber SS, Porch-Curren C. Unproved diagnostic and therapeutic approaches to food allergy and intolerance. *Curr Opin Allergy Clin Immunol* 2003; 3: 217–221.

56. Skolnick HS, Conover-Walker MK, Koerner CB, et al. The natural history of peanut allergy. *J Allergy Clin Immunol* 2001; 107: 367–374.

57. Asmus MJ, Sherman J, Hendeles L. Bronchoconstictor additives in bronchodilator solutions. *J Allergy Clin Immunol* 1999; 104: S53–S60

58. Weber RW, Hoffman M, Rane DA, Nelson HS. Incidence of bronchoconstrictions due to aspirin, azo dyes, non-azo dyes, and preservatives in a population of perennial asthmatic. *J Allergy Clin Immunol* 1979; 64: 32–37.

59. Stevenson DD, Simon RA, Lumry WR, Mathison DA. Adverse reactions to tartrazine. *J Allergy Clin Immunol* 1986; 78: 182–191.

60. Pleskow WW, Stevenson DD, Mathison DA, et al. Aspirin-sensitive rhinosinusitis/asthma: spectrum of adverse reactions to aspirin. *J Allergy Clin Immunol* 1983; 71: 574–579.

61. Simon RA. Specific challenge procedures: experimental methodology for studies of adverse reactions to foods and food additives. *J Allergy Clin Immunol* 1990; 86: 428–436.

62. Kochen J. Sulfur dioxide, a respiratory tract irritant, even if ingested (letter). *Pediatrics* 1973; 52: 145.

63. Taylor SL, Bush RK, Nordlee JA. Sulfites. In Metcalfe DD, Sampson HA, Simon RA (eds.). *Food Allergy: Adverse Reactions to Food and Food Additives.* Blackwell Scientific, Boston, 1997, pp. 339–357.

64. Simon RA, Green L, Stevenson DD. The incidence of ingested metabisulfite sensitivity in an asthmatic population [abstract]. *J Allergy Clin Immunol* 1982; 69: 118.

65. Bush RK, Taylor SL, Holden K, Nordlee JA, Busse WW. The prevalence of sensitivity to sulfiting agents in asthmatics. *Am J Med* 1986; 81: 816–820.

66. Sokol WN, Hydick IB. Nasal congestion, urticaria, and angioedema caused by an IgE-mediated reaction to sodium metabisulfite. *Ann Allergy* 1990; 65: 233–237.

67. Yang WH, Purchase ECR, Rivington RN. Positive skin tests and Prausnitz-Kustner reactions in metabisulfite sensitive subjects. *J Allergy Clin Immunol* 1986; 78: 443–449.

68. Wright W, Zhang YG, Salome CM, Woolcock AJ. Effect of inhaled preservatives on asthmatic subjects. I. Sodium metabisulfite. *Am Rev Respir Dis* 1990; 141: 1400–1404.

69. January 23, 1985. Sulfites on shrimp. *Fed Regist* 1985; 50: 2957.

70. July 9, 1986. Sulfiting agents; revocation of Generally Recognized as Safe status for use on fruits and vegetables intended to be served or sold raw to consumers. *Fed Regist* 1986; 51: 25021.

71. September 30, 1986. Labeling of sulfites in alcoholic beverages. BATF Notice No. 566. *Fed Regist* 1986; 51: 34706.

72. Nagy SM, Teuber SS, Loscutoff SM, Murphy PJ. Clustered outbreak of adverse reactions to a salsa containing high levels of sulfites. *J Food Prot* 1995; 58: 95–97.

73. Timbo B, Koehler KM, Wolyniak C, Klontz KC. Sulfites—a food and drug administration review of recalls and reported adverse events. *J Food Prot* 2004; 67: 1806–1811.

74. Taylor SL, Bush RK, Selner JC, et al. Sensitivity to sulfited foods among sulfite-sensitive subjects with asthma. *J Allergy Clin Immunol* 1982; 69: 335–338.

75. Vally H, Thompson PJ. Role of sulfite additives in wine induced asthma: single doses and cumulative dose studies. *Thorax* 2001; 56: 763–769.

76. Boushey HA. Bronchial hyperreactivity to sulfur dioxide: physiologic and political implications. *J Allergy Clin Immunol* 1982; 69: 335–338.

77. Delohery J, Simmul R, Castle WD, Allen DH. The relationship of inhaled sulfur dioxide reactivity to ingested metabisulfite sensitivity in patients with asthma. *Am Rev Respir Dis* 1984; 130: 1027–1032.

78. Simon R, Goldfarb G, Jacobsen D. Blocking studies in sulfite-sensitive asthmatics (SSA) [abstract]. *J Allergy Clin Immunol* 1984; 73: 136.

79. Bellofiore S, Caltagirone F, Pennisi A, et al. Neutral endopeptidase inhibitor, thiorphan, increases airway narrowing to inhaled sodium metabisulfite in normal subjects. *Am J Respir Crit Care Med* 1994; 150: 853–856.

80. Simon RA. Sulfite sensitivity. *Ann Allergy* 1986; 56: 281–288.

81. Bush RK. Sulfite and aspirin sensitivity: who is most susceptible? *J Respir Dis* 1987; 8: 23–32.

82. Allen DH, Delohery J, Baker GJ. Monosodium L-glutamate induced asthma. *J Allergy Clin Immunol* 1987; 80: 530–537.

83. Filer LJ, Steginkt LD, eds. A report of the proceeding of a MSG workshop held August 1991. *Crit Rev Food Sci Nutr* 1994; 34: 159–174.

84. Woessner KM, Simon RA, Stevenson DD. Monosodium glutamate sensitivity in asthma. *J Allergy Clin Immunol* 1999; 104: 305–310.

85. Stevenson DD. Monosodium glutamate and asthma. *J Nutr* 2000; 130: 1067S–1073S.

86. Stevenson DD, Simon RA, Lumry WR, Mathison DA. Adverse reactions to tartrazine. *J Allergy Clin Immunol* 1986; 78: 182–191.

87. Murdoch D, Pollock I, Young E, Lessof MH. Food additive induced urticaria: studies of mediator release during provocation tests. *J Royal College Phys* 1987; 4: 262–266.

88. Spector SL, Wangaard CH, Farr RS. Aspirin and concomitant idiosyncrasies in adult asthmatic patients. *J Allergy Clin Immunol* 1979; 64: 500–506.

89. Stenius BSM, Lemola M. Hypersensitivity to acetylsalicylic acid (ASA) and tartrazine in patients with asthma. *Clin Allergy* 1976; 6: 119–127.

90. Virchow C, Szczeklik A, Bianco S, et al. Intolerance to tartrazine in aspirin-induced asthma: results of a multicenter study. *Respiration* 1988; 53: 20–23.

91. Stevenson DD, Simon RA, Lumry WR, Mathison DA. Pulmonary reactions to tartrazine. *Pediatr Allergy Immunol* 1992; 3: 222–227.

92. Caucino JA, Armenaka M, Rosensteich DL. Anaphylaxis associated with a change in Premarin dye formulation. *Ann Allergy* 1994; 72: 33–35.

93. Gross PA, Lance K, Whitlock RJ, et al. Additive allergy: allergic gastroenteritis due to yellow dye #6. *Ann Intern Med* 1989; 111: 87–88.

94. Jacobsen DW. Adverse reactions to benzoates and parabens. In: *Food allergy: Adverse Reactions to Foods and Food Additives*. 2nd ed. Metcalfe DD, Sampson HA, Simon RA (eds.). Blackwell Science, Cambridge, MA, 1997, pp. 375–386.

95. Hoffman M. Challenges with aspirin, FD and C dyes and preservatives in asthma [abstract]. *J Allergy Clin Immunol* 1976; 57: 206–207.

96. Tarlo SM, Broder I. Tartrazine and benzoate challenge and dietary avoidance in chronic asthma. *Clin Allergy* 1982; 12: 303–312.

97. Nagel JE, Fuscaldo JT, Fireman P. Paraben allergy. *JAMA* 1977; 237: 1594–1595.

98. Goodman DL, McDonnell JT, Nelson HS, Vaughan TR, Weber RW. Chronic urticaria exacerbated by the antioxidant food addives, butylated hydroxyanisole (BHA) and butylated hydroxytoluene (BHT). *J Allergy Clin Immunol* 1990; 86: 570–575.

99. Kim SH, Ahn Y. Anaphylaxis caused by benzalkonium in a nebulizer solution. *J Korean Med Sci* 2004; 19: 289–290.

100. Beasley CRW, Rafferty P, Holgate ST. Bronchoconstrictor properties of preservatives in ipratropium bromide (Atrovent) nebulizer solution. *Br Med J* 1987; 294: 1197–1198.

101. Hedman J, Kaprio J, Poussa T, Nieminen MM. Prevalence of asthma, aspirin intolerance, nasal polyposis and chronic obstructive pulmonary disease in a population-based study. *Int J Epidemiol* 1999; 28: 717–722.

102. Kasper L, Stadek K, Duplaga M, et al. Prevalence of asthma with aspirin hypersensitivity in the adult population of Poland. *Allergy* 2003; 58: 1064–1066.

103. Vally H, Taylor ML, Thompson PJ. The prevalence of aspirin-intolerant asthma (AIA) in Australian asthmatic patients. *Thorax* 2002; 57: 569–574.

104. Szczeklik A, Nizankowska E, Duplaga M on behalf of the AIANE Investigators. Natural history of aspirin-induced asthma. *Eur Respir J* 2000; 16: 432–436.

105. Berges-Gimeno MP, Simon RA, Stevenson DD. The natural history and clinical characteristics of aspirin exacerbated respiratory disease. *Ann Allergy Asthma Immunol* 2002; 89: 472–478.

106. Szczeklik A, Stevenson DD. Aspirin-induced asthma: advances in pathogenesis, diagnosis, and management. *J Allergy Clin Immunol* 2003; 111: 913–921.

107. Picado C, Fernandez-Morata JC, Juan M, et al. Cyclooxygenase-2 mRNA is downexpressed in nasal polyps from aspirin-sensitive asthmatics. *Am J Respir Crit Care Med* 1999; 160: 291–296.

108. Cowburn AS, Sladek K, Soja J, et al. Overexpression of leukotriene C4 synthase in bronchial biopsies from patients with aspirin-intolerant asthma. *J Clin Invest* 1998; 101: 834–846.

109. Pierzchalska M, Szabo Z, Sanak M, Soja J, Szczeklik A. Deficient prostaglan E2 production by bronchial fibroblasts of asthmatic patients with special reference to aspirin-induced asthma. *J Allergy Clin Immunol* 2003; 111: 1041–1048.

110. Gylifors P, Bochenek G, Overholt J, et al. Biochemical and clinical evidence that aspirin intolerant asthmatic subjects tolerate the cyclooxygenase 2-selective analgetic drug celecoxib. *J Allergy Clin Immunol* 2003; 111: 1116–1121.

111. Stevenson DD, Simon RA. Lack of cross-reactivity between rofexocib and aspirin-sensitive patients with asthma. *J Allergy Clin Immunol* 2001; 108: 47–51.

112. Jinnai N, Sakagami T, Kakihara M, et al. Polymorphisms in the prostaglandin E2 receptor subtype 2 gene confer susceptibility to aspirin-intolerant asthma: a candidate gene approach. *Hum Mol Genet* 2004; 13: 3203–3217.

113. Daffern PJ, Muilenburg D, Hugli TE, Stevenson DD. Association of urinary leukotriene E4 excretion during aspirin challenges with severity of respiratory responses. *J Allergy Clin Immunol* 1999; 104: 559–564.

114. Christie PE, Tagari P, Ford-Hutchinson AW, et al. Urinary leukotriene E4 concentrations increase after aspirin challenges in aspirin-sensitive asthmatic subjects. *Am Rev Respir Dis* 1991; 143: 1025–1029.

115. Arm JP, O'Hickey SP, Spur BW, et al. Airway responsiveness to histamine and leukotriene E4 in subjects with aspirin-induced asthma. *Am Rev Respir Dis* 1989; 140: 148–153.

116. Sousa AR, Parkih A, Scadding G, Corrigan CJ, Lee TH. Leukotriene-receptor expression on nasal mucosal inflammatory cells in aspirin-sensitive rhinosinusitis. *N Engl J Med* 2002; 347: 1493–1499.

117. Stevenson DD. Oral challenge: aspirin, NSAIDs, tartrazine and sulfites. *N Engl Regional Allergy Proc* 1984; 5: 111–118.

118. Melillo G, Balzano G, Bianco S, et al. Oral and inhalation provocation tests for the diagnosis of aspirin-induced asthma. *Allergy* 2001; 56: 899–911.

119. Stevenson DD, Hougham AJ, Schrank PJ, Goldlust MB, Wilson RR. Salsalate cross-sensitivity in aspirin-sensitive patients with asthma. *J Allergy Clin Immunol* 1990; 86: 749–758.

120. Settipane RA, Stevenson DD. Cross-sensitivity with acetaminophen in aspirin-sensitive subjects with asthma. *J Allergy Clin Immunol* 1989; 84: 26–33.

121. Settipane RA, Shrank PJ, Simon RA, et al. Prevalence of cross-sensitivity with acetaminophen in aspirin sensitive subjects. *J Allergy Clin Immunol* 1995; 96: 480–485.

122. Bavbek S, Celik G, Ozer F, Mungan D, Misirligil Z. Safety of selective COX-2 inhibitors in aspirin/nonsteroidal anti-inflammatory drug-intolerant patients: comparison of nimesulide, meloxicam, and rofecoxib. *J Asthma* 2004; 41: 67–75.

123. Dahlen SE, Malmstrom K, Nizankowska E, et al. Improvement of aspirin-intolerant asthma by montelukast, a leukotriene antagonist. *Am J Respir Crit Care Med* 2002; 165: 9–14.

124. Dahlen B, Nizankowska E, Szczeklik A, et al. Benefits from adding the 5-lipoxygenase inhibitor zileuton to conventional therapy in aspirin-intolerant asthmatics. *Am J Respir Crit Care Med* 1998; 157: 1187–1194.

125. Berges-Gimeno M, Simon RA, Stevenson DD. Treatment with aspirin desensitization in patients with aspirin exacerbated respiratory disease. *J Allergy Clin Immunol* 2003; 111: 180–186.

126. Berges-Gimeno MP, Simon RA, Stevenson DD. Early effects of aspirin desensitization treatment in asthmatic patients with aspirin-exacerbated respiratory disease. *Ann Allergy Asthma Immunol* 2003; 90: 338–341.

13 Allergic Bronchopulmonary Aspergillosis

An Evolving Challenge in Asthma

Brian M. Morrissey, MD, and Samuel Louie, MD

CONTENTS

KEY POINTS

- Allergic bronchopulmonary aspergillosis (ABPA) represents an immunoglobulin E-mediated hypersensitivity to fungal antigens in patients with asthma.
- Consider the possibility of ABPA in difficult-to-control asthma cases.
- Reactive airway disease is commonly present in patients with ABPA.
- ABPA is not an invasive fungal infection but may occasionally mimic invasive diseases.
- Uncontrolled ABPA leads to progressive bronchiectasis and respiratory decline.
- Early recognition of ABPA—before bronchiectasis becomes permanent and severe—may alter the clinical course.
- Chest imaging can assist in early diagnosis.
- Computed tomography (CT) imaging can define the extent and severity of bronchiectasis and identify ABPA complications.
- Control of the acute and chronic inflammatory response is central to the treatment of ABPA.
- Antifungal therapy is an important adjunct to corticosteroids and may be steroid-sparing.

From: *Current Clinical Practice: Bronchial Asthma:*
A Guide for Practical Understanding and Treatment, 5th ed.
Edited by: M. E. Gershwin and T. E. Albertson © Humana Press Inc., Totowa, NJ

INTRODUCTION

Allergic bronchopulmonary aspergillosis (ABPA) describes a syndrome in which patients with asthma harbor the saprophytic growth of *Aspergillus* species, most often *Aspergillus fumigatus,* within their airways. An intense allergic inflammation results in response to fungal antigens, leading to clinical disease. ABPA represents an immunoglobulin (Ig)E-mediated hypersensitivity to *A. fumigatus* antigens, as well as non-Aspergillus fungal antigens in patients with asthma with persistent cough, wheezing, dyspnea, and, occasionally, fever. Recurring clinical exacerbations can lead to bronchiectasis, pulmonary fibrosis, and even death. ABPA is present in 1–2% of all patients with asthma and up to 15% of patients with cystic fibrosis (CF). Although the initial manifestations of disease may be subtle, more severe disease may be dramatic and, at times, life-threatening. The understanding of ABPA is evolving: recognition and treatment earlier in its natural history, certainly before bronchiectasis becomes permanent and severe, may alter the course of disease. ABPA is commonly unrecognized, because the early clinical course may mimic a chronically indolent case of moderate to severe persistent asthma requiring frequent oral corticosteroid (CS) therapy. Unrecognized and untreated ABPA can progress to repeated and prolonged periods of clinical asthma exacerbations. ABPA, like rhinosinusitis, gastroesophageal reflux disease (GERD), and chronic obstructive pulmonary disease (COPD) should be included whenever considering an asthma diagnosis. Assiduous therapy in ABPA can decrease the frequency of exacerbations and may slow the progressive lung damage, which can lead to pulmonary fibrosis and death.

ABPA DEFINED

ABPA represents a specific hypersensitivity to *Aspergillus* species growing within the lung manifested immunologically by elevated immunoglobulins, i.e., IgE specific to this fungus' antigens. An initial inoculum of fungal spores is believed to enter and seed the respiratory airways. Subsequently, the fungus grows branching, septated hyphae in a saprophytic manner within the susceptible airways. Susceptibility for ABPA may arise from a genetic predisposition or abnormal mucociliary clearance (e.g., areas of scarring, bronchiectasis) *(1,20)*. *Aspergillus* species are ubiquitous in the soil and are not limited to any particular geographic region, as are *coccidioides, Paracoccidioides,* blastomycetes, and histoplasma. Virtually everyone has been exposed to *Aspergillus,* and clinical disease likely requires predisposing factors. Because the fungi are fully contained within the airways—without invasion or penetration to the submucosa—they are not considered invasive *(3)*. However, even without invasive growth, an intense and perhaps overly exuberant, allergic and T-helper 2 (Th2)-dominant inflammatory response are stimulated. The characteristic ABPA inflammation contains large numbers of eosinophils, as well as neutrophils, Curschmann's spirals, desquamated epithelial cells, and mucous *(3)*. The often-associated parenchymal infiltrates are similar in character to those of eosinophilic pneumonia and are believed to arise in areas distal to mucous-obstructed airways. Unchecked, chronic inflammation leads to the progressive airway damage and bronchiectasis typically found in ABPA. As bronchiectasis becomes more severe, the density and number of inflammatory cells increases *(4)*, which parallel the development of chronic symptoms of cough, wheezing, and sputum production. The inflammation persists, and fibrotic changes can result.

Table 1
Reported Causes of Allergic Bronchopulmonary Mycosis

Fungi	Reference
Aspergillus sp.	—
Candida sp.	*39*
Fusarium	*40,41*
Pseudoallescheria boydii	*42*
Scedosporium apiospermum	*43*

The inflammatory and interleukin (IL) profile of inflammation in ABPA has an asthma-like Th2 dominant pattern *(5)*, with relatively low levels of IL-10 *(6)*. *Aspergillus* as a type II allergen is believed to produce proteases that impair tolerance—T-cell activity *(7)*. An increased sensitivity of the peripheral blood monocytes cells to IL-4 is also observed in ABPA *(8)*.

Because other non-*Aspergillus* species may cause similar clinical manifestations, an alternative more encompassing name, allergic bronchopulmonary mycosis (ABPM), may better describe the syndrome. ABPA is a more widely recognized term than ABPM. Nonetheless, other fungi should be considered as potentially causative. Clinicians should look for other fungi in the appropriate clinical scenarios, particularly when there is no objective evidence for *Aspergillus* (*see* Table 1).

Beyond this allergic lung disease, *Aspergillus* and other fungi may cause other pulmonary diseases, including pulmonary aspergilloma, chronic necrotizing aspergillosis, and invasive pulmonary aspergillosis. These invasive infections resulting from *Aspergillus* should not be confused with ABPA, because the clinical significance and therapies are different *(9)*. Selected cases of true infection may be difficult to differentiate from ABPA. Uncommonly, cases of ABPA may progress to include features of or progress into invasive disease *(10,11)*. The clinical setting and radiographic findings are often adequate to distinguish these invasive infections from ABPA. However, empiric antifungal treatment is used when invasive disease is suspected to prevent rapid progression while further diagnostic evidence is being gathered.

Other Pulmonary Syndromes Resulting From Aspergillus

Aspergillus is notorious for the variety of clinical presentations and extent of disease possible. Invasive or noninvasive growth depends largely on the host's immune system. Aspergilloma, chronic necrotizing pulmonary aspergillosis, and invasive pulmonary aspergillosis complete the clinical syndromes beyond ABPA caused by *Aspergillus*.

Pulmonary aspergilloma, or more generically pulmonary mycetoma, is an anatomically opportunistic fungal infection. A mycetoma typically forms within a cavity previously created by granulomatous lung disease (e.g., sarcoidosis or tuberculosis) or other cavitary lung diseases (e.g., site of lung abscess). Within the remaining cavity, inflammatory cells, fungi, and cellular debris combine to form a sphere or fungus ball. A posterior–anterior chest radiograph (CXR) or CT of the chest may incidentally reveal such a mass as the first indication of disease. A suggestive and nearly pathognomonic crescent-shaped radiolucency (Monod sign) or even a mobile sphere within the cavity may be detected. *(12)*. Most patients do not develop overt clinical disease, but should significant hemoptysis

(>50–200 mL/episode) or growth occur, hospitalization in a critical care unit and immediate surgical consultation or interventional radiology consultation are indicated.

Chronic necrotizing pulmonary aspergillosis, or so-called "semi-invasive" aspergillosis, describes a progressive fungal infection causing lung parenchymal destruction and, in most cases, locally limited. A cavity within the lung may form, and a secondary mycetoma can develop. Radiographically, chronic necrotizing aspergillosis may have similar characteristics as ABPA, and when they are not clinically distinct, bronchoscopy or biopsy may be necessary *(9)*. Treatment with systemic antifungal therapy has greatly reduced the need for surgical resection *(13)*.

Invasive fungal disease with *Aspergillus* is difficult to recognize early, but it is the most life-threatening pulmonary aspergillosis. Fortunately, this severe disease is rare outside of patients with serious immune compromise, e.g., persistent neutropenia, leukemia, or organ transplant-related immune suppression. The illness may be severe and acute, but the signs and symptoms are not distinct: profound respiratory distress with severe dyspnea and chest pain (that can be pleuritic), with or without fever. Nonetheless, in the at-risk neutropenic patient, these findings are often adequate enough to justify empiric antifungal treatment. Unlike in the case of ABPA, *Aspergillus* mycelia from either *A. fumigatus* or *A. flavus* invade through lung tissue and cause thrombosis of blood vessels, leading to area of pulmonary infarction. The radiographic changes of invasive disease can be focal or diffuse but typically do not have the characteristic central airway findings seen in ABPA, i.e., bronchiectasis. The clinical circumstances and symptoms in aspergilloma are distinct. Given the high mortality among at-risk individuals, any evidence of fungus should prompt a presumptive diagnosis of invasive disease and initiation of therapy—more definitive diagnosis requires lung biopsy.

MAKING THE DIAGNOSIS

At its essence, a diagnosis of active ABPA requires three elements be present: (1) reactive airway disease (asthma), (2) noninvasive fungi, and (3) an active allergic response to the fungus. Although some authors also call for bronchiectasis to be present, the authors of this chapter prefer not to require this for diagnosis.

Since the first case series descriptions of the syndrome, various diagnostic criteria have been developed. The variations in diagnostic criteria reflect clinician preferences and the serological testing available to them. In his initial description of ABPA in 1952, Hinson identified patients who had fungus in their airways, recurrent fevers, CXR changes, and blood eosinophilia *(3)*. In the 1970s, Safirstein (1973) and Rosenberg (1977) proposed similar criteria, which called for major (required) and minor (supportive) diagnostic information *(see* Table 2). They added serological testing data beyond peripheral blood eosinophilia (high serum IgE, immediate skin reaction to *Aspergillus* antigen, and precipitating antibodies) and called for central bronchiectasis to be present. Rosenberg includes serum precipitins to *Aspergillus* antigens and uses of IgE levels (>1000 ng/mm^3) as major criteria *(14,15)*.

The approach taken by the authors of this chapter to the diagnosis of ABPA uses standard criteria for asthma as outlined by regional societies (e.g., British or American Thoracic Society). To establish the presence of fungus, they obtain a culture of a high-quality expectorated sputum specimen. Rarely, a bronchoscopy will be necessary to obtain culture material or airway assessments. They use total serum IgE levels—in a

Table 2
Diagnostic Criteria

Safirstein et al. *(14)*
Major and minor criteria in 50 patients with ABPA

Major	Recurrent pulmonary densities in chest radiographs
	Eosinophilia in sputum and blood
	Asthma
	Allergy to *Aspergillus fumigatus* (Type 1 or Type 3)
Minor	Recovery of *A. fumigatus* from sputum
	A. fumigatus serum precipitins
	History of recurrent pneumonia
	History of plugs in expectorated sputum

Rosenberg et al. *(46)*
Major and minor criteria

Major	History of pulmonary infiltrates
	Peripheral blood eosinophilia
	Asthma
	Immediate skin reactivity to *Aspergillus*
	Precipitins to *Aspergillus* antigens
	Central bronchiectasis
	Elevated serum immunoglobulin (Ig) E
Minor	Recovery of *Aspergillus* from sputum
	History of expectoration of brown plugs or flecks
	Arthus reaction to *Aspergillus* antigen (Type 3)

All patients fulfilled major criteria, and 66–88% of patients fulfilled one or more minor criteria.

similar manner as recommended for patients with CF—as a screening test in patients who are at risk. When this general marker of allergic inflammation exceeds 1000 ng/mm^3, they perform further specific testing.

Radioallergoabsorbent testing (RAST), or serum precipitins specific for *Aspergillus* species' antigens, identify specific hypersensitivity in patients with ABPA (as alternatives to skin-prick testing) to *Aspergillus*-specific antigens. A diagnosis of ABPA or flare of existing disease is made when there is evidence of a specific allergic response to fungus and total IgE levels are more than 1000 ng/mL or twice a patient's baseline.

Bronchiectasis, which is found in the preponderance (>80%) of cases of ABPA, is best detected by noncontrast high-resolution CT and may not be apparent on posterior–anterior CXRs. Bronchiectasis should be considered a late finding in ABPA. Waiting for bronchiectasis to become apparent may significantly delay the recognition of early ABPA and thwart efforts at preventing the permanent airway damage.

Clinical Manifestations

Individuals with asthma or CF are at risk for ABPA. Nearly 2% of patients with asthma have ABPA. In patients with asthma who require oral CSs, the incidence triples to 6% *(16)*. Initially, these patients may have few distinguishing findings other than difficult-to-control or persistent asthma. With progression of disease, patients may report intense bouts of coughing and production of sputum with grit or small bits of

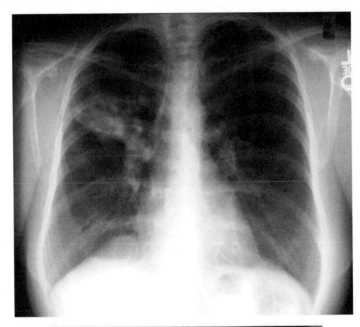

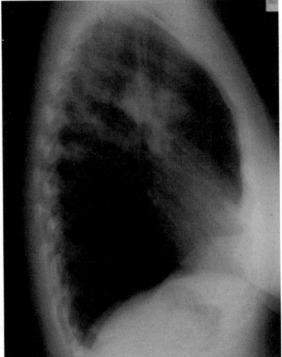

Fig. 1. Posterior–anterior and lateral chest radiographs of a woman with severe ABPA. Dense airway filling and parenchymal infiltrate are present. The companion computed tomography images show finger-in-glove finding of mucous-filled and grossly dilated airways and findings of bronchiectasis (dilated, thickened, and irregular bronchi).

brown hard matter. These represent mucous plugs or small casts of the airways and often contain fungal elements when examined by microscopy. Unusual presentations and manifestations of ABPA include eosinophilic pleural effusions, hemoptysis, and

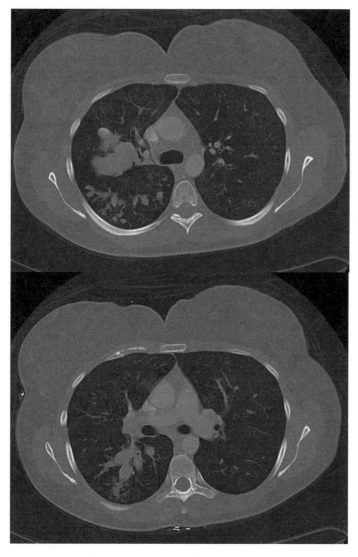

Fig. 1. *(Continued)*

the development of super infections *(17)*. Hemoptysis in ABPA from bronchiectasis is often minimal and rarely massive.

Radiology

CXRs of patients with ABPA may be normal or show signs of bronchiectasis, mucous plugging, or focal infiltrates in an alveolar filling pattern suggestive of eosinophilic infiltration and inflammation *(14,15)* *(see* Fig. 1). Central airway bronchiectasis—third- to fifth-generation bronchi (thickened, dilated, or distorted airways)—is characteristic of ABPA. Chest radiographic patterns include circular shadows, parallel nontapering lines (ectatic airways), dense cylindrical shadows (mucous plugs), finger-in-glove (mucous plugs), or signet ring patterns (increased bronchus:artery ratio) *(12,18)*. Bronchiectasis is most clearly identified by high-resolution/thin-cut CT scan. Distal to an obstructed airway, an alveolar pattern or infiltrate may develop. These diffuse or "fleeting infiltrates"

Table 3
Selected Antifungal Therapy Reports in ABPA

Drug (dosing)	Description	Outcome (reference)
Ketoconazole (400 mg/d)	12 months	Decreased immunoglobulin (Ig) E and symptoms (44)
Itraconazole (400 mg/d)	RDBPC, n = 29, 16 wk	Decreased IgE, fewer exacerbations (35)
Itraconazole (400 mg/d)	RDBPC, n = 55, 16 wk	Decrease of corticosteroid dose and improved x-rays and PFTs (33)
Itraconazole	Open, n = 14, 2 yr	Decrease of corticosteroid dose, total IgE (34)
Itraconazole (≥200 mg/d)	Observational, n = 14	Decreased corticosteroid use, decreased eosinophilia, decreased exacerbations (34)
Itraconazole (no corticosteroids)	Case reports	Resolution of symptoms (45)

of ABPA may be wedge shaped in a pattern representing the affected segment or subsegment obstructed by mucous plugging or intense eosinophilic inflammation. Although chest CT is more sensitive and specific for APBA, it is not routinely required. Serial imaging by CXRs or CT is important in assessing response to therapy and monitoring for progression of disease or complications (19). Clinical correlation is necessary. This is particularly important because radiographs may reveal focal infiltrates, mucous plugs, or bronchiectasis even in the patient who is asymptomatic (14).

Serology

Serological measures, such as total IgE and specific IgE (RAST and immunoprecipitins) are helpful in diagnosing and managing ABPA. Immunoprecipitin testing or RAST may detect *Aspergillus* precipitins and specific IgE antibodies against the fungus in the patient with ABPA. For both diagnosis and to monitor response to therapy, most clinicians use total serum IgE levels. Levels more than 1000 ng/mL in patients with CF or others are considered consistent with a diagnosis of ABPA or poorly controlled disease. IgE levels often correlate well with clinical status and identify response to therapy (20). Serial measurements of IgE thus may guide therapeutic efforts. However, elevated serum IgE levels are not specific to ABPA and may also be elevated in other fungal infections, asthma without ABPA, parasitic infections, and allergic rhinosinusitis. Total and specific IgE levels can be elevated in the absence of ABPA when bronchiectasis is present—some 11% of patients with CF and 17% of those with idiopathic bronchiectasis may have elevated levels with or without the other diagnostic criteria for ABPA (21,22).

CLASSIFICATIONS OF ABPA

At least two different classification schemes have been proposed for assessing the ABPA severity. The first, a staging system, separates patients into stages I–V and reflects the various manifestations of ABPA but may not necessarily reflect the progression of disease. The stages reflect a combination of disease response to corticosteroids, severity of disease, time course, and radiographic changes (23) (see Table 4).

Table 4
Classifications of ABPA

Stage (23)
- I Acute—meets diagnostic criteria and is responsive to corticosteroid therapy
- II Remission—free of significant symptoms or asthma after corticosteroid therapy
- III Exacerbation—characterized by periods of worsened symptoms, radiographs,
  orincreased serum immunoglobulin (Ig) E
- IV Corticosteroid-dependent asthma—patients unable to discontinue corticosteroid therapy
- V Fibrotic disease—significant structural changes (radiographic) and irreversible airflow
  obstruction with corticosteroid-dependent asthma

Severity
- Mild—"ABPA-serological"
    Aspergillus skin test (+), elevated serum IgE, and eosinophilia
- Moderate—"ABPA central bronchiectasis" (CB)
    Serological diagnosis
    Central bronchiectasis on chest computed tomography
- Severe—"ABPA-CB-other radiological features" (ORF)
    Serological diagnosis
    Central bronchiectasis
    Other radiological features, including pulmonary fibrosis, blebs,
      bullae, pneumothorax, pleural effusion, or collapse *(24)*

The second classification system orders patients into groups based on radiographic abnormalities. This method, classifying patients based on varying degrees of structural lung damage (no changes, central bronchiectasis, central bronchiectasis, and more), orders patients by severity of disease (mild, moderate, or severe) *(24)* (Table 4).

A third classification system, using solely a radiographic scoring system, has also been devised, which roughly correlates with clinical disease *(25)*.

Classifications are likely most important to the study of the disease or populations with ABPA. Most helpful to the authors' patients and to the authors—for planning therapy and anticipating complications—are the degree of respiratory impairment and structural lung disease.

ABPA MIMICS

Allergic fungal sinusitis may be confused with ABPA, particularly because many patients with asthma have concurrent sinus disease. Allergic fungal sinusitis is similar to ABPA, but the sinus cavities are the site of saprophytic infection and may be coincident with ABPA. (In one study, 13% of patients with ABPA had findings of sinusitis on CT [18]). Serological measures (RAST, IgE, and immunoprecipitins) will not distinguish ABPA from allergic sinusitis. Radiographic imaging (sinus CT) and suggestive findings on history and physical examination may identify this ABPA look-alike.

Individuals with CF, an autosomal recessive genetic disease, have a relatively high incidence of ABPA (6–15%) as compared to the general population *(2,26)*. Whether this reflects a genetic predisposition or an increased risk resulting from the associated bronchiectasis remains uncertain. Rarely, the onset of ABPA may represent the first sign of CF. Based on retrospective analyses of patients with ABPA, some investigators suggest that CF genes are more common in individuals with ABPA *(27)*. They suggest that individuals who are heterozygotic for a gene that causes CF are predisposed to develop ABPA. However, there are no prospective population studies to confirm this interpretation.

Other eosinophilic pneumonias should be remembered when considering ABPA. These loosely describe a collection of pulmonary pathologies associated with elevated serum eosinophil levels. Of these diseases, Churg-Strauss and infectious eosinophilic pneumonias bear some resemblance to ABPA. Both may be associated with wheezing, eosinophilic pulmonary infiltrates, and blood eosinophilia.

The allergic granulomatous, angiitis, and periarteritis nodosa of Churg-Strauss syndrome often manifests systemic findings owing to small vessel vasculitis. The eosinophilia, although nonspecific, is often greater than typically seen in ABPA. Definitive diagnosis relies on pathological examination of a lung biopsy for eosinophilic pneumonia and, most important, small vessel angiitis *(28)*. Infectious eosinophilic pneumonias, which may result from infection with an endemic parasite (or fungi, e.g., *Coccidioides immitis*), characteristically present with high levels of eosinophilia, an exposure to an infectious agent, and prominent systemic infectious manifestations *(28)*.

TREATMENT

The related goals of therapy, preservation of pulmonary function and control of symptoms, guide therapeutic decisions. Total serum (i.e., not *Aspergillus*-specific), IgE levels provide measures of immunological activity and response to therapy. Additionally, pulmonary function testing, patient symptoms, other markers of inflammation, and radiographs are used singly and in combination to adjust therapy.

Unchecked inflammation ultimately results in progressive bronchiectasis and potentially other complications, including pulmonary fibrosis. This concern supports the use of primary therapy with corticosteroids aimed at controlling inflammation. Because asymptomatic patients may have progressive disease *(14)*, the authors also follow total IgE levels aiming to decrease the total IgE level by at least 50%. CXRs and pulmonary function tests forced expiratory volume in 1 s and forced vital capacity, including carbon monoxide-diffusing capacity, may be used to monitor disease activity. In stable patients, quarterly or semiannual assessments with improvement prompt a decrease in CS dosing. Despite control of pulmonary function, symptoms, and radiographic abnormalities, some patients will have persistently elevated IgE levels. Thus, a 50% decrease in total IgE has been proposed as an alternate measure of significant response to therapy. Patients with worsened findings trigger increased or resumption of CS therapy and consideration of antifungal medication. In patients whose disease remains recalcitrant to the authors' treatment plan, they pursue a thorough reevaluation within a period of days or weeks, not months, for invasive non-*Aspergillus* fungal infection, superinfection with bacteria or alternative *Aspergillus* clinical syndromes, and even lung cancer.

Corticosteroids

For decades, the treatment of ABPA has been directed at the host's immune response to the fungi in the airways. However, a recent addition to this treatment paradigm stems from the introduction of antifungal azoles. Oral CSs remain the mainstay of ABPA therapy. The use of CSs in ABPA has moderate case-based data and empiric clinical evidence as support. In a 1973 review of 50 patients with ABPA, Safirstein found that CS therapy (average daily dose: 10.5 mg) decreased the frequency of exacerbations *(14)*. Common practice initiates therapy with a daily dose of 0.5 mg/kg. In acute cases, CSs are administered for 2–8 wk, followed by a gradual reduction. Symptoms, serology, pulmonary function testing, and radiographs guide the reduction of CSs. The sequential tapering of corticosteroids may be to lower daily doses or more commonly to every-other-day dosing.

In an effort to decrease the adverse effects of systemic CSs, inhaled CSs are often proposed as possible adjuncts to disease control. Although many clinicians may prescribe inhaled CSs, they are routinely employed primarily as therapy for the coincident asthma. A few case series suggest some efficacy in control of symptoms using inhaled CSs *(29)*. More formal prospective trials have *only* shown better asthma control without significant benefit in other ABPA disease manifestations *(30)*.

Allergen avoidance is a long-standing therapeutic recommendation for allergic diseases. Unfortunately, this is not easily accomplished in the case of ABPA and has not proven clinically beneficial. *Aspergillus* is a nearly ubiquitous organism such that environmental control is unlikely to ever be fully efficacious. Additionally, the patient harbors the antigen source within his or her own airways. Because the offending organism/allergen has taken up residence in the patient, antifungal medications have been used in an attempt to decrease the allergen load and saprophytic organisms.

Antifungal Medications

For several decades, antifungal medications have been considered and used in patients with ABPA in attempts to decrease the antigen burden and need for CS therapy. Initial trials of inhaled antifungals, such as natamycin, and more recent efforts failed to show clinical efficacy *(31,32)*. Inhaled, instilled, and systemic delivery of amphotericin has been used without formal assessments. However, the azoles, a newer group of antifungal medications, may have some use in ABPA and have been the subject of several ABPA studies (Table 2).

Ketoconazole, the first azole studied, showed some clinical improvements but the associated risk of liver toxicity and adrenal suppression has prevented it from gaining much use in ABPA. Itraconazole, with moderately good oral preparations, a better safety profile, and excellent activity against *Aspergillus* species, has shown an ability to decrease the average CS dose (14 mg/d) needed for ABPA *(33,34)*. Most reports are of case–control studies, but recent blinded prospective trials have shown modest benefits with the use of itraconazole *(35)*. The mechanism of these ascribed benefits may be through inhibition of fungal growth, interference with CS metabolism, or some other yet-unrecognized process. Voriconazole, another azole with a good oral preparation and excellent efficacy against aspergillus, may also prove useful, but it remains clinically untested *(36)*.

For patients who respond rapidly and remain stable after moderate courses of CSs, the added expense, monitoring, and additional risks of oral azole therapy may not be justifiable. On the other hand, for patients in whom the adverse effects of CSs are severe and have disease severe enough to need prolonged daily therapy, the CS-sparing effects of adjunctive azole therapy appears worthwhile.

Other Management Issues

The associated bronchiectatic airways of ABPA thwart the normal mucociliary clearance of the lung. Devices and maneuvers to improve airway clearance have become a standard in the management of bronchiectasis *(37)*. As an adjunct to chemotherapy, sputum clearance may be beneficial to patients with ABPA, particularly if they have already developed significant bronchiectasis.

Invasive disease should always be considered. Albeit rare in the typical immuno-competent patient with asthma with ABPA, when increasing dosages of or prolonged therapy with CSs are required, invasive disease must be reconsidered *(38)*. Radiographic imaging, particularly high-resolution chest CT scanning, can usually distinguish an invasive radiologic pattern from patterns that are more typical of aspergilloma or other diagnoses, e.g., sarcoidosis.

The damaged bronchiectatic airways of the patient with ABPA bring increased risk for other airway infections as well. Bacterial superinfection should be considered in the patient with ABPA who worsens or has increased symptoms despite appropriate therapy. Probable pathogens are numerous but are likely to be those most commonly implicated in nonspecific bronchiectasis: *Haemophilus influenza*, *Staphylococcus aureus*, *Pseudomonas aeruginosa*, and mycobacterial species. Intermittent surveillance with sputum cultures may identify the probable pathogens and the chronically infected at-risk patient.

An increased risk of hemoptysis accompanies most diseases with chronic lung infec-tions or bronchiectasis. ABPA is no exception. Small amounts of bloody sputum may be present with cases of more severe ABPA disease usually from the severe bronchiectasis. Nonetheless, should severe hemoptysis develop, a bronchial artery source should be considered and definitive therapy with bronchial artery embolization offered. Chest CT imaging can usually identify an aspergilloma that may require definitive treatment with surgical resection *(11)*.

SUMMARY

ABPA represents an IgE-mediated hypersensitivity to *A. fumigatus* antigens, as well as non-*Aspergillus* fungal antigens. ABPA is a potentially severe and destructive lung disease, but milder forms of the disease most often accompany patients with moderate to severe persistent asthma and in patients with CF. The diagnosis of ABPA should always be suspected in patients with asthma who have difficult-to-control symptoms, require systemic CSs for control, have sputum production, or have abnormal CXRs. The diagnosis of ABPA requires evidence of a specific and intense allergic response to *Aspergillus* species in a patient with asthma without evidence of invasive fungal disease. Serum IgE levels (>1000 ng/mm^3) are sensitive for diagnosis and helpful in chronic disease man-agement, particularly response to pharmacotherapy. Treatment aims to preserve lung function, maintain quality of life, and reduce exacerbation rate through the control of the inflammatory response with prednisone and decreasing antigen exposure. Antifungal azole antibiotics are an adjunctive therapy to CSs and can decrease the need for high dosages of systemic CSs. ABPA management is evolving such that earlier diagnosis and intervention may prevent or forestall bronchiectasis.

REFERENCES

1. Aron Y, Bienvenu T, Hubert D, et al. HLA-DR polymorphism in allergic bronchopulmonary aspergillosis. *J Allergy Clin Immunol* 1999; 104(4 Pt 1): 891–892.
2. Mastella G, Rainisio M, Harms HK, et al. Allergic bronchopulmonary aspergillosis in cystic fibrosis. A European epidemiological study. Epidemiologic Registry of Cystic Fibrosis. *Eur Respir J* 2000; 16: 464–471.

3. Hinson KF, Moon AJ, Plummer NS. Broncho-pulmonary aspergillosis: a review and a report of eight new cases. *Thorax* 1952; 7: 317–333.

4. Wark PA, Saltos N, Simpson J, et al. Induced sputum eosinophils and neutrophils and bronchiectasis severity in allergic bronchopulmonary aspergillosis. *Eur Respir J* 2000; 16: 1095–1101.

5. Skov M, Poulsen LK, Koch C. Increased antigen-specific Th-2 response in allergic bronchopulmonary aspergillosis (ABPA) in patients with cystic fibrosis. *Pediatr Pulmonol* 1999; 27: 74–79.

6. Grunig G, Corry DB, Leach MW, et al. Interleukin-10 is a natural suppressor of cytokine production and inflammation in a murine model of allergic bronchopulmonary aspergillosis. *J Exp Med* 1997; 185: 1089–1099.

7. Kheradmand F, Kiss A, Xu J, et al. A protease-activated pathway underlying Th cell type 2 activation and allergic lung disease. *J Immunol* 2002; 169: 5904–5911.

8. Khan S, McClellan JS, Knutsen AP. Increased sensitivity to IL-4 in patients with allergic bronchopulmonary aspergillosis. *Int Arch Allergy Immunol* 2000; 123: 319–326.

9. Stevens DA, Kan VL, Judson MA, et al. Practice guidelines for diseases caused by Aspergillus. Infectious Diseases Society of America. *Clin Infect Dis* 2000; 30: 696–709.

10. Chung Y, Kraut JR, Stone AM, Valaitis J. Disseminated aspergillosis in a patient with cystic fibrosis and allergic bronchopulmonary aspergillosis. *Pediatr Pulmonol* 1994; 17: 131–134.

11. Bodey GP, Glann AS. Central nervous system aspergillosis following corticosteroidal therapy for allergic bronchopulmonary aspergillosis. *Chest* 1993; 103: 299–301.

12. Reiff DB, Wells AU, Carr DH, Cole PJ, Hansell DM. CT findings in bronchiectasis: limited value in distinguishing between idiopathic and specific types. *Am J Roentgenol* 1995; 165: 261–267.

13. Saraceno JL, Phelps DT, Ferro TJ, Futerfas R, Schwartz DB. Chronic necrotizing pulmonary aspergillosis: approach to management. *Chest* 1997; 112: 541–548.

14. Safirstein BH, D'Souza MF, Simon G, Tai EH, Pepys J. Five-year follow-up of allergic bronchopulmonary aspergillosis. *Am Rev Respir Dis* 1973; 108: 450–459.

15. Rosenberg M, Mintzer R, Aaronson DW, Patterson R. Allergic bronchopulmonary aspergillosis in three patients with normal chest x-ray films. *Chest* 1977; 72: 597–600.

16. Kumar R, Gaur SN. Prevalence of allergic bronchopulmonary aspergillosis in patients with bronchial asthma. *Asian Pac J Allergy Immunol* 2000; 18: 181–185.

17. O'Connor TM, O'Donnell A, Hurley M, Bredin CP. Allergic bronchopulmonary aspergillosis: a rare cause of pleural effusion. *Respirology* 2001; 6: 361–363.

18. Panchal N, Bhagat R, Pant C, Shah A. Allergic bronchopulmonary aspergillosis: the spectrum of computed tomography appearances. *Respir Med* 1997; 91: 213–219.

19. Munro NC, Han LY, Currie DC, Strickland B, Cole PJ. Radiological evidence of progression of bronchiectasis. *Respir Med* 1992; 86: 397–401.

20. Rosenberg M, Patterson R, Roberts M. Immunologic responses to therapy in allergic bronchopulmonary aspergillosis: serum IgE value as an indicator and predictor of disease activity. *J Pediatr* 1977; 91: 914–917.

21. Pasteur MC, Helliwell SM, Houghton SJ, et al. An investigation into causative factors in patients with bronchiectasis. *Am J Respir Crit Care Med* 2000; 162(Pt 1): 1277–128.

22. Nepomuceno IB, Esrig S, Moss RB. Allergic bronchopulmonary aspergillosis in cystic fibrosis: role of atopy and response to itraconazole. *Chest* 1999; 115: 364–370.

23. Patterson R, Greenberger PA, Radin RC, Roberts M. Allergic bronchopulmonary aspergillosis: staging as an aid to management. *Ann Intern Med* 1982; 96: 286–291.

24. Kumar R, Singh P, Arora R, Gaur SN. Effect of itraconazole therapy in allergic bronchopulmonary aspergillosis. *Saudi Med J* 2003; 24: 546–547.

25. Kiely JL, Spense L, Henry M, et al. Chest radiographic staging in allergic bronchopulmonary aspergillosis: relationship with immunological findings. *Eur Respir J* 1998; 12: 453–456.

26. Mroueh S, Spock A. Allergic bronchopulmonary aspergillosis in patients with cystic fibrosis. *Chest* 1994; 105: 32–36.

27. Marchand E, Verellen-Dumoulin C, Mairesse M, et al. Frequency of cystic fibrosis transmembrane conductance regulator gene mutations and 5T allele in patients with allergic bronchopulmonary aspergillosis. *Chest* 2001; 119: 762–767.

28. Cordier J. Eosinophilic pneumonias. In M. I. A. K. Schwarz, T. E. (ed.). *Intersitial lung disease*, 4th ed. B C Decker, Inc., Hamilton, Ontario, 2003, pp. 657–700.

29. Seaton A, Seaton RA, Wightman AJ. Management of allergic bronchopulmonary aspergillosis without maintenance oral corticosteroids: a fifteen-year follow-up. *QJM* 1994; 87: 529–537.

30. Inhaled beclomethasone dipropionate in allergic bronchopulmonary aspergillosis. Report to the Research Committee of the British Thoracic Association. *Br J Dis Chest* 1979; 73: 349–356.
31. Henderson AH, Pearson JE. Treatment of bronchopulmonary aspergillosis with observations on the use of natamycin. *Thorax* 1968; 23: 519–523.
32. Currie DC, Lueck C, Milburn HJ, et al. Controlled trial of natamycin in the treatment of allergic bronchopulmonary aspergillosis. *Thorax* 1990; 45: 447–450.
33. Stevens DA, Schwartz HJ, Lee JY, et al. A randomized trial of itraconazole in allergic bronchopulmonary aspergillosis. *N Engl J Med* 2000; 342: 756–762.
34. Salez F, Brichet A, Desurmont S, et al. Effects of itraconazole therapy in allergic bronchopulmonary aspergillosis. *Chest* 1999; 116: 1665–1668.
35. Wark PA, Hensley MJ, Saltos N, et al. Anti-inflammatory effect of itraconazole in stable allergic bronchopulmonary aspergillosis: a randomized controlled trial. *J Allergy Clin Immunol* 2003; 111: 952–957.
36. Murphy M, Bernard EM, Ishimaru T, Armstrong T. Activity of voriconazole (UK-109,496) against clinical isolates of Aspergillus species and its effectiveness in an experimental model of invasive pulmonary aspergillosis. *Antimicrob Agents Chemother* 1997; 41: 696–698.
37. Morrissey BM, Evans SJ. Severe bronchiectasis. *Clin Rev Allergy Immunol* 2003; 25: 233–247.
38. Sancho JM, Ribera JM, Rosell A, Munoz C, Feliu E. Unusual invasive bronchial aspergillosis in a patient with acute lymphoblastic leukemia. *Haematologica* 1997; 82: 701–702.
39. Pinson P, Van der Straeten M. Fibrotic stage of allergic bronchopulmonary candidiasis. *Chest* 1991; 100: 565–567.
40. Saini SK, Boas SR, Jerath A, Roberts M, Greenberger PA. Allergic bronchopulmonary mycosis to Fusarium vasinfectum in a child. *Ann Allergy Asthma Immunol* 1998; 80: 377–380.
41. Backman KS, Roberts M, Patterson R. Allergic bronchopulmonary mycosis caused by *Fusarium vasinfectum*. *Am J Respir Crit Care Med* 1995; 152(Pt 1): 1379–1381.
42. Miller MA, Greenberger PA, Amerian R, et al. Allergic bronchopulmonary mycosis caused by *Pseudallescheria boydii*. *Am Rev Respir Dis* 1993; 148: 810–812.
43. Cimon B, Carrere J, Vinatier JF, et al. Clinical significance of Scedosporium apiospermum in patients with cystic fibrosis. *Eur J Clin Microbiol Infect Dis* 2000; 19: 53–56.
44. Shale DJ, Faux JA, Lane DJ. Trial of ketoconazole in non-invasive pulmonary aspergillosis. *Thorax* 1987; 42: 26–31.
45. Fujimori Y, Tada S, Kataoka M, et al. Allergic bronchopulmonary aspergillosis effectively treated with itraconazole. *Nihon Kokyuki Gakkai Zasshi* 1998; 36: 781–786.
46. Rosenberg M, Patterson R, Mintzer R, Cooper BJ, Roberts M, Harris KE. Clinical and immunologic criteria for the diagnosis of allergic bronchopulmonary aspergillosis. *Ann Intern Med* 1977; 86: 405–414.

14 Occupational Asthma

A Special Environmental Interaction

Nicholas J. Kenyon, MD, Brian M. Morrissey, MD, and Timothy E. Albertson, PhD, MD, MPH

CONTENTS

KEY POINTS

- Occupational asthma is the most common occupational lung disease.
- Occupational asthma and work-aggravated asthma are the two forms of asthma causally related to the workplace.
- Reactive airways dysfunction syndrome is a separate entity and a subtype of occupational asthma.

From: *Current Clinical Practice: Bronchial Asthma:*
A Guide for Practical Understanding and Treatment, 5th ed.
Edited by: M. E. Gershwin and T. E. Albertson © Humana Press Inc., Totowa, NJ

- The diagnosis of occupational asthma is most often made on clinical grounds; the gold-standard test, specific inhalation challenge, is rarely used.
- Low-molecular-weight isocyanates are the most common compounds that cause occupational asthma.
- Workers with occupational asthma secondary to low-molecular-weight agents may not have elevated specific immunoglobulin E levels. The mechanisms of occupational asthma associated with these compounds are partially described.
- Not all patients with occupational asthma will improve after removal from the workplace.

INTRODUCTION

Occupation-related asthma is the most common lung disease found in the workplace today. It has surpassed silicosis and other pneumoconioses both in incidence and in attention from the National Institute of Occupation Safety and Health (NIOSH). There are two major subtypes of work-related asthma: occupational asthma (OA)—the most common form—and work-aggravated asthma. Diagnosing patients with either subtype is difficult, in part, because the gold-standard diagnostic test—specific inhalation challenge—is neither readily available nor commonly used. More than 400 proteins, glycoproteins, and chemicals in the workplace can cause asthma. Although the mechanisms leading to the development of occupational asthma are not fully outlined, significant advances have been made in the past decade. High-molecular-weight (HMW) agents classically trigger the production of specific immunogobulin (Ig)E, whereas low-molecular-weight (LMW) agents generally do not, and cause occupational asthma through a host of pathways. The explosion in genomic and proteomic technologies will greatly improve our understanding of the role of these molecules in the development of occupational asthma. Treatment of occupational asthma centers on removing the worker from the workplace and prescribing standard controller medications, such as inhaled corticosteroids (CSs) and long-acting β-agonists. Unfortunately, a subset of individuals who develop asthma at work will not improve, and this group is the focus of intense study.

EPIDEMIOLOGY

There are 25 million people with asthma in the United States, but estimates of the fraction that has OA vary widely. The reported prevalence of OA among all adults with asthma ranges from 2 to 36% (1–3). One explanation for these varied prevalence rates is that the OA diagnosis may not be as stringent in some retrospective studies as it is in documented worker compensation cases. In a comprehensive meta-analysis of OA studies from 1966 to 1999, Blanc and Toren concluded that 1 in 10 adults with asthma had an occupational trigger for their disease (4). Therefore, the more conservative estimate is that the prevalence of OA is 5–10% of all adult asthma cases.

Despite improved reporting systems, the true incidence of OA remains unknown. Twenty-five new cases of OA per million population were reported annually in the United Kingdom in the 1990s, whereas 3–18 cases per million were reported in the United States (5–7). Several large organizations track incident cases, including the Surveillance of Work-related and Occupational Respiratory Diseases (SWORD) (8) in the United Kingdom and Sentinel Event Notification System for Occupational Risks (SENSOR) (6) in the United States. The SENSOR program documents occupational diseases in four states (California,

Table 1
Estimated Prevalence of Occupational Asthma Among
Nonsmoking Workers by Industry—US Residents Aged 17 Yr
and Older, 1988–1994

Industry	Prevalence, % (95% CI)
Hospitals	14.4 (8.1,20.7)
Apparel/accessory stores	11.5 (4.1,18.9)
Machinery	11.2 (0.6,21.8)
Paper products, printing	9.7 (0.0,22.4)
Chemicals, petroleum	8.4 (0.2,16.6)
Transportation equipment	7.5 (2.4,12.6)
Food stores	6.8 (3.1,10.5)
Overall	6.7 (3.2,10.2)

Source: National Health and Nutrition Examination Survey
(NHANES) III (1999).

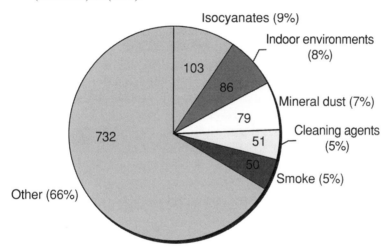

Fig. 1. Distribution of occupational asthma cases in the United States, by most frequently associated agent, 1993–1995.

Michigan, Massachusetts, and New Jersey) and is a rich source of epidemiological data. Overall, OA is common and must be considered in adult patients with asthma with difficult-to-control disease. Given these prevalence and incidence figures, it is estimated that there are roughly 1 million people with OA in the United States (*see* Table 1).

The economic effect of OA is substantial, which reflects the costs from lost productivity, costs of treatment, employer and employee health insurance costs, and legal fees. Of all people with asthma, 5–20% suffer partial disability that affects their ability to work *(9)*, and 40–80% lose considerable income as a consequence of their disease *(10,11)*. Using a proportional attributable risk of 15% for both asthma and chronic obstructive pulmonary disease (COPD), Leigh and colleagues estimated the 1996 US costs of OA at $1.6 billion and the COPD costs at $5 billion (*see* Fig. 1) *(12)*. Clearly, both OA and COPD are diseases that place considerable financial burdens on patients, employers, and public health systems. Prevention strategies likely will be the only cost-effective intervention to tackle this problem.

DEFINITIONS

The terminology and definitions for asthma in the workplace are not standardized, and they differ considerably among consensus statements *(6,8,13–15)*. Therefore, we have used the term OA to refer to all patients suffering from asthma in the workplace. This is not technically correct because other forms exist. Almost all consensus opinions agree that two major entities exist of asthma causally related to the work environment: OA and work-aggravated asthma.

The term "occupational asthma" encompasses all workers who develop new respiratory symptoms and obstructive airways physiology consistent with the diagnosis of asthma, for which the cause can be directly attributed to an exposure in the workplace. The key element is that OA is asthma caused by an organic protein, a chemical, or another compound unique to the workplace. OA is further split into two separate subtypes–sensitizer-induced OA (>90% of the cases) and irritant-induced asthma, such as reactive airway dysfunction syndrome (RADS).

Work-aggravated asthma refers to previously diagnosed asthma that is worsened, but not caused, by agents found in the workplace. The distinction between these two entities is not superfluous because it affects treatment strategies and medico-legal decisions. Millions of people with established asthma work, and exacerbations of disease can occur in the workplace. Clearly, these patients should not have their work eligibility affected by their chronic disease and, in general, their symptoms should be completely controllable. Patients with preexisting asthma whose disease becomes uncontrolled in a new work environment should be evaluated as a new case of OA. OA, therefore, represents the majority of asthma cases caused by an agent in the workplace, and the evaluation and diagnosis of this entity must follow established protocols and guidelines.

REACTIVE AIRWAY DYSFUNCTION SYNDROME

RADS, initially described by Brooks et al., refers to an asthma-like respiratory syndrome resulting from irritating vapors, fumes, or smoke in individuals with no prior respiratory disease *(16)*. The incidence of RADS as a portion of OA ranges as high as 25% *(17)*, with 9.3–10% *(18)* as a more typically reported range. Scenarios that lead to RADS often involve inadvertent exposure to multiple workers. It is likely that any mucosal irritant may lead to RADS if administered at a high enough exposure level. Some of the identified agents are listed in Table 2.

The initial respiratory symptoms of RADS may manifest within minutes or hours of exposure to the implicated irritant. Previous exposure or previous sensitization is neither required nor characteristic of this syndrome. Rather, a rapid time course to symptoms, no exposure history, and good prior respiratory health are characteristic of the syndrome. The nonimmunological, lymphocyte-predominant response that is characteristic of this syndrome is attributed to direct airway injury caused by the inhaled irritant. Although most individuals with RADS will have a single identifiable exposure, some may have multiple exposures to the irritant. Most criteria for RADS also require the symptoms to be present 1 mo after exposure to distinguish RADS from the direct toxin-mediated pathology. Persistent respiratory symptoms are typically managed with bronchodilators and assiduous irritant avoidance. The course of disease may resolve over weeks to years or, in some cases, persist indefinitely.

Table 2
Selected Reports of Reactive Airways Dysfunction Syndrome
and Causative Agents

Agent	Setting
Glacial acetic acid	Hospital chemical spill
Phthalic anhydride	Truck tanker spill
Hydrogen sulfide	Swine confinement building; police at chemical spill
Various	World Trade Center site
Methyl isocyanate	Bhopal chemical plant
Dinitrogen tetroxide	Railroad tanker spill
Hydrofluoric acid	Household exposure

Historically, noteworthy exposures include the Bhopal chemical plant toxic gas release in India and the World Trade Center (WTC) collapse in New York (19,20). In Bhopal, India, 30 tons of methyl isocyanate were accidentally released overnight on December 3, 1984. Approximately 2500 people died acutely, with many more sustaining less-than-lethal injuries. Retrospective evaluations found persistent respiratory complaints and RADS-like patterns in exposed individuals (21).

In New York, rescue personnel were exposed to various inhaled irritants during the rescue efforts after the destruction of the WTC. In prospective study and monitoring, Prezant with others (20) recognized WTC cough and RADS among the exposed individuals. This work represents the best prospective evaluation of RADS under study.

DIAGNOSIS

Making an accurate OA diagnosis requires that several key relationships between asthma and work be established. The 1995 American College of Chest Physicians diagnosis of OA is detailed in Table 3. In essence, the following three criteria need to be met:

- A worker receives a new diagnosis of asthma.
- A worker is exposed to an agent in the workplace that is known to cause OA.
- A sufficient causal relationship is established between the causative agent and the worker's symptoms.

Several tools should be employed to investigate the potential causal relationship between asthma and the workplace, including symptom diaries, employment questionnaires, lung function testing performed at and away from work, immunological testing, and occasional workplace site visits. Oddly, the gold-standard test for diagnosing OA, the specific inhalation challenge, is not included because it is performed at only a few specialized centers. The specific inhalation challenge (SIC) test and others are discussed as they pertain to making a clinical diagnosis of OA.

CLINICAL PRESENTATION

Episodic wheezing, dyspnea, cough, and nocturnal awakenings are the typical presenting complaints of an adult patient with OA. Shortness of breath with or without wheezing was the chief complaint of 36% of workers exposed to wood products

Table 3
1995 ACCP Case Definition of Occupational Asthma[a]

A	Diagnosis of asthma
B	Onset of asthma after entering workplace
C	Association between work and asthma symptom
D1	Workplace exposure to agent known to cause OA
D2	Work-related changes in FEV_1 or PEFR
D3	Work-related changes in bronchial hyperresponsiveness
D4	Onset of asthma with a clear association with work exposure

[a]Occupational asthma (OA) case definition: A+B+C+D2 orD3 or D4 or D5.
Likely OA definition: A+B+C+D1.
Adapted from Chan-Yeung. *See* ref. *13.*

containing methylene diphenyl diisocyanate for 8 mo, and this figure increased to 45% by 20 mo *(22)*. The second most common symptom in this cohort was chest tightness, which occurred in 30% of workers at 8 mo and 38% at 20 mo. These two symptoms plus cough, phlegm production, and sudden attacks of shortness of breath occurred in at least 25% of all workers by 20 mo.

Although the chief complaints in OA may not differ from those with other forms of asthma, the temporal nature of them may. Patients with OA may report that their symptoms are better on the weekends and worse at the end of the workday or at night. Asking direct questions regarding the timing of the symptoms is the key to eliciting an OA clinical history.

WORK-SITE EVALUATION

Questionnaires can help determine the extent of a worker's exposure to specific compounds, but a workplace visit and an on-site investigation may be necessary in some instances. The focus of these assessments is twofold. First, is the person with asthma exposed to a single agent in the workplace that is known to cause asthma? Second, is there a clear temporal association between the patient's symptoms and the workplace exposure to this agent?

Examples of potential questions for use in OA questionnaires are listed in Table 4. In general, questions should address the time of day that symptoms develop and whether these symptoms resolve during extended breaks from work (e.g., weekends or vacations). One study reported that only 50% of pulmonologists and allergists asked about the association between asthma symptoms and work habits *(23)*. A failure to ask such questions may lead to the wrong diagnosis.

Approximately 250 or more agents have been causally linked to OA, but most cases of OA are caused by only a handful of compounds. Table 5 lists the major classes of compounds that cause OA and the industries that often employ them. Clinicians must elicit a detailed work history from patients with adult-onset asthma. Specific job duties, date of hire, and job environment should be asked directly and documented in an evaluation. Occasionally, workers are unaware of all the products used in their industrial plant and clinicians can ask that the worker bring in copies of the material safety data sheets (MSDS) from their employers and any reports from work-site visits.

Table 4
Five Questions That Can Help Elicit History of Occupational Asthma

1. Have you ever had to leave your job because it affected your breathing?
2. Is your asthma worse at work or in the evening after work?
3. Do your symptoms resolve or improve on the weekends or vacation?
4. Do symptoms develop within minutes of entering the workplace or performing a specific job?
5. Did the symptoms begin after starting a new job?

Adapted from Balmes. *See* ref. *23a.*

Table 5
Common Low- and High-Molecular-Weight Compounds That Cause Occupational Asthma

Low-molecular-weight compounds	*Occupations*
Isocyanates	Plastics workers, painters, and insulators
Anhydrides	Plastics and resins workers
Amines	Lacquer and shellac workers
Metals (e.g., platinum, vanadium salts)	Platers, welders, and chemical workers
Chloramine-T	Cleaners

High-molecular-weight compounds	*Occupations*
Animal proteins (e.g., lipocalins)	Animal handlers
Latex	Health care workers
Gums	Carpet workers and pharmaceuticals workers
Seafood	Food-industry workers
Cereals	Bakers, millers, and textile workers
Wood products	Carpenters and loggers
Dyes	Textile workers

Adapted from ref. *13.*

Inhalation is the primary portal of entry for chemicals and other compounds, and repeated exposure leads to systemic sensitization. An evaluation of the exposure risk for a worker often cannot be done efficiently without help from outside experts. Occupational hygienists or occupational medicine professionals specialize in sampling techniques and sensitive assays, such as liquid chromatography, gas chromatography, and mass spectrometry, to measure concentrations of particulate airborne compounds. Unless trained in this highly specialized area, clinicians should focus their efforts on the patient's complaints as they pertain to the work site.

LUNG FUNCTION TESTING

Once clinicians suspect a temporal relationship between a patient's asthma symptoms and the workplace, they should order lung function testing. Measurements of lung function must be performed both at and away from the work site. The simplest, least expensive tests are serial peak expiratory flow rate (PEFR) measurements. Newer patient-activated, portable devices store full spirometry data, including forced expiratory volume in 1 s (FEV_1) readings, but they remain expensive. These devices record and log spirometry readings and reduce the problem of falsified records. Training in the forced vital capacity maneuver and adherence to PEFR and spirometry measurement diaries is essential.

One formal study of serial PEFR during and after work is named the "stop–resume work test" (24). Essentially, this test asks that the worker monitor and record serial peak flow data while at work and at home. Workers with asthma caused by an occupational agent will demonstrate significant peak flow variability (20–30%), with higher readings on weekends and lower readings during and after work. It is important that clinicians ask that measurements be recorded for several days, including nonworking days. Good peak flow data are recorded at the same times each day, such as in the early morning, during lunch, at the end of the work shift, and at bedtime. Adherence to this regimen can be difficult.

In addition to spirometry, repeated airway hyperresponsiveness measurements with methacholine challenge testing (MCT) provide strong evidence for OA. MCT changes depend on whether the patient with OA has been recently exposed to the agent that caused his or her OA or whether he or she has been away from work for an extended period. A threefold difference in the methacholine dose required to trigger a positive response is strongly indicative of OA. The American Thoracic Society recommendations for MCT need to be adhered to closely (25).

An OA diagnosis can be wrong even when it is based on accurate symptom data, spirometry readings, and MCT results. Several studies published in the mid-1980s to early 1990s showed a discrepancy between the clinical diagnosis of OA and the diagnosis confirmed by specific inhalation challenge, the gold-standard test (26–28). In one study, when diagnosed by specialist physicians, 63 workers with OA secondary to isocyanate exposure underwent inhalation challenge testing to isocyanate (27). Only 48% of the workers demonstrated airway hyperresponsiveness to isocyanates, although most workers reported respiratory symptoms during the test. Forty-three percent of the workers had no response to isocyanate but showed airway hyperresponsiveness to methacholine. This reinforces the distinction between asthma and OA. Proving a causal relationship between a specific compound and a worker's asthma is not straightforward.

SPECIFIC INHALATION CHALLENGE TESTING

SIC mirrors other inhalation challenge testing, except that we aerosolize known occupational antigens. Although considered the gold-standard test to document OA, SIC is not performed commonly in the United States and cannot be considered part of the standard evaluation. In many countries, clinicians order SIC routinely. A recent survey of 123 US and Canadian pulmonary and allergy medicine training programs found that only 15 centers performed SIC tests (29). Of 2065 patients diagnosed in the United States with OA in the preceding years, only 130 (6%) had been diagnosed with the help of SIC testing. In contrast, 130 of 308 (42%) patients with OA in Canada underwent SIC testing. Sixty percent (74 of 123) of the training programs believed SIC was useful, but only 55% of the respondents could order the test. A list of the 15 centers performing SIC in the United States and Canada can be found in the 2002 article by Ortega and colleagues (29).

As with most gold standards, problems exist with SIC. False-negative tests with SIC occur if the wrong compound (e.g., wrong isocyanate) is chosen or if SIC is performed long after the worker has left the workplace. Sastre and colleagues demonstrated that 5 of 22 workers with apparent isocyanate-induced OA had a negative SIC, but 3 of these 5 workers were subsequently positive when tested a second time *(30)*. Despite these deficiencies, SIC remains the gold-standard test for diagnosing OA in as many as 50% of patients in Canada and throughout much of the world. The same cannot be said for the Unites States, where SIC is rarely ordered and performed.

IMMUNOLOGICAL TESTING

Skin-prick testing and radioallergosorbent testing (RAST) can determine if a worker has developed an antibody response to a HMW protein or glycoprotein in the workplace. This type of immunological testing is often the next step in the evaluation of OA, but as shown in Table 2, RAST or skin testing is not required to make the diagnosis. Skin-prick testing and RAST using a panel of common occupational antigens is a sensitive, but not specific, marker for occupational rhinitis, dermatitis, and asthma. Testing for an IgG- and IgE-mediated response to a panel of common HMW proteins is relatively straightforward, whereas testing for LMW antigens, such as diisocyanate, is not. Diisocyanate, for example, may lead to elevated IgE levels in only 20–30% of exposures where it appears to act as a hapten *(31)*. Newer in vitro assays are becoming available to detect isocyanate and other LMW agent-induced OA. For example, the production of monocyte chemotactic protein-1 by peripheral blood mononuclear cells in patients with diisocyanate-induced OA can distinguish them from workers without asthma *(31)*. In the authors' experience, skin-prick tests and RAST provide important supporting data demonstrating sensitization to occupational antigens.

MISCELLANEOUS DIAGNOSTIC TESTS

Surrogates of airway inflammation, such as sputum eosinophilia and exhaled nitric oxide (NO), contribute to the management of patients with asthma, and these markers are now being evaluated in OA. Green and colleagues showed that the number of exacerbations of asthma in a population of people with asthma decreased significantly when sputum eosinophil counts were maintained less than 3% or exhaled NO concentrations less than 5.0 ppb *(32)*. Peripheral blood and airway eosinophilia is evident in all forms of OA, including RADS, and induced sputum eosinophils and neutrophils increase after exposure to specific work-related compounds, such as isocyanates *(33–35)*. In one study, serial spirometry measurements plus induced sputum eosinophil counts improved the accuracy of the OA diagnosis compared with spirometry testing alone *(36)*.

Compared with sputum eosinophil counts, data with exhaled nitric oxide in OA are scant. One study documented that exhaled NO levels increased in workers with a positive inhalation challenge and not in those with negative tests in a small cohort of 40 workers *(37)*. The potential strength of the exhaled NO test lies in its use for disease management. At this juncture, limited evidence suggests that induced sputum eosinophil counts, but not exhaled NO, may aid in supporting the diagnosis of OA.

GENETICS OF OCCUPATIONAL ASTHMA

Nucleotide polymorphisms are a research focus in asthma and this focus has spilled over to OA as well. Clearly, a gene marker that signals a predisposition to OA would be of interest in certain industries with high incidences of OA (e.g., animal care and food industries). Although no such gene has been identified to date, researchers continue to focus on two candidate families: the glutathione-*S*-transferase (GST) and human leukocyte antigen (HLA) family. The GST family of genes involves a host of enzymes that protect the host lung epithelium from oxidative stress. The GSTP1 Val/Val genotype has been associated with both allergic asthma and toluene diisocyanate (TDI)-induced OA *(38,39)*. In one study, the presence of GSTP1 Val/Val had a protective effect against OA in workers exposed to TDI for 10 yr *(40)*. In turn, other genes in the GST family confer an increased risk of OA, including GSTM1, GSTM3 AA, and GSTP1 Ile/Ile.

The second class of genes of interest in OA is the HLA class II molecules—part of the major histocompatibility complex (MHC)—that are involved in antigen presentation. Young and colleagues demonstrated a strong correlation between increased expression of HLADR3 and the development of OA after exposure to trimellitic anhydride *(41)*. However, this correlation is not apparent with exposures to other compounds *(42)*.

MECHANISMS OF OCCUPATIONAL ASTHMA

As with all asthmas, the mechanisms leading to the development of OA are not fully known. Two major classes of agents—HMW and LMW agents—cause OA, and the mechanisms appear to differ significantly. As shown in Table 3, common HMW organic proteins that cause OA include grains, latex, animal-derived proteins, and seafood. More than 140 LMW chemicals and compounds trigger sensitization in humans, and this list includes isocyanates (e.g., TDI), anhydrides, dyes, and smaller organic compounds.

HMW antigens (>5000 kDa in size) act like other environmental antigens that lead to sensitization and IgG and IgE antibody production. In general, months to years of exposure are necessary to develop this allergic response, and latency helps distinguish OA from RADS. HMW organic proteins can trigger a vigorous immune response, and the period of latency may be less than 1 yr. A recent prospective study following 118 apprentice bakers and new animal workers found that 64% of the new hires developed positive skin-prick test responses to grains and animal proteins and 12% developed asthma symptoms *(43)*. The incidence of occupational rhinitis in this study was higher than OA, which is consistent with most studies.

The pathways leading to systemic sensitization to HMW proteins and polysaccharides do not differ significantly from the pathways involved in the development of environmental asthma. Briefly, an HMW antigen, such as an animal dander protein, will associate with an MHC II molecule on a dendritic cell, and will be transported to a lymph node. An allergenic peptide sequence will interact with naïve T-cells, and some undergo transformation to T-helper (Th) 2 or 1 cells. Cytokines (interleukins [IL]-4, -5, and -13) from these cells then stimulate IgE production from B cells and eosinophil recruitment from the bone marrow. The pathological sequence in IgE-mediated OA resembles that of more common forms of asthma, except the sequence of events can occur more rapidly.

The development of OA from LMW compounds can result in a type I, IgE-mediated immune response by acting as haptens, but in most cases, it does not. Admittedly, evidence supporting the concept that LMW agents act as haptens is slim. One investigator suggested that the degree of hydrophilicity of the LMW compound may affect its function and determine whether it stimulates a type I immune response *(14)*. Hydrophilic LMW compounds, for example, may cross the respiratory epithelial membrane more readily, bind lung proteins, and trigger IgE production, whereas more hydrophobic compounds may not.

Most LMW agents, like TDI, cause a delayed type III, cell-mediated immune response by binding to organic macromolecules at the airway–epithelium interface. This inflammatory response occurs more rapidly than with HMW compounds *(44)* and is characterized, in part, by increased numbers of airway CD8+ lymphocytes. Affinity of certain LMW compounds for various organic proteins and other adducts has been shown. Trimellitic anhydride, for example, can bind with amino groups, alcohols, and epithelial cell proteins *(45)*. Intracellular glutathione may also act as a transfer molecule for LMW agents and serve as an intermediary in the development of the allergic response *(46,47)*.

Another factor that may enhance sensitization to LMW compounds is tobacco smoke. Workers exposed to second-hand environmental tobacco smoke at work have a higher incidence of work-related asthmatic symptoms *(48)*. The risk of sensitization to platinum salts in refinery workers is higher in workers who smoked, for example *(49)*. Overall, the diverse mechanisms involved in the development of LMW antigen-associated OA are interesting, and further investigation will provide information to determine the relevance to all asthma.

DISEASES OF INTEREST IN THE MEDICAL FIELD

Based on surveys from NIOSH, the prevalence of OA in hospital and biomedical workers is as high as 15% *(50)*. Two types of exposures in workers in the biomedical field that commonly present to clinicians for evaluation of respiratory symptoms are discussed: (1) hospital staff exposed to latex and (2) laboratory workers who handle animals.

Latex Allergy and Asthma

Allergy and OA related to latex and natural rubber compounds represent a significant and illustrative example of occupational illness. Latex-related allergy and asthma was recognized first in the 1970s in patients who were exposed to latex, such as those with spina bifida. It gained prominence during the late 1980s and 1990s with the implementation of NIOSH/Centers for Disease Control and Prevention (CDC) universal precautions for blood-borne infections. The CDC precautions increased the use of latex gloves and led to more worker exposure to natural rubber products. As with other examples of HMW agent-related OA, the incidence and severity of disease correlates with exposure level. Currently, latex-related OA represents some 4% of all work-related asthma cases (10.3% in Michigan). Diagnosis is similar to other OA cases, with the exception of immunological testing. RAST is less sensitive in the case of latex allergy and OA, with nearly a 30% false-negative rate as compared to patch or skin-prick testing.

Although latex allergy and OA are present in other industries (e.g., food handling and manufacturing) the incidence is twice as high in health care workers (5–18%) as in the general populace *(51)*, and it is more prevalent in work areas with high-level exposures to latex gloves and glove dust. With the recognition of latex allergy as a problem, NIOSH implemented recommendations to decrease the incidence of latex-related allergy and OA by decreasing workplace latex antigen exposures. In hospitals where these recommendations are implemented (the use of powderless gloves, nonlatex gloves, and gloves of higher quality manufacturing techniques) the incidence of latex-related OA and allergy has decreased *(8)*.

Occupational Asthma in Animal Workers

The incidence of atopic sensitization to small laboratory animals and pets is reported to be between 15 and 40% *(52)* and preexisting atopy to environmental allergens is the primary risk factor for developing animal allergy *(43)*. Two million people work in jobs that expose them constantly to animals *(53)*. Inhalation of animal proteins in dander, fur, feces, urine, and saliva can lead to sensitization. Proteins isolated in the urine of rodents, called lipocalins, for example, trigger an IgE-mediated response. Lipocalin sequences are now added to skin-prick and RAST panel tests. Although low exposure to these proteins can lead to sensitization and OA, high exposure time increases these risks significantly. Implementation of prevention strategies that decrease total exposure to inhaled animal proteins remains a key goal for NIOSH and should be for all medical centers and industries.

PREVENTION

Screening for preexisting atopic conditions in new workers is not legal; therefore, employer interventions must be aimed at limiting exposures to certain airborne antigens. The Occupational Safety and Health Administration (OSHA) and NIOSH regulations regarding worker contact with specific compounds often appear burdensome to industry, but these regulations will remain the primary strategy to combat OA. One example of specific recommendations made by NIOSH can be found in the publication on animal health, *Preventing Asthma in Animal Handlers (50)*. Five of the top recommendations are as follows:

1. Modify ventilation and filtration systems.
   - Increase the ventilation rate and humidity in animal housing areas.
   - Ventilate animal handling areas separately from the rest of the facility.
   - Install ventilated animal cage racks or filter-top animal cages.
2. Perform animal manipulations within ventilated hoods when possible.
3. Decrease animal density (number of animals per cubic foot of room volume).
4. Avoid wearing street clothes when working with animals. Leave work clothes at the workplace to avoid potential exposure problems for family members.
5. Provide training to educate workers about animal allergies and steps for risk reduction.

These recommendations encourage employers to formulate their own policies and procedures regarding this issue. Ventilation and individual protection strategies are near the top of many NIOSH recommendations for specific worker groups. A proactive employer will institute these guidelines and a workplace screening program. Small studies have shown that such measures can decrease the incidence of OA. In one recent example, Grammer and colleagues offered personal protective masks to 66 workers newly hired in a plant producing an acid anhydride *(54)*. For 7 yr, the workers who used the protective masks decreased their absolute risk of developing rhinitis or OA from 10 to 2%. Preventing exposure to airborne agents should decrease the incidence of OA, but installation of new ventilation systems is costly for employers, and personal protective industrial masks and helmet respirators do not seem practical to many workers.

TREATMENT

Minimizing allergen exposure is an essential component of every asthma treatment plan. Similarly, quitting work or avoiding the work site exposure is the primary treatment in OA. Inhaled CSs, long-acting β_2-agonists, and rescue-drug medications should be prescribed according to the guidelines of the National Asthma Education and Prevention Program (55,56), but the efficaciousness of these therapies in OA is less well established.

Two studies have shown that patients who remain in the workplace after an OA diagnosis suffer worsening lung function despite appropriate steroid therapy (10). In one crossover study, Malo and colleagues found that the addition of inhaled CSs to work site removal did improve asthma symptoms, airway hyperresponsiveness, and quality-of-life measures more than work removal alone (56). In another recent study, Marabini and colleagues treated 20 patients with OA who remained at their job with beclomethasone dipropionate (500 µg bid) and salmeterol (50 µg bid) for 3 yr (58). At the time of enrollment, their FEV_1 percentage predicted was mildly reduced at 80.2%. After 3 yr, lung function remained the same, as did airway hyperreactivity, symptoms, and rescue β_2-agonist drug usage. Although lung function and symptoms did not improve with inhaled CS treatment, neither did they worsen. The authors surmised that the outcome in these 20 workers might be the same with adequate controller therapy, whether they quit or continued to work. At this time, this approach cannot be recommended. Larger prospective studies needed to evaluate this question may never be performed.

Management of work-aggravated asthma, where asthma is a preexisting condition and the disease flares with work exposures, differs from that of OA. Avoidance of work-site exposures is important, but pharmacotherapy can control symptoms. In general, fewer workers with work-aggravated asthma lose their jobs than do workers with OA. This practice may be influenced both by the medico-legal complexities associated with OA and the belief that work-aggravated asthma represents a milder form of the disease (59). Like work-aggravated asthma, irritant-induced asthma or RADS is amenable to drug therapy and workers often return to their jobs.

OUTCOMES

Unfortunately, asthma symptoms and airway hyperresponsiveness (AHR) persist in many patients after removal from the work site and, in this sense, OA mirrors environmental asthma. More than 50% of workers with OA have persistent asthma symptoms and AHR in the years succeeding their quit date (14). Malo and colleagues found that lung function, as measured by FEV_1, stabilized approx 1 yr after leaving work (60). As expected, specific IgE to the offending compound that caused the OA decreases significantly once the worker leaves. Immune cell memory does not fade completely, however, and rechallenge with the same compound 2 yr later will trigger an asthmatic attack in the majority of those affected.

Biologically, it makes sense that once an insult—be it an environmental, infectious, or occupational one—triggers structural airway changes, such as airway wall thickening and smooth muscle hypertrophy, the disease will not abate completely in all patients.

Simple avoidance alleviates, but does not necessarily cure, the disease. Nonetheless, early removal from the workplace portends a better prognosis.

COMPENSATION AND DISABILITY

The economic realities of OA for a worker can be overwhelming and life-changing. Several groups have studied the economic impact of OA on workers, and an interesting review on this topic has recently been published *(59)*. In one study, of 55 US workers with OA, 69% remained unemployed an average of 2.5 yr after the diagnosis *(61)*. In Vandenplas and colleagues' meta-analysis of six studies from three European countries and Canada, approximately one-third of workers with OA reported prolonged unemployment or work disruption and one-half to two-thirds reported significant lost income *(59)*.

Diagnoses of OA inherently lead to decisions regarding the impairment, disability, and compensation of workers. Physicians should advocate for workers diagnosed with OA and adopt a proactive approach by reporting the diagnosis to compensation boards, surveillance organizations (e.g., SENTINEL), and possibly employers. Impairment and disability programs are exceedingly complex and differ significantly among states and countries. The 1993 American Thoracic Society guidelines on this topic serve as the primary reference *(62)*. In general, impairment is based on the degree of lung function compromise. Workers with objectively recorded and diagnosed OA should receive temporary disability immediately and decisions regarding permanent disability should be made after some period of observation and review. Most workers receive complete, permanent disability for the job that caused their OA and for any job where they might be exposed to the same product or compound. Physicians' roles should focus on making an objective and accurate diagnosis. If the diagnosis of OA is established, physicians should initiate appropriate controller drug therapy, remove patients from the work environment, request temporary disability from that job, and report the case to the appropriate monitoring and surveillance boards.

CONCLUSION

OA is the primary lung disease in the workplace and is of increasing importance to OSHA, state regulatory boards, and employers. Every measure must be taken to prevent sensitization to occupational antigens that commonly cause OA and occupational rhinitis. Studies in the past 10 yr have helped to elucidate some of the mechanisms leading to asthma secondary to HMW and some LMW compounds, but other pathways need exploring. Many workers remain symptomatic and suffer continued loss of lung function after being removed from the work environment. Disability and compensation issues will become increasingly common, and the specialist will need to remain updated on this important disease.

REFERENCES

1. Johnson AR, Dimich-Ward HD, Manfreda J, et al. Occupational asthma in adults in six Canadian communities. *Am J Respir Crit Care Med* 2000; 162: 2058–2062.
2. Ng TP, Hong CY, Goh LG, Wong ML, Koh KT, Ling SL. Risks of asthma associated with occupations in a community-based case-control study. *Am J Ind Med* 1994; 25: 709–718.

3. Brooks SM, Hammad Y, Richards I, Giovinco-Barbas J, Jenkins K. The spectrum of irritant-induced asthma: sudden and not-so-sudden onset and the role of allergy. *Chest* 1998; 113: 42–49.

4. Blanc PD, Toren K. How much adult asthma can be attributed to occupational factors? *Am J Med* 1999; 107: 580–587.

5. Meredith S, Nordman H. Occupational asthma: measures of frequency from four countries. *Thorax* 1996; 51: 435–440.

6. Jajosky RA, Harrison R, Reinisch F, et al. Surveillance of work-related asthma in selected U.S. states using surveillance guidelines for state health departments—California, Massachusetts, Michigan, and New Jersey, 1993–1995. *MMWR CDC Surveill Summ* 1999; 48: 1–20.

7. Henneberger PK, Kreiss K, Rosenman KD, et al. An evaluation of the incidence of work-related asthma in the United States. *Int J Occup Environ Health* 1999; 5: 1–8.

8. McDonald JC, Keynes HL, Meredith SK. Reported incidence of occupational asthma in the United Kingdom, 1989–1997. *Occup Environ Med* 2000; 57: 823–829.

9. Balder B, Lindholm NB, Lowhagen O, et al. Predictors of self-assessed work ability among subjects with recent-onset asthma. *Respir Med* 1998; 92: 729–734.

10. Marabini A, Dimich-Ward H, Kwan SY, et al. Clinical and socioeconomic features of subjects with red cedar asthma. A follow-up study. *Chest* 1993; 104: 821–824.

11. Dewitte JD, Chan-Yeung M, Malo JL. Medicolegal and compensation aspects of occupational asthma. *Eur Respir J* 1994; 7: 969–980.

12. Leigh JP, Romano PS, Schenker MB, Kreiss K. Costs of occupational COPD and asthma. *Chest* 2002; 121: 264–272.

13. Chan-Yeung M, Malo JL. Occupational asthma. *N Engl J Med* 1995; 333: 107–112.

14. Chan-Yeung M, Malo JL, Tarlo SM, et al. Proceedings of the first Jack Pepys Occupational Asthma Symposium. *Am J Respir Crit Care Med* 2003; 167: 450–471.

15. Guidelines for assessing and managing asthma risk at work, school, and recreation. *Am J Respir Crit Care Med* 2004; 169: 873–881.

16. Brooks SM, Weiss MA, Bernstein IL. Reactive airways dysfunction syndrome (RADS). Persistent asthma syndrome after high level irritant exposures. *Chest* 1985; 88: 376–384.

17. Wheeler S, Rosenstock L, Barnhart S. A case series of 71 patients referred to a hospital-based occupational and environmental medicine clinic for occupational asthma. *West J Med* 1998; 168: 98–104.

18. Rosenman KD, Reilly MJ, Kalinowski DJ. A state-based surveillance system for work-related asthma. *J Occup Environ Med* 1997; 39: 415–425.

19. Banauch GI, Alleyne D, Sanchez R, et al. Persistent hyperreactivity and reactive airway dysfunction in firefighters at the World Trade Center. *Am J Respir Crit Care Med* 2003; 168: 54–62.

20. Prezant DJ, Weiden M, Banauch GI, et al. Cough and bronchial responsiveness in firefighters at the World Trade Center site. *N Engl J Med* 2002; 347: 806–815.

21. Nemery B. Late consequences of accidental exposure to inhaled irritants: RADS and the Bhopal disaster. *Eur Respir J* 1996; 9: 1973–1976.

22. Wang ML, Petsonk EL. Symptom onset in the first 2 years of employment at a wood products plant using diisocyanates: some observations relevant to occupational medical screening. *Am J Ind Med* 2004; 46: 226–233.

23. Milton DK, Solomon GM, Rosiello RA, Herrick RF. Risk and incidence of asthma attributable to occupational exposure among HMO members. *Am J Ind Med* 1998; 33: 1–10.

23a. Balmes JR. Surveillance for occupational asthma. *Occ Med* 1991; 6: 101–110.

24. Moscato G, Godnic-Cvar J, Maestrelli P, et al. Statement on self-monitoring of peak expiratory flows in the investigation of occupational asthma. Subcommittee on Occupational Allergy of the European Academy of Allergology and Clinical Immunology. American Academy of Allergy and Clinical Immunology. European Respiratory Society. American College of Allergy, Asthma and Immunology. *Eur Respir J* 1995; 8: 1605–1610.

25. Crapo RO, Casaburi R, Coates AL, et al. Guidelines for methacholine and exercise challenge testing-1999. This official statement of the American Thoracic Society was adopted by the ATS Board of Directors, July 1999. *Am J Respir Crit Care Med* 2000; 161: 309–329.

26. Karol MH, Tollerud DJ, Campbell TP, et al. Predictive value of airways hyperresponsiveness and circulating IgE for identifying types of responses to toluene diisocyanate inhalation challenge. *Am J Respir Crit Care Med* 1994; 149: 611–615.

27. Banks DE, Sastre J, Butcher BT, et al. Role of inhalation challenge testing in the diagnosis of iso-cyanate-induced asthma. *Chest* 1989; 95: 414–423.

28. Moller DR, Brooks SM, McKay RT, et al. Chronic asthma due to toluene diisocyanate. *Chest* 1986; 90: 494–499.

29. Ortega HG, Weissman DN, Carter DL, Banks D. Use of specific inhalation challenge in the evaluation of workers at risk for occupational asthma: a survey of pulmonary, allergy, and occupational medicine residency training programs in the United States and Canada. *Chest* 2002; 121: 1323–1328.

30. Sastre J, Fernandez-Nieto M, Novalbos A, et al. Need for monitoring nonspecific bronchial hyperresponsiveness before and after isocyanate inhalation challenge. *Chest* 2003; 123: 1276–1279.

31. Bernstein DI, Cartier A, Cote J, et al. Diisocyanate antigen-stimulated monocyte chemoattractant protein-1 synthesis has greater test efficiency than specific antibodies for identification of diisocyanate asthma. *Am J Respir Crit Care Med* 2002; 166: 445–450.

32. Green RH, Brightling CE, McKenna S, et al. Asthma exacerbations and sputum eosinophil counts: a randomised controlled trial. *Lancet* 2002; 360: 1715–1721.

33. Lemiere C, Chaboillez S, Malo JL, Cartier A. Changes in sputum cell counts after exposure to occupational agents: what do they mean? *J Allergy Clin Immunol* 2001; 107: 1063–1068.

34. Maestrelli P, Calcagni PG, Saetta M, et al. Sputum eosinophilia after asthmatic responses induced by isocyanates in sensitized subjects. *Clin Exp Allergy* 1994; 24: 29–34.

35. Park HS, Jung KS, Hwang SC, Nahm DH, Yim HE. Neutrophil infiltration and release of IL-8 in airway mucosa from subjects with grain dust-induced occupational asthma. *Clin Exp Allergy* 1998; 28: 724–730.

36. Lemiere C. The use of sputum eosinophils in the evaluation of occupational asthma. *Curr Opin Allergy Clin Immunol* 2004; 4: 81–85.

37. Piipari R, Piirila P, Keskinen H, et al. Exhaled nitric oxide in specific challenge tests to assess occupational asthma. *Eur Respir J* 2002; 20: 1532–1537.

38. Fryer AA, Bianco A, Hepple M, et al. Polymorphism at the glutathione S-transferase GSTP1 locus. A new marker for bronchial hyperresponsiveness and asthma. *Am J Respir Crit Care Med* 2000; 161: 1437–1442.

39. Mapp CE, Pozzato V, Pavoni V, Gritti G. Severe asthma and ARDS triggered by acute short-term exposure to commonly used cleaning detergents. *Eur Respir J* 2000; 16: 570–572.

40. Mapp CE, Fryer AA, De Marzo N, et al. Glutathione S-transferase GSTP1 is a susceptibility gene for occupational asthma induced by isocyanates. *J Allergy Clin Immunol* 2002; 109: 867–872.

41. Young RP, Barker RD, Pile KD, Cookson WO, Taylor AJ. The association of HLA-DR3 with specific IgE to inhaled acid anhydrides. *Am J Respir Crit Care Med* 1995; 151: 219–221.

42. Rihs HP, Barbalho-Krolls T, Huber H, Baur X. No evidence for the influence of HLA class II in alleles in isocyanate-induced asthma. *Am J Ind Med* 1997; 32: 522–527.

43. de Meer G, Postma DS, Heederik D. Bronchial responsiveness to adenosine-5'-monophosphate and methacholine as predictors for nasal symptoms due to newly introduced allergens. A follow-up study among laboratory animal workers and bakery apprentices. *Clin Exp Allergy* 2003; 33: 789–794.

44. Malo JL, Ghezzo H, D'Aquino C, et al. Natural history of occupational asthma: relevance of type of agent and other factors in the rate of development of symptoms in affected subjects. *J Allergy Clin Immunol* 1992; 90: 937–944.

45. Griffin P, Allan L, Beckett P, Elms J, Curran AD. The development of an antibody to trimellitic anhydride. *Clin Exp Allergy* 2001; 31: 453–457.

46. Lange RW, Day BW, Lemus R, et al. Intracellular S-glutathionyl adducts in murine lung and human bronchoepithelial cells after exposure to diisocyanatotoluene. *Chem Res Toxicol* 1999; 12: 931–936.

47. Karol MH, Macina OT, Cunningham A. Cell and molecular biology of chemical allergy. *Ann Allergy Asthma Immunol* 2001; 87: 28–32.

48. Radon K, Busching K, Heinrich J, et al. Passive smoking exposure: a risk factor for chronic bronchitis and asthma in adults? *Chest* 2002; 122: 1086–1090.

49. Calverley AE, Rees D, Dowdeswell RJ, Linnett PJ, Kielkowski D. Platinum salt sensitivity in refinery workers: incidence and effects of smoking and exposure. *Occup Environ Med* 1995; 52: 661–666.

50. *Preventing asthma in animal handlers*. Bethesda, MD. U.S. Department of Health and Human Services. NIOSH Alert 1998; Publication No. 97-116.

51. Amr S, Suk WA. Latex allergy and occupational asthma in health care workers: adverse outcomes. *Environ Health Perspect* 2004; 112: 378–381.

52. Bush RK, Stave GM. Laboratory animal allergy: an update. *Ilar J* 2003; 44: 28–51.

53. Alberts WM, Brooks SM. Advances in occupational asthma. *Clin Chest Med* 1992; 13: 281–302.

54. Grammer LC, Harris KE, Yarnold PR. Effect of respiratory protective devices on development of antibody and occupational asthma to an acid anhydride. *Chest* 2002; 121: 1317–1322.

55. National Heart, Lung and Blood Institute, National Asthma Education and Prevention Program. *Guidelines for the diagnosis and management of asthma*. US Department of Health and Human Services, Bethesda, MD, Expert Panel Report 2 1997; Publication No. 97-405.

56. National Heart, Lung and Blood Institute, National Asthma Education and Prevention Program. *Update on Selected Topics 2002*. Bethesda, MD: U.S. Department of Health and Human Services. Expert Panel Report 2002; Publication No. 02-5074.

57. Malo JL, Cartier A, Cote J, et al. Influence of inhaled steroids on recovery from occupational asthma after cessation of exposure: an 18-month double-blind crossover study. *Am J Respir Crit Care Med* 1996; 153: 953–960.

58. Marabini A, Siracusa A, Stopponi R, Tacconi C, Abbritti G. Outcome of occupational asthma in patients with continuous exposure: a 3-year longitudinal study during pharmacologic treatment. *Chest* 2003; 124: 2372–2376.

59. Vandenplas O, Toren K, Blanc PD. Health and socioeconomic impact of work-related asthma. *Eur Respir J* 2003; 22: 689–697.

60. Malo JL, Cartier A, Ghezzo H, et al. Patterns of improvement in spirometry, bronchial hyperresponsiveness, and specific IgE antibody levels after cessation of exposure in occupational asthma caused by snow-crab processing. *Am Rev Respir Dis* 1988; 138: 807–812.

61. Gassert TH, Hu H, Kelsey KT, Christiani DC. Long-term health and employment outcomes of occupational asthma and their determinants. *J Occup Environ Med* 1998; 40: 481–491.

62. Guidelines for the evaluation of impairment/disability in patients with asthma. American Thoracic Society. Medical Section of the American Lung Association. *Am Rev Respir Dis* 1993; 147: 1056–1061.

15 Anesthesia for Patients With Asthma

Dennis L. Fung, MD

CONTENTS

KEY POINTS

- Anesthesia poses unique risks for the patient with asthma.
- A preoperative assessment of patients with asthma is essential in order to establish baseline conditions and identify correctable points.
- The patient's own subjective assessment of his or her asthma is unreliable.
- Endotrachial tube intubation frequently promotes brochospasm.
- Although the pharmacology of anesthetic agents is similar in all patients, there are very few clinical studies in patients with hyperreactive airways.
- Fortunately, bronchoconstriction is not a common occurrence during surgery.
- The use of inhaled anesthetics during status asthmaticus remains a controversial issue.

INTRODUCTION

This chapter covers basic issues in perioperative anesthesia as they relate to the management of the patient with asthma. Anesthesia presents unique risks for the patient with reactive airway disease (*see* Table 1). The concepts and information presented are intended to aid nonanesthesia practitioners in providing perioperative care and medical consultation. The particulars of general anesthesia and regional anesthesia are discussed. Airway management techniques, with emphasis on methods that limit bronchospasm, are reviewed. The induction agents that initiate anesthesia and the drugs that maintain

From: *Current Clinical Practice: Bronchial Asthma:*
A Guide for Practical Understanding and Treatment, 5th ed.
Edited by: M. E. Gershwin and T. E. Albertson © Humana Press Inc., Totowa, NJ

Table 1
Risks of Anesthesia for Asthmatics

Anesthetic effect	Risk
Exposure to multiple drugs	Possible airway effects resulting in bronchoconstriction
	Possible drug interaction
Endotracheal intubation	Stimulation of reflex bronchoconstriction
Depression of protective airway reflexes	Aspiration
Respiratory depression	Hypoventilation and need for artificial ventilation
Depression of inspiratory and expiratory effort	Atelectasis and retained secretions
Limited access to the patient for diagnosis and treatment	Delayed diagnosis
	Ineffective treatment

Note. These are generic risks of anesthesia that have special significance for asthmatic patients.

anesthesia, as well as muscle relaxants, are also reviewed. The various inhaled anesthetic agents, including more recently developed drugs, are discussed with respect to their potential to either provoke or alleviate bronchospasm. Pain relief for the patient with asthma, including the use of spinal opiates, is briefly explained. Various methods of regional anesthesia techniques are explained, so the medical provider will have a familiarity with them. Preoperative preparation of the patient with asthma as an outpatient or inpatient is essential, and this is explained to guide medical optimization of the surgical patient with asthma. The conduct of anesthesia for the patient with asthma is explained with case scenarios. The management of acute intraoperative bronchospasm is also explained. The important differential diagnosis of wheezing in the operating room is likewise explained. Important measures of postoperative care in the immediate postanesthesia recovery period, intensive care unit (ICU), and ward are reviewed. Finally, the critical periods of intensive care, requiring airway management for endotracheal intubation, and the more rare, but more complex, use of inhaled anesthetics for management of status asthmaticus are described in detail. This chapter is not a manual for anesthesia care of the patient with asthma, but, as a starting point, it should impart significant information, so that the medical care provider will have insight into the pertinent anesthesia care of the patient with asthma. A review of asthma management directed at anesthesiologists has been authored by Gal *(1)*.

PREOPERATIVE ASSESSMENT OF THE PATIENT WITH ASTHMA

All patients with any form of reactive airway disease will be referred to here as "patients with asthma." There is usually no practical way to subcategorize a particular patient, nor is there a difference in the anesthetic management. Preoperative assessment of patients with asthma should establish the patient's baseline condition under medical management and identify correctable conditions. Symptomatic patients, who are untreated or are not compliant with medical management, should have elective surgery postponed until they are stable under therapy. Not every patient can be symptom free, but an increase in symptom severity that does not respond to therapy should result in delay

Table 2
Preoperative Anesthetic Evaluation of Asthma Patients

Presentation	Concern	Risks
Asymptomatic asthma	Minimal concerns	Possible onset of wheezing treated or untreated triggered by drugs or airway intubation.
Asthma with acute symptoms	Possibility of poor compliance with therapy or onset of respiratory tract infection	Possible postoperative pulmonary complications, especially if the surgical site is thoracic or upper abdominal. Risk may be reduced by delay for preoperative treatment.
Chronic asthma	Possibility of irreversible airway disease and chronically decreased reserve	Possible postoperative pulmonary complications, especially if the surgical site is thoracic or upper abdominal.
Unexpected preoperative wheezing (not previously diagnosed as asthmatic)	Undiagnosed medical problem	Possible mistaken diagnosis of asthma and incorrect treatment.
	No prior treatment	Risk of severe bronchospasm and excessive airway mucus, if it is necessary to proceed in an emergency. Risk may be reduced by delay for preoperative diagnosis and treatment. Possible postoperative pulmonary complications, especially if the surgical site is thoracic or upper abdominal.

of elective surgery until the patient's condition improves to baseline. In an emergency, there may be little time for preoperative control of bronchial hyperreactivity or airway inflammation. Table 2 briefly lists some of the preoperative concerns that arise, based on the clinical presentation of the patient with asthma.

PREOPERATIVE PREPARATION OF THE PATIENT WITH ASTHMA

Prevention of perioperative anesthetic complications depends on assessment and appropriate preoperative preparation of patients with asthma. Neither the patient's own subjective assessment nor the physician's physical examination is unfailingly reliable in identifying the need for additional preoperative treatment (2). Consequently, it is reasonable to try to improve the condition of every patient with asthma, except those who are free of asthma signs and symptoms. In pediatric patients, preoperative preparation is believed to reduce the risk of asthma complications to a level comparable to children without asthma (3). For some patients, the need for adherence to their bronchodilator therapy and smoking cessation must be stressed. This should be done well in advance of the surgical date. In patients who are judged to be at high risk for perioperative

Table 3
American Society of Anesthesiologist's Physical Status and NIH Asthma Guidelines

ASA physical status	Description	Asthma severity step
1	Healthy, or localized disease	—
2	Mild disease and well compensated	1 and 2 (mild intermittent or persistent)
3	Severe disease, or poorly compensated	3 (moderate persistent with daily symptoms)
4	Life threatening disease	4 (severe persistent with continual symptoms)
5	Moribund	—

bronchospasm, a brief course of corticosteroid therapy may be indicated. There is little risk of wound complications or adrenal insufficiency *(4)*. The patient's physical status will usually be summarized using the American Society of Anesthesiologists' classification (*see* Table 3). The last table column gives the approximate Asthma Severity step. If the patient has additional problems, the physical status may be higher than shown in the table.

GENERAL AND REGIONAL ANESTHESIA: ISSUES PERTINENT TO ASTHMA

The property of general anesthetic agents to obtund the laryngeal and pharyngeal reflexes and reduce bronchomotor tone are certainly beneficial to patients with asthma who are undergoing general anesthesia. There are, however, several aspects of general anesthesia that put the patient with asthma at risk. One risk is potential aspiration of gastric contents, which, although a rare occurrence in patients who have fasted, is a significant concern in the patient who presents without having fasted. Other patients who are at risk for gastric aspiration syndrome are those in whom there is gastroesophageal reflux, marked obesity, bowel obstruction, gastroparesis (trauma or diabetes), pregnancy, or other factors increasing intragastric pressure. As a result of these risks, general anesthesia requires protection of the airway, which is generally accomplished by endotracheal intubation.

The airway, even in those without a risk for aspiration, must be supported to avoid airway obstruction. This is increasingly being achieved by the use of devices, such as the laryngeal mask airway (LMA) that, although it does not protect the airway from gastric aspiration, can be highly effective in supporting the airway during spontaneous ventilation and general anesthesia. It is used in the patient who has fasted who is not otherwise at risk for gastric aspiration. In a limited fashion during brief periods, it has also been used during controlled ventilation and general anesthesia. For the patient with asthma, endotracheal intubation will trigger a bronchospastic response unless this response is obtunded by anesthetic and other pharmacological agents. The use of the laryngeal mask airway is discussed because in the patient with asthma, a device for airway management that does not pass the vocal cords into the trachea is beneficial. If positive pressure ventilation in severe asthma is required, however, controlled ventilation will require an endotracheal tube (ET). The ET tube is uncuffed in small children but cuffed in adults to reduce or eliminate leak and prevent aspiration. When high inflation pressures are required (>25 mmHg), even a cuffed ET will leak during peak inspiration, resulting in tidal volume loss (*see* the following heading).

If the patient with asthma can be comfortably and safely managed for surgical care with regional anesthesia block, then the method of regional anesthesia will be dictated by the site of the operation and the willingness and suitability of the patient to undergo the surgical procedure using a regional anesthetic technique. In certain circumstances, local anesthesia in concert with sedation may be appropriate. Benefits of a regional anesthesia technique include the lack of necessity for the use of an airway device. Whenever a regional anesthetic is used, the patient and anesthesia care provider should be fully prepared to convert to general anesthesia, including endotracheal intubation. Conversion from a regional anesthetic to general anesthesia is necessary if the regional method does not provide sufficient analgesia; immobility of the surgical field cannot be achieved so that the surgical technique is hampered, or the hemodynamic/and or respiratory status of the patient mandates conversion to a general anesthetic technique. As mentioned, such general anesthesia will then necessarily require airway management. This may simply entail manual positioning of the airway (positioning the jaw forward and placing the neck in a sniffing position) and using a mask anesthesia. Airway management under these circumstances may require the use of an LMA or commonly will necessitate endotracheal intubation, with significant potential for stimulation of bronchospasm, or at least some airway reactivity in the patient with asthma.

GENERAL ANESTHESIA
Airway Management

MASK ANESTHESIA

Airway management during general anesthesia can require simply the placement of a mask over the patient's face, with appropriate positioning of the jaw and neck to avoid airway obstruction by the tongue. Mask anesthesia obviates the need for placement of an airway device in many cases; however, some patients may not have an adequate airway without the placement of a nasal or oral airway during the conduct of this method of general anesthesia. Some patients may even require the placement of an LMA (*see* Subheading entitled "Laryngeal Mask") or ET during intended mask anesthesia. Occasionally, emergency airway insertions have to be performed because of unanticipated airway obstruction, and this may provoke or exacerbate asthma-related bronchospasm.

SEDATION, INCLUDING DEEP SEDATION WITH INTRAVENOUS PROPOFOL

Certain procedures can be accomplished with sedation only, e.g., when local anesthesia is injected by the surgeon for limited surgical procedures, including breast biopsy, minor excisions of other lesions, certain eye surgeries, and certain other facial surgeries. Combinations of short-acting benzodiazepines (midazolam) and synthetic opiates (fentanyl) are most commonly used for sedation during such surgical procedures. When an anesthesiologist is present, this is referred to as "monitored anesthesia care."

The advent of the short-acting anesthetic agent propofol has made it possible also to use deep sedation to accomplish many surgeries without the need for inhaled anesthetics. This frequently used form of anesthesia uses either propofol general anesthesia during spontaneous ventilation for placement of local anesthesia by the surgeon or sometimes more prolonged infusion of propofol to provide profound sedation or general anesthesia. This often can be accomplished without the need for airway adjuncts; however, as noted and as with any anesthetic technique, unanticipated airway management may be needed, and this can have significant consequences for the patient with asthma. Opiates, such as fentanyl, sufentanil, and remifentanil, with short-elimination half-lives are now used in concert with propofol in some circumstances to design total intravenousanesthesia. An advantage of opiates is prompt emergence from anesthesia, not requiring inhalation anesthesia. For the patient with asthma, the inhalation agents, because of their bronchodilating properties, have been preferred, but intravenous anesthesia may also have a role in management patients with asthma.

LARYNGEAL MASK

The LMA is a silicone rubber airway device that is made of a tube, much like an ET onto which is incorporated an elliptical mask with an inflatable rim *(5)*. LMA devices are made in sizes ranging from neonate to large adult. The LMA is passed through the mouth of the patient, after suitable anesthesia, into the hypopharynx, where it straddles the glottic opening, without passing through the vocal cords. It is available in sizes that can accommodate age ranges from neonate to large adult. Although it does not protect the lungs from aspiration of gastric secretions, it does form a seal to limit aspiration of secretions from the oropharynx *(6)*. As a result, perhaps, and because of its efficacy in maintaining the airway, laryngospasm is an uncommon occurrence during general anesthesia using the LMA.

For the patient with asthma, this less invasive option for airway management relative to endotracheal anesthesia can help to avoid stimulating airway reactivity. Some anesthesia practitioners prefer it to endotracheal intubation for management of the asthmatic surgical patient. Exceptions are patients who are at risk for aspiration or need for muscle relaxation with prolonged positive pressure ventilation. An important use of the LMA in the ICU or emergency room is the management of the difficult airway and during resuscitation after failed intubation. The LMA is part of the difficult airway algorithm of the American Society of Anesthesiologists. In the patient who is critically ill, it can be lifesaving, pending the insertion of a more definitive airway, such as an endotracheal intubation or tracheostomy *(7)*.

ENDOTRACHEAL INTUBATION

The placement of an ET into the airway of a patient with asthma frequently provokes bronchospasm. The likelihood of this occurring is greater if the patient has not been adequately preoperatively prepared for general endotracheal anesthesia by the administration of bronchodilators, preferably β_2-selective adrenergic agonists. At the author's facility, this is most commonly achieved by instruction in the preoperative clinic that the patient use his or her inhaler in the hours preceding their surgery. The use of longer acting inhaled bronchodilators is also advisable, particularly if the patient requires them to prevent nocturnal asthmatic symptoms or breakthrough bronchospasm. At the author's facility, it is common for the patient with asthma to present with the history that he or she uses a twice- or thrice-daily regimen of salmeterol and uses an albuterol inhaler for breakthrough symptoms. For patients with the most severe asthma, perioperative steroid therapy must be considered in concert with the primary care provider or pulmonary consultant on an individual basis.

Also, the likelihood of bronchospasm developing in response to endotracheal intubation will depend on the extent to which the induction and administration of inhalation anesthesia will sufficiently obtund airway reflexes. In the case of the intravenous and inhaled agents, the various agents differ in their effects and are discussed below.

ANESTHETIC DRUGS IN PATIENTS WITH ASTHMA

The pharmacology of anesthetic drugs is significant from two perspectives: the effect of the anesthetic on airway mechanics, and the interaction of anesthetics with drugs that are used to manage asthma. Unfortunately, most of the science is not based on studies in humans with hyperreactive airways.

Preinduction and Intravenous Induction Agents

The initiation of general anesthesia is usually preceded by the administration of sedation, often in the form a benzodiazepine. A short-acting drug, such as midazolam, is preferred to avoid postoperative respiratory depression and somnolence. It is during this preinduction period that the patient with asthma should also be asked if a recent dose of an inhaled bronchodilator has been administered. If not, it is generally advisable that the patient use a metered-dose inhaler at this time. If the patient is too young or, for other reasons, incapable of using the metered-dose inhaler, then a nebulizing device and a face mask can be applied in the anesthesia preoperative staging area for administration of a bronchodilator. In the author's facility, albuterol is most commonly used because it is generally free of unwanted systemic side effects, such as tachycardia.

For patients who are obese, a nonparticulate antacid is administered orally to neutralize the gastric acid pH and often an additional intravenous dose of metoclopramide is administered to expedite gastric emptying. These measures, in concert with compression of the cricoid cartilage against the sixth cervical vertebrae during induction, are used to decrease the likelihood of gastric aspiration of secretions into the lung once protective airway reflexes are lost during the induction of general anesthesia.

Selection of the appropriate intravenous anesthetic induction agent for the patient with asthma is important, because the agents have different pharmacokinetic and pharmacodynamic profiles (8). Short-acting sedative hypnotics are typically used. The induction thiobarbiturates thiopental and thiamylal are short acting and, as with most intravenous induction agents, produce loss of consciousness within one arm-to-brain circulation time (usually within <30 s). Their safety for induction in patients with asthma is questionable. Laboratory and clinical evidence suggest that thiobarbiturates can induce the release of histamine (9). Methohexital, an oxybarbiturate, does not release histamine in this fashion. Anesthesia with barbiturates, if profound, does suppress airway reactivity. Nevertheless, profound barbiturate anesthesia (such as in the usual clinical induction of anesthesia) has been complicated by a significant incidence of bronchospasm in patients with asthma. The phencyclidine derivative ketamine has been recommended in the patient with asthma because of its tendency to cause release of catecholamines. However, ketamine can produce unfavorable psychotropic effects, such as night terrors, and, therefore, it is not an ideal choice. The imidazole etomidate is an intravenous agent that is not generally associated with the provocation of bronchospasm, and it lends hemodynamic stability during anesthesia induction, as well. Propofol has been clinically effective as an agent that is promptly eliminated, as well as having a favorable profile for the patient with asthma. It is uncommonly associated with intraoperative provocation of bronchospasm. In patients both with and without asthma, propofol induction is accompanied by less wheezing than induction with thiopental or methohexital *(10)*.

NEUROMUSCULAR-BLOCKING DRUGS

When neuromuscular blockade is needed for airway management, ventilation, or operative procedures, drugs such as succinylcholine and vecuronium may be required. The neuromuscular-blocking drugs, commonly referred to as "relaxants," differ not only in potency, duration, and mechanism of elimination but also in their side effects and drug interactions. Should some of these drugs be avoided in asthmatic patients?

Although there may be some theoretical concerns about histamine release by the benzylisoquinolinium class of relaxants (atracurium and mivacurium), there is little evidence for a significant or frequent problem in asthmatics. Intravenous injection of drugs, such as atracurium and mivacurium, can produce flushing and blood pressure reduction by causing histamine release from mast cells. Bronchospasm is seldom observed. The risk of histamine release is reduced by slow injection, prophylactic anti-histamines, and small doses. The risk is avoided by using a steroidal relaxant, such as pancuronium, vecuronium, or rocuronium. Anaphylactic reactions to relaxants are rare but have been reported. None of the newer relaxants has a reputation for producing ana-phylaxis. A more likely cause of bronchospasm than histamine after a muscle relaxant is mechanical airway stimulation from introduction of an ET.

The only significant interaction between relaxants and bronchodilators is a single case report of marked tachycardia when pancuronium, which has a vagolytic effect and blocks adrenergic reuptake, was given to a child who had been treated with adrenergic agonists.

Inhaled Anesthetic Agents

All of the currently used potent inhaled anesthetics (sevoflurane, desflurane, isoflu-rane, and less commonly now, halothane) are bronchodilators at clinical concentrations. Unfortunately, the inhaled anesthetics have many side effects, including respiratory and myocardial depression, sensitization to catecholamines, and, in susceptible patients, malignant hyperthermia. These side effects may limit the ability to use an inhaled agent despite its bronchodilating effects. Both sevoflurane and desflurane produce rapid induction and recovery, but sevoflurane is preferred in patients with asthma because desflurane causes airway irritation when inhaled.

Of particular interest to the nonanesthesiologist is whether the inhaled anesthetics can be used to facilitate recovery from status asthmaticus and, if so, whether use of an inhaled anesthetic is safer or more effective than other methods for managing status asthmaticus. Numerous clinical reports attest to the efficacy of inhalation anesthetics in the successful management of status asthmaticus. However, it is difficult to imagine that this therapy does more than provide prolonged bronchodilation with mechanical ventilation and reduction of metabolic demands. All of these can be provided by other pharmacological agents. There are no comparative studies on which to base a choice. The logistical problem of providing continuous anesthesia significantly limits the use of this method.

Opiate Analgesia

Opiate drugs have a central role as perioperative analgesics. The older, longer-acting opiates, such as morphine and meperidine, given intravenously have been associated with histamine release and the appearance of urticaria proximal to the site of injection. This is considered a pharmacologically induced rather than immunologically induced (allergic) release. The clinical significance is questionable. Newer synthetic opiates, such as fentanyl, sufentanil, and remifentanil, are short acting and potent, and they have not been associated with histamine release.

The past two decades have seen an increasing use of opiates administered via a variety of routes for perioperative analgesia. They are administered intravenously, epidurally, intrathecally, intraarticularly, transcutaneously, and transmucosally. There is little risk of respiratory impairment, compared with intravenous administration. The exceptions are inadvertent migration of an epidural catheter into the intrathecal space or the delayed respiratory depression from cephalad migration of a single intrathecal morphine dose. Progressive sedation is a warning sign of respiratory depression when opiates are given continuously. Therefore, it is advisable to limit the use of sedative drugs, such as benzodiazepines and minor tranquilizers, so that progressive sedation can be recognized for serious consequences. One other possible exception is epidurally administered fentanyl. Because of its high lipid solubility, blood concentrations of epidural fentanyl are similar to those obtained by intravenous infusion of fentanyl. Current practice frequently combines opiate infusions with low concentrations of local anesthetics to augment the analgesia and to permit reduction in the amount of opiate that is necessary to produce satisfactory analgesia.

REGIONAL ANESTHESIA

If appropriate for the surgical procedure, regional local anesthetic techniques, such as spinal anesthesia, epidural anesthesia, and peripheral nerve blocks, avoid exposing the patient to the risk of bronchial stimulation from endotracheal intubation. As expected, sporadic case reports of bronchospasm occurring during regional anesthesia have appeared. In the absence of a convincing mechanism or causal relationship to regional anesthesia, such reports should not weigh strongly against the use of regional anesthesia in patients with asthma. As with all patients undergoing regional anesthesia, judicious sedation will help to control the side effects of anxiety.

In patients with asthma, anxiety control may be particularly important in preventing perioperative exacerbation of symptoms.

Brachial Plexus Block

Anesthesia of the hand, arm, and shoulder is produced by injection of local anesthetic within the fibrous sheath that contains the brachial plexus. The injection can be performed at a variety of sites, from the base of the neck (interscalene) to the axilla. These approaches differ slightly in technical difficulty, risk, and distribution of analgesia, so the anesthesiologist will need to determine the most appropriate approach for a given patient and procedure. In patients with asthma, surgery on an upper extremity can be performed without the need for airway and ventilation management if brachial plexus anesthesia is appropriate and successful. The interscalene approach can cause transient hemidiaphragmatic paralysis, and supraclavicular approaches have some risk of inducing pneumothorax. The anesthesiologist will assess the risk and benefits in formulating his or her recommendations for a particular block technique.

A single injection into the brachial plexus produces anesthesia for 2 h or more, depending on the particular local anesthetic that is used. Brachial plexus block duration can be extended by the placement of a catheter for repeated injections or continuous infusions. However, the surface anatomy and mobility of the shoulder girdle area make it difficult to keep a brachial plexus catheter in position for extended periods of time.

Intravenous Regional (Bier) Block

Intravenous regional block can be used to provide rapid anesthesia of the hand and forearm. The technique requires only the placement of an intravenous catheter in a hand vein and the application of an effective double tourniquet. Recovery is rapid when the tourniquet is released. Unfortunately, because of the gradual onset of tourniquet pain, this method of anesthesia is limited to operations not longer than 1 h. Although there is a transient increase in local anesthetic and products of tissue metabolism when the tourniquet is released, there are no specific disadvantages for patients with asthma.

Epidural (Peridural) Block

Anesthesia below the upper abdomen can be produced by local anesthetic injection into the epidural space, the compartment between the dura and boney spinal canal and concentric to the dural compartment. In patients with asthma, this method of anesthesia is used to advantage for obstetrical, gynecological, lower extremity orthopedic, urological, and lower body superficial operations. Of particular advantage is the ability to continue epidural blockade for postoperative pain relief by placement of a catheter in the epidural space. Intermittent doses or continuous infusion of local anesthetic and/or opiates can provide many days of postoperative pain analgesia. Anticoagulation is a significant contraindication to the use of epidural block. A significant contraindication to continuous postoperative epidural analgesia is the use of postoperative anticoagulation, which introduces the risk of epidural hematoma.

Spinal (Intrathecal, Subarachnoid) Block

Spinal or intrathecal anesthesia is used for the same types of operations as epidural block. Onset is more rapid, duration can be prolonged, and muscle relaxation is more significant with intrathecal injection of local anesthetics. Spinal headache is a well-known complication of dural puncture. The headache is worse in the upright position and decreases or disappears with recumbence. Postdural puncture headache is usually self-limited, but slow recovery is sometimes inconvenient when a patient needs to be upright and active. Remedies, such as increasing fluid intake, wearing an abdominal binder, oral or intravenous caffeine, and epidural fluid infusion can provide effective, but often transient, relief. In patients with asthma who take theophylline-containing drugs and β-adrenergic agonists, there may be risk of toxicity if caffeine is used to treat the headache. The relief of postdural puncture headache by epidural autologous blood injection ("blood patch") is usually effective and enduring.

Lower Extremity Blocks

For operations involving one extremity, particularly the distal part, a variety of peripheral nerve blocks can be used to provide the same advantages as a spinal or

Table 4
Advantages and Disadvantages of Anesthetic Technique for Asthma Patients

Anesthetic technique	Advantages	Disadvantages/risks

General anesthesia
  Inhaled agents
  Intravenous agents
  Neuromuscular block
	Inhaled agents are
	  bronchodilators
		Airway and ventilation effects
		  require management that may
		  precipitate bronchospasm.
		Inhaled agents lower the threshold for
		  arrhythmias from β-adrenergic
		  bronchodilators.
		Depressed expiratory muscle activity
		  may result in hypoventilation.

Regional anesthesia
  Epidural block
  Subarachnoid block
  Brachial plexus block
  IV regional block
  Peripheral nerve block
	Usually able to avoid
	  airway and ventilation
	  management.
	
	Post-operative analgesia is
	  possible with some
	  blocks that can be
	  continued by infusion
		Epinephrine-containing local
		  anesthetics may contribute to
		  side effects from β-adrenergic
		  bronchodilators.
		Anxiety may need to be managed
		  with drugs that can lead to
		  respiratory depression.
		Paralyzed expiratory muscles may
		  result in hypoventilation.

Local anesthesia	Minimal interference
	  with airway or
	  ventilation.
		Epinephrine-containing local
		  anesthetics may contribute to
		  side effects from β-adrenergic
		  bronchodilators.

Note. There are advantages, disadvantages, and risks that are not mentioned here, because they do not specifically relate to asthma patients.

epidural block but without the risk of spinal cord injury or sympathetic block. On the other hand, the use of a tourniquet is a problem when only part of an extremity is blocked. Discomfort from tissue ischemia may require supplemental doses of intravenous opiates and eventually general anesthesia. Because peripheral nerve blocks can also provide a measure of postoperative analgesia, recent years have seen a growing interest in developing and improving the techniques of peripheral blocks.

CONDUCT OF ANESTHESIA FOR THE PATIENT WITH ASTHMA

General and regional anesthetic techniques have been discussed in preceding subheadings. Table 4 summarizes some of the advantages, disadvantages, and risks that are associated with the different anesthetic techniques. Despite careful selection of technique and drugs, the patient with asthma may experience an exacerbation during surgery. Table 5 lists some special considerations in selected surgical patient populations.

Intraoperative Management of Acute Bronchospasm

Bronchoconstriction is not a common occurrence during surgery *(11)*, but it is the most likely cause of wheezing under anesthesia in a patient with asthma. In a patient who has not been preoperatively identified as asthmatic, the onset of wheezing and/or increasing ventilation pressures is less easily assigned to bronchoconstriction. In

Table 5
Asthmatic Patient Groups With Special Considerations

Group	Problems	Management considerations for general anesthesia
Pregnancy and cesarean section patients	Aspiration risk requiring rapid induction and intubation if general anesthesia is needed. Consequent risk of triggering bronchospasm.	Preinduction anticholinergic drug, such as glycopyrrolate. Ketamine or propofol induction.
Pediatric patients	May have frequent/continuous respiratory tract infections. Inhaled induction frequently used.	Immediate preinduction evaluation for possible new symptoms. Sevoflurane for inhaled induction.
Geriatric patients	Other chronic diseases, such as coronary artery disease. Diminished reserve resulting in sensitivity to depressant drugs.	Cautious use of prophylactic β-adrenergic blockers. Cautious use of inhaled agents that produce respiratory and myocardial depression.
Trauma victims	Unknown history of medical problems, including possible asthma. Undiagnosed pulmonary injury that can mimic asthma. Unknown drug history leading to risk of adverse drug interactions.	Maintain a level of suspicion for the presence of asthma or asthma mimics.
Malignant hyperthermia (MH) susceptible patients	Inhaled agents can trigger an MH episode	Total intravenous anesthesia.

patients who are unanesthetized, other causes of wheezing include airway secretions, airway foreign body, pulmonary aspiration, pulmonary edema, pneumothorax, and anaphylactic drug reactions. During anesthesia, light anesthesia, ET obstruction, and bronchial intubation must be added to the list. The latter two causes of intraoperative wheezing can lead to rapid hypoxemia and are therefore high priorities on the list of possible problems. If the presence of immediately life-threatening problems can be eliminated, it is common practice to offer a trial of bronchodilator therapy or to deepen the level of anesthesia. Even if light anesthesia is present, it may not always be appropriate to deepen the anesthesia if the patient cannot tolerate the side effects of deeper anesthesia or if the operation is ending.

Perioperative Bronchodilators

Bronchodilators that can be given by aerosol or injection can be given during anesthesia. Aerosolized β₂-adrenergic agonists are usually used for perioperative bronchodilation. A variety of methods have been proposed for administering bronchodilators into the anesthetic breathing circuit. It is common to give 10 or more puffs of a bronchodilator. Measurement of drug delivered in a laboratory model suggests that this method is efficient *(12)*. Intravenous bronchodilators are rarely used, except when severe bronchospasm prevents the effective delivery of aerosolized drugs. Intravenous aminophylline probably produces no reduction in airway resistance beyond what is obtained from an inhaled anesthetic. Furthermore, theophylline is associated with cardiac arrhythmias in the presence of inhaled anesthetics. If aminophylline is given intraoperatively, it should be given at half the usual infusion rate to compensate for reduced clearance under anesthesia, and the electrocardiogram should be monitored for signs of cardiac irritability.

Postoperative Management

On arrival in the postanesthesia care unit, patients may have residual muscle relaxation and central respiratory depression. A sustained head lift is the best clinical sign of recovery from neuromuscular blockade. Signs of respiratory fatigue, asthma exacerbation, or secretion retention require intervention. Anticholinesterase inhibitors, such as neostigmine, are used to reverse the effects of muscle relaxants. The resulting parasympathomimetic effects may worsen the condition of the patient with asthma by increasing bronchial tone and increasing the volume of airway secretions. Bronchodilator treatments, and possibly intravenous corticosteroids, may be necessary for postoperative exacerbation of asthma. Some patients are better managed initially with continued intubation and mechanical ventilation. This is the case with patients who are at high risk for postoperative pulmonary complications. Risk factors include patients whose asthma is poorly controlled, patients whose surgical incision is in the upper abdominal or thoracic region, and patients who will require large doses of postoperative opiates.

The level of postoperative care may require placement in the ICU. The critical care management of patients with asthma is not discussed here. Some commonly used anesthetic drugs are used as adjuncts in the management of asthmatics in the ICU. Considerations are similar to the immediate postoperative concerns about adequate recovery from neuromuscular blockade and central respiratory depressants.

There are few restrictions on postoperative analgesia in the patient with asthma. The two greatest concerns are retention of tenacious mucous, because of poor cough effort, or respiratory depression and hypoventilation from central respiratory depression or fatigue. Some of the common methods of analgesia, with their advantages and risks, are summarized in Table 6. Epidural infusion of opiate with or without low concentrations of local anesthetic is particularly recommended for thoracic and upper abdominal procedures in asthma patients. The risk of sedation and respiratory depression is low, and the patient should be able to generate an effective cough. However, the use of anticoagulation to prevent postoperative thromboembolism is an important contraindication to the use of continuous epidural infusions.

EMERGENCY INTERVENTION

Intubation of the Patient With Asthma Who is Decompensating

The patient with asthma who is decompensating and who requires intubation presents a dangerous challenge.

Bronchodilators may have been given until the adrenergic side effects have become a problem. The patient may already be hypercarbic and hypoxemic. In this situation,

Table 6
Postoperative Analgesia Considerations in the Asthma Patient

Analgesia technique	Advantages	Disadvantages/risks
Oral medication	Patient-controlled (within limits) with limited potential for respiratory depression.	Risk of precipitating bronchospasm in patients who are sensitive to aspirin, but otherwise minimal risk.
Patient-controlled analgesia	Patient-controlled within limits.	No disadvantages specific for asthma patients.
Continuous epidural infusion	Analgesia with little risk of impairment of respiration and ability to cough.	No disadvantages specific for asthma patients.
Continuous brachial plexus infusion	Analgesia with little risk of impairment of respiration and ability to cough.	No disadvantages specific for asthma patients.

Note. There are advantages, disadvantages, and risks that are not mentioned here because they do not specifically relate to asthma patients.

the use of paralyzing muscle relaxants is particularly hazardous because, if intubation is unsuccessful, the patient's high airway resistance will probably make attempts with mask ventilation ineffective. If on examination the patient appears to be a potentially difficult intubation, awake intubation with topical anesthesia may be the safest method. Correct placement of the ET can be difficult to verify by auscultation, particularly if the patient suffers a transient, reflex bronchoconstriction as a result of airway stimulation by the ET. This may be partially preventable by four puffs of inhaled albuterol 3 min before intubation. Intravenous lidocaine, once considered useful for preventing reflex bronchoconstriction, seems not to be effective.

Status Asthmaticus

The efficacy of inhaled anesthetics as bronchodilators has motivated their use in the management of status asthmaticus. Several case reports describe the successful use of inhaled agents. Endotracheal intubation and mechanical ventilation are required, because the inhaled anesthetics depress respiratory drive and airway protective reflexes. Additionally, several practical issues must be addressed. An anesthesiologist should be in continuous attendance, and an anesthesia machine must be provided for several hours. Although halothane has an established reputation as a potent bronchodilator, isoflurane is probably just as effective and has less risk of adverse interaction with β-adrenergic bronchodilators. Because there are no definitive guidelines for the anesthetic concentration or duration of treatment, the patient is treated until improvement or toxicity occurs. Neuromuscular blocking drugs with appropriate sedation may be used to facilitate mechanic ventilation. Some advantages of neuromuscular block are minimization of oxygen consumption and no misinterpretation of coughing and straining as increases in bronchoconstriction. Possible disadvantages include loss of negative pleural pressure generated by inspiratory effort and risk of disconnect from the ventilator, particularly when high airway pressures or frequent suctioning are needed. Finally, the possible role of muscle relaxants, corticosteroids, and immobility in producing myopathy and difficulty weaning from mechanical ventilation *(13)*.

REFERENCES

1. Gal TJ. Bronchial hyperresponsiveness and anesthesia: physiological and therapeutic perspectives. *Anesth Analg* 1994; 78: 559–573.
2. Alario AJ, Lewander WJ, Dennehy P, Seifer R, Mansell AL. The relationship between oxygen saturation and the clinical assessment of acutely wheezing infants and children. *Pediatr Emerg Care* 1995; 11: 331–339.
3. Zachary CY, Evans R 3rd. Perioperative management for childhood asthma. *Ann Allergy Asthma Immunol* 1996; 77: 468–472.
4. Kabalin CS, Yarnold PR, Grammer LC. Low complication rate of corticosteroid-treated asthmatics undergoing surgical procedures. *Arch Intern Med* 1995; 155: 1379–1384.
5. Brain AIJ. The development of the laryngeal mask: a brief history of the invention, early clinical studies and experimental work from which the laryngeal mask evolved. *Eur J Anaesthesiol* 1991; 4: 5–17.
6. John RE, Hill S, Hughes TJ. Airway protection by the laryngeal mask: a barrier to dye placed in the pharynx. *Anaesthesia* 1991; 46: 366–367.
7. American Society of Anesthesiologists Task Force on Management of the Difficult Airway. Practice guidelines for management of the difficult airway anesthesiology. *Anesthesiology* 1993; 78: 597–602.
8. Rooke GA, Choi J-H, Bishop MJ. The effect of isoflurane, halothane, sevoflurane, and thiopental/nitrous oxide on respiratory system resistance after tracheal infection. *Anesthesiology* 1997;86: 1294–1299.
9. Hirshman CA, Edelstein RA, Ebertz JM, Hanifin JM. Thiobarbiturate-induced histamine release in human skin mast cells. *Anesthesiology* 1985; 63: 353–356.
10. Pizov R, Brown RH, Weiss YS, et al. Wheezing during induction of general anesthesia in patients with and without asthma. A randomized, blinded trial. *Anesthesiology* 1995; 82: 1111–1116.
11. Warner DO, Warner MA, Barnes RD, et al. Perioperative respiratory complications in patients with asthma. *Anesthesiology* 1996; 85: 460–467.
12. Peterfreund RA, Niven RW, Kacmarek RM. Syringe-activated metered dose inhalers: a quantitative laboratory evaluation of albuterol delivery through nozzle extensions. *Anesth Analg* 1994; 78: 554–558.
13. Behbehani NA, Al-Mane F, D'yachkova Y, Paré P, Fitzgerald JM. Myopathy following mechanical ventilation for acute severe asthma. The role of muscle relaxants and corticosteroids. *Chest* 1999; 115: 1627–1631.

16 How Recreational Drugs Affect Asthma

Timothy E. Albertson, PhD, MD, MPH,
Steve Offerman, MD,
and Nicholas J. Kenyon, MD

CONTENTS

KEY POINTS

- Because of the recent epidemic, drugs of abuse have more opportunity to interact with a common disease such as asthma.
- Drugs of abuse have not been proven to cause asthma, but they may exacerbate pre-existing asthma.
- Case reports of asthma exacerbations after recreational drug abuse continue to increase.
- Abuse of cocaine and the opioid heroin have the richest literature supporting an interaction with asthma and offer possible pathophysiological mechanisms.
- Marijuana use, like tobacco use, can lead to a progressive decline in lung function.
- Tobacco use, but not nicotine addiction, is associated with worsening of asthma and obstructive pulmonary function changes.
- Healthcare providers need to specifically question their patients with asthma about recreational drug use and educate them about potential interactions.
- The only definitive treatment to eliminate any potential interaction between drug abuse and asthma is abstinence.

From: *Current Clinical Practice: Bronchial Asthma:*
A Guide for Practical Understanding and Treatment, 5th ed.
Edited by: M. E. Gershwin and T. E. Albertson © Humana Press Inc., Totowa, NJ

INTRODUCTION

Drug abuse in the United States remains a significant medical and social problem. There are many areas of health and disease that are potentially affected by the misuse of drugs. The more common a specific disease is, the more likely an interaction between the disease and drug abuse will be seen in clinical practice. In this chapter, the experience and literature available on the interaction of the most common drugs and chemicals abused and the increasingly common disease asthma are reviewed. For most drugs of abuse, little scientific data exist. Because the majority of experience with these agents is based on case reports and small series, conclusions regarding the incidence and prevalence of asthma associated with specific drugs are difficult to make. Therefore, proposed mechanisms of disease and drug interaction are often speculative. Recreational drug abuse is an epidemic problem and places a significant burden on healthcare resources in the United States and many other countries *(1)*. In addition to effects on asthma, recreational drug use has been associated with several other respiratory toxicities *(2,3)* (*see* Table 1). This chapter limits its discussion to major categories of frequently abused drugs, including the stimulants (tobacco/nicotine, cocaine, and amphetamine derivatives), the opioids (heroin), the depressants (marijuana), the hallucinogens, and inhaled volatile solvents. The use of recreational drugs should be considered by the primary care or emergency department physician in patients with difficult-to-control asthma or with atypical features of asthma. Patients should be questioned by their health care providers regarding such habits and educated about the importance of abstinence in gaining better asthma control.

COCAINE

Cocaine, an alkaloid from the plant *Erythroxylon coca,* has continued to be a significant drug of abuse with wide negative health effects. Cocaine, like amphetamines and other similar stimulants, has a multitude of complex pharmacological effects. Peripherally, cocaine prevents the neuronal reuptake of epinephrine and norepinephrine, resulting in higher synaptic catecholamine levels. In the central nervous system (CNS), cocaine increases norepinephrine release from presynaptic nerve terminals and prevents dopamine and serotonin reuptake. Unlike amphetamines, cocaine also blocks fast sodium channels at the cell membrane level, giving it a profound local anesthetic effect.

During the 19th century, patent medicines, such as the oral "Dr. Tucker's Asthma Specific" (420 mg of cocaine/oz), claimed to treat asthma. The Harrison Narcotics Act of 1914 later prohibited the sale of cocaine-containing elixirs, and the use of cocaine decreased until about 1970, when the illicit use of cocaine developed. Because of the relatively recent popularity of smoking free-base and crack cocaine, increased interest exists in the pulmonary complications of cocaine use. Smoking "crack" or "rock" cocaine is favored because of its rapid absorption and high serum concentrations, resulting in a pronounced, although short-lived, "high." When street cocaine is smoked, not only is the alkaloid cocaine (benzoylecgonine) involved but also the pyrolysis of its metabolites, contaminants, and the fuel used to burn the cocaine. Each of these components of burned or vaporized street cocaine may affect the patient with asthma. Numerous initial clinical reports have led to more sophisticated studies, particularly investigating the mechanism and role of cocaine abuse in asthma and pulmonary function.

Table 1
Nonasthma Respiratory Tract Complications Associated With Recreational Drug Abuse

Drugs of abuse	Complication
Cocaine	Nasal septal perforation
	Chronic sinusitis
	Pulmonary hypertension
	Noncardiogenic pulmonary edema
	Barotrauma—pneumothorax, pneumomediastinum
	Bronchiolitis obliterans with organizing pneumonia
	"Crack lung"—pulmonary infiltrates
	Pulmonary granulomatosis
	Nonspecific interstitial pneumonitis
	Pulmonary infiltrates with eosinophilia
	Pulmonary hemorrhage
	Hemoptysis
	Tracheal stenosis
	Foreign body aspiration
	"Cancerization effects" on bronchial epithelium
Amphetamines	Pulmonary hypertension
	Noncardiogenic pulmonary edema
	Panlobular emphysema
	Tracheal stenosis
	Foreign body aspiration
	Barotrauma—pneumomediastinum
Opioids	Barotrauma
	Foreign body embolization
	Bullous emphysema
	Pulmonary hypertension
	Eosinophilic pneumonia
	Granulomatous changes
	Respiratory depression/hypoventilation
	Bronchiectasis
Marijuana	Malignancy—bronchogenic, oropharyngeal, laryngeal
	"Cancerization effects" on bronchial epithelium
	Chronic bronchitis
	Barotrauma—pneumothorax, pneumomediastinum
	Noncardiogenic pulmonary edema
	Mild chronic airflow obstruction
	Bullous emphysema
	Possible predisposition for invasive pulmonary Aspergillus and other opportunistic infections in immunocompromised patients
Nicotine/tobacco	Malignancy—bronchogenic, oropharyngeal, laryngeal
	"Cancerization effects" on bronchial epithelium
	Chronic bronchitis
	Emphysema
	Bullous emphysema
	Eosinophilic granuloma
	Bronchiolitis-associated interstitial lung disease
Volatile substance abuse	Asphyxiation
	Pulmonary fibrosis
	Chronic rhinitis

Adapted from refs. 2–4.

Association With Asthma

Asthma has been linked with cocaine for several decades, although its causality in this disease process remains unproven. The first known report *(5)* discussing cocaine's potential association with asthma was published in 1932. This case report described the apparent precipitation of an asthma exacerbation in a patient using cocaine as a local anesthetic. The advent of smoked cocaine abuse has drawn significantly more attention to asthma, particularly in the inner cities. In 1990, 21% of all asthma deaths in the 5- to 34-yr-old age group in the United States were in New York City and Cook County, IL *(6)*. This astounding fact sparked investigations of the asthma deaths, including the potential association with cocaine abuse. A preliminary study in Chicago *(7)* found drug abuse to be a significant variable in asthma deaths. When 102 cases of fatal asthma and respiratory arrest of indeterminate cause in patients under 45 yr old were investigated *(8)*, mucous plugging or lung hyperinflation consistent with fatal asthma was identified at autopsy in 70% of the patients. Of these patients, 92 had significant toxicology for illicit drugs or alcohol. Cocaine and its metabolites was the most common illicit drug identified, occurring in 44% of these cases *(8)*. Studies like this are potentially complicated by confounders such as cocaine serving as a marker for other environmental and social economic factors. A similar conclusion was drawn in a smaller New York City case–control study of 59 consecutive patients presenting to the hospital emergency department with new-onset wheezing or a recrudescence of asthma after five symptom-free years *(9)*. When compared to 53 age- and gender-matched controls, 36% of the new-onset asthma group and 15% of the controls had positive urine screens for cocaine metabolites. A multivariate analysis, adjusting for age and sex, suggested that cocaine abuse was associated with a threefold-higher prevalence of asthma *(9)*. Another small inner-city emergency department study *(10)* noted that 36% of the 22 patients with new-onset wheezing had positive urine levels for cocaine, whereas only 13% of the 22 controls had positive urine for cocaine. A more recent emergency department study of 103 patients with severe asthma symptoms who consented to toxicology testing found that 13% had positive urine screens for cocaine metabolite (baseline for population estimated to be 2%), and twice as many (38%) with positive screens required hospitalization than those with negative screens *(11)*.

A host of case reports and small series attempt to more closely tie cocaine use, particularly smoked free-base cocaine, with asthma attacks. Six patients were described who presented to a New York City hospital with severe, life-threatening asthma after smoking cocaine *(12)*. Although many had concomitant use of tobacco and/or marijuana or upper respiratory tract infections, the authors believed that cocaine was the precipitating factor in each case. Rebhun *(13)* described three patients with asthma symptoms that only presented after smoking cocaine, despite a habit of previous cocaine snorting. One fatal case of asthma associated with cocaine has been reported again from New York *(14)*. Ironically, the patient's family reported that the patient's brother used crack cocaine and also died from a severe asthma exacerbation.

A case report of a 32-yr-old woman with preexisting asthma presented with severe bronchospasm and respiratory failure requiring intubation several hours after snorting cocaine. This was believed to be the first case of near-fatal asthma associated with nasal insufflation of cocaine and has been followed by several others *(12,15,16)*.

Pulmonary Function Abnormalities

Pulmonary function testing (PFT) and methacholine challenge testing (MCT) provide some objective evidence of variable expiratory flow limitation, its severity, and response to treatment. It is understandable, therefore, that a series of studies have focused on the use of PFT to further understand the relationship between crack or snorted cocaine use and asthma. In general, the results of these studies are inconclusive and somewhat inconsistent. Several spirometry studies (17–21) have documented near-normal forced expiratory volume in 1 s (FEV_1) and FEV_1 divided by forced vital capacity (FVC) ratios in free-base cocaine smokers. Tashkin (3,22) studied 14 former intravenous cocaine users without asthma who were given smoked and intravenous cocaine. Similar increases in heart rate and self-reported levels of intoxications were seen, but only the smoked cocaine alkaloid caused a decrease in airway specific conductance (SGaw) at 5 min (22). Similarly airway resistance (Raw) was significantly increased in the smoked cocaine group compared with the intravenous group, an effect that persisted for 30 min. The study demonstrated a bronchoconstrictive effect related solely to inhaled crack cocaine. Because there were no observable differences noted in SGaw and Raw in the intravenous group compared with control groups, it appears that a local irritant effect of the drug, its metabolites or contaminants after pyrolysis, may be responsible for many of the asthmatic exacerbations reported (22). A gas diffusion abnormality, specifically reduced diffusion capacity (DLCO), is reported more commonly in habitual cocaine smokers (3). Adrenergically mediated pulmonary vasoconstriction and a reduction in circulating pulmonary blood volume have been postulated as possible mechanisms to explain these reductions, which have not been universally reported (3).

Potential Mechanisms

Although several potential mechanisms of cocaine-induced effects on asthma have been postulated, no definitive single cause has been defined. One case may shed light on the potential multiple mechanisms involved (23). A 47-yr-old woman developed a syndrome of wheezing, shortness of breath, and cough, requiring hospitalization three times in a 6-mo period, after smoking crack cocaine. Each time, she had fleeting pulmonary infiltrates, fever, a peripheral eosinophilia, and a markedly elevated immunoglobulin (Ig)E level. Transbronchial biopsy specimens revealed nondiagnostic interstitial collections of lymphocytes, plasma cells, and eosinophils. These findings were called "crack lung" and were temporally related to her inhaled cocaine use and indicate a probable immunological mechanism for her respiratory syndrome (23). Whether cocaine-related allergens can prompt an IgE-mediated response, and if so, whether it occurs commonly is unclear. The syndrome this patient experienced may well be idiosyncratic, but clearly a spectrum of potential mechanisms for reactive airways after smoking cocaine exist.

In Levenson's previously noted autopsy study linking unexplained asthma deaths with illicit drug use (mostly cocaine), the majority of patients (69%) had the usual asthmatic findings of mucous plugging and hyperinflation, suggesting the chronic inflammatory nature of the disease (8). The observation that eosinophils, key inflammatory promoter cells in asthma, have been found in the sputum of free-base smokers with asthma supports the claim that cocaine smoking potentiates the airway inflammation of asthma but does not eliminate the possibility that the smokers had underlying quiescent asthma (12).

Another theory proposed to explain cocaine associated severe asthma attacks focuses on a study that reported that patients with near-fatal asthma had a blunted response to hypoxia and an impaired sensation of dyspnea *(24)*. This blunted response may be further augmented by the local anesthetic effect of inhaled cocaine. Finally, an uncommon mimic of an acute asthma exacerbation was reported when an adult patient presented with "wheezing" and respiratory failure requiring mechanical ventilation. On chest computed tomography (CT) scan, it was found that he had aspirated several bags of cocaine during a confrontation with police *(25)*.

AMPHETAMINES

Amphetamines are CNS stimulants with pharmacological properties similar to cocaine without the local anesthetic effects. They were first synthesized in 1927. By the 1930s, inhaled nasal products, such as Benzedrine Nasal Inhaler, were commonly used and abused stimulants. The Controlled Substance Act of 1970 greatly curtailed the legal distribution of most amphetamines outside of prescription use. The illegal production of methamphetamine and designer amphetamine derivatives have created the current demographics of stimulant abuse, causing amphetamine to be more popular than cocaine in many parts of the United States. A more pure and potent form of methamphetamine known as "ice" is volatile and allows a strong rapid high when inhaled or smoked.

Association With Asthma

Despite the similar pharmacological properties and frequent pyrolysis of methamphetamine, no significant link has yet been made to exacerbations of asthma. To date, two cases have been reported in the medical literature *(26,27)*. One report *(26)* describes a young man found dead with a bronchodilator inhaler in his hand, autopsy findings of severe acute asthma, and significant levels of the designer amphetamine methylenedioxymethamphetamine (MDMA). Another case reported a 30-yr-old male truck driver found dead at the side of the road with a nebulizer in his hand *(27)*. His autopsy suggested asthma as the cause of death, with hair and blood levels suggesting chronic methamphetamine use. A causal link was suggested in both case reports but could not be proven. Two small series *(28,29)* described 13 patients who abused iv methylphenidate and had panlobular emphysema with significant airflow obstruction. Oral methylphenidate has not been associated with emphysema, and it was postulated that the pathological changes were likely secondary to talc and other embolic material. Formal PFT in amphetamine abusers has not been systematically reported.

OPIOIDS

Naturally occurring opioids derive from the poppy, *Papaver somniferum,* with heroin remaining the most widely abused semisynthetic form. As with other recreational drugs of abuse, users have devised several means of heroin self-administration, including injection, inhalation, smoking, nasal insufflation, and ingestion.

Association With Asthma

Although the association between opioids and asthma was first described in the 1960s, a host of case reports from England in the mid-1980s noted an apparent association between asthma, including severe and fatal cases, and recent heroin use *(30–36)*. For example, one report of three chronic heroin inhalers ("chasing the dragon") noted the sudden onset of bronchospasm, respiratory failure, and anoxic encephalopathy in two of three patients after using heroin *(33)*. Survey studies *(9,34,35)* have provided further indirect evidence linking heroin use with asthma. Of 29 young asthma deaths in an urban setting, 7 had a toxicological screen positive for opioids *(8)*. In a study of 2276 mostly intravenous heroin abusers, 5% were identified as asthmatic from reviewing medical records and 31 of these addicts with asthma had reported temporal relationship between their heroin use and the onset of an asthma attack *(35)*. The authors concluded that this 1.4% of opioid users who demonstrated reactive airways to heroin represented a significant percentage of the burden on health care services from this addiction *(35)*. Heroin-induced bronchospasm may be more severe in those with previously recognized asthma. A case of asthma associated with diffuse pulmonary infiltrates and alveolar eosinophils has been reported that resolved rapidly with steroids and abstinence from heroin *(37)*.

Pulmonary Function Abnormalities

The results of PFTs evaluating the potential link between asthma and opioid abuse have been contradictory. One study reported four out of six young men who presented with new-onset wheezing and dyspnea after inhaling heroin vapor had either a positive carbachol challenge test or spirometry, suggesting airway obstruction *(30)*. However, they had peripheral or sputum eosinophilia that also strongly suggested an atopic association to their asthma, drawing into question the association with heroin. Other PFT studies refute these results *(37–40)*. In a study of 512 consecutive hospitalized intravenous drug users with positive opioid screens at admission *(40)*, 6% had evidence of airway obstruction on PFT, 7% had restriction, and 42% had an abnormally low DLCO. Krantz *(41)* has reported a series of inner-city intensive care unit admissions for asthma in which 41.3% had a positive history of use and urine toxicological screen positive for opioids on admission, compared with a 12.5% positive rate ($p = 0.006$) for patients with diabetic ketoacidosis admitted to the same unit. However, other studies *(42–44)* have demonstrated that the administration of morphine or modulation of the opioid receptors can ameliorate bronchoconstriction caused by noxious stimuli in patients with asthma.

Potential Mechanisms

Several proposed mechanisms exist for opioid interaction with asthma. Morphine and codeine caused wheezing as the result of the release histamine from mast cells in animal and some human studies. Decrease in airway SGaw has been shown when μ-opioid receptor agonists, such as codeine, are inhaled in patients with asthma who are histamine sensitive but not when taken orally. Whether this is a direct effect of the μ receptor agonist on mast cells or an indirect effect perhaps through stimulation of cholinergic J-receptors is unknown. The development of an allergic response to opioids is suggested by the demonstration of IgG and IgM antibodies to morphine in some pharmaceutical industry workers, many of whom have atopic dermatitis and asthma *(45,46)*. None of these specific mechanisms has been proven to be causative, and one or more could contribute to a patient's opioid-associated asthma.

MARIJUANA

Marijuana comes from the *Cannabis sativa* plant. The word "marijuana" is derived from the Mexican word meaning "inebriant plant." Marijuana is the most commonly used illicit recreational drug in this country. The cannabinoid, Δ^9-tetrahydrocannabinol (THC), is primarily responsible for the intoxicating properties of the marijuana cigarettes, commonly known as "joints" or "reefers." Marijuana cigarettes contain 5% THC, which stimulates CNS cannabinoid-1 (CB-1) receptors or peripheral immune CB-2 receptors *(3)*.

Association With Asthma

The interaction between marijuana abuse and asthma is a complex one. The acute effects of marijuana or THC inhalation have been reviewed extensively by Tashkin *(3)*. A decrease in Raw and an increase in SGaw have been reported after smoking marijuana or inhaling THC in healthy patients and patients with asthma, with the peak bronchodilator effects seen at 15 to 20 min and persisting for 60 min. Paradoxically high-dose exposure to THC has a bronchoconstrictor effect, and tolerance to the bronchodilator effect also occurs within several weeks of exposure *(3)*.

Population studies of regular users of marijuana have shown significant increases in cough, sputum production, wheeze, exertional dyspnea, and acute bronchitic episodes compared to nonsmokers *(3,47–49)*. Some investigators *(48)* suggest that the inhaled irritants in the marijuana smoke account for these observed symptoms. The complex interaction between asthma and marijuana appears at this time to be only indirect.

Pulmonary Function Abnormalities

Studies investigating the effects of marijuana smoke on PFTs are conflicting. As mentioned, initial bronchodilator effect with improved FEV_1 is seen after marijuana or THC inhalation. Tashkin has shown significant increase at 2–4 h in SGaw in 10 subjects after they smoked marijuana or ingested THC pills *(50)*. Tachyphylaxis develops to this bronchodilation in habitual users, with air flow obstruction being reported in heavy users *(3)*. Tashkin *(51)* has also reported that airway hyperresponsiveness by the MCT, a key feature of asthma, is not more common in marijuana smokers. Currently, there is no evidence that the long-term changes seen in airflow with chronic marijuana are related to THC but more likely related to the off-gas from the pyrolysis products.

Potential Mechanisms

If marijuana smoke or inhaled THC interacts with asthma, there are several potential mechanisms. As noted, the immediate bronchodilation seen with marijuana smoke or inhaled THC is probably from stimulation of the G protein-coupled CB-1 receptors either causing CNS modulation of bronchial tone or through direct effects. The CB-1 receptors have been found to be in proximity to airway smooth muscle cells *(3)*.

Although tachyphylaxis eventually can negate the bronchodilation, actual bronchoconstriction may be triggered by irritants in the marijuana smoke. It has also been postulated that THC has immunosuppressive properties by interacting with the CB-2 receptor on natural-killer lymphocytes *(52,53)*. This may allow an exaggerated inflammatory response to the irritant gases, which then contributes to airway injury.

TOBACCO AND NICOTINE

Cigarette smoking is endemic in the United States, and nicotine use remains the most common legal and overall recreational drug of abuse. There are at least 48 million smokers in this country alone, with prevalence use among high school students ranging as high as 35% in 1995 *(54)*. A recent report found large racial variations with prevalence among youths aged 12–17 yr, ranging from 27.9% in Native Americans to 5.2% in Japanese American youths *(55)*. Tobacco is one of the most deadly and expensive drugs of abuse. Annual estimates in the United States alone are more than 430,000 direct deaths and direct health care costs that exceed an astronomical $50 billion as the result of cigarette smoking *(56)*.

It is clear that tobacco contains, in addition to nicotine, numerous toxins and carcinogens that contribute to the development of chronic bronchitis, emphysema, and malignancy. Nicotine is a powerful central- and peripheral-acting agent that contributes to cigarette smoking addiction, but a direct link to these other pathophysiological processes is less clear. Despite the many studies on nicotine, the drug's direct effects on the lungs are not well defined.

Association With Asthma

In numerous studies *(57–61)*, either direct (active) or indirect (passive) exposure to environmental tobacco smoke has been proven to be a risk factor for the development and worsening of childhood asthma. This association has been shown even with fetal exposure by maternal smoking *(58,62)*. Risk-factor analysis for children with who require intubation for acute respiratory failure showed that exposure to secondhand tobacco smoke had the highest odds ratio of 22.4 ± 7.4 (95% CI) *(63)*. The association of tobacco smoke with worsening asthma has also been shown repeatedly in adults *(64)*. Although the evidence does not prove causality, the association is robust and has been consistently shown in many studies. Repeated exposure to tobacco smoke triggers inflammatory responses in certain children and adults that may initiate the development or worsening of asthma symptoms. No such association has been shown for nicotine alone.

Pulmonary Function Abnormalities

Although long-term active and passive exposure to tobacco smoke is associated with PFT changes showing worsening airways obstruction in numerous long-term smokers *(62)*, the data for patients with asthma are not as convincing *(60,65,66)*. At least one study in children with asthma reported that passive smoke exposure was associated with a decline in peak flow and an increase in respiratory symptoms *(67)*. In children, an increase in airway hyperresponsiveness as determined by the MCT was not associated with passive tobacco exposure, whereas an increase in asthma symptoms were *(61)*.

Potential Mechanisms

Tobacco smoke contains many respiratory irritants, including ammonia, sulfur dioxide, and formaldehyde, as well as numerous carcinogens. Different compounds found in cigarette smoke may be injurious to given predisposed individuals, leading to a triggering of or lowering of the threshold for asthma. Smoking is also associated with increased airway inflammation. The interaction of tobacco smoke and asthma is likely to be multifactorial even for individuals. Smoking may also modulate immunological responses. Active smoking is associated with an increase in total IgE. An increase in IgE is also seen in first-degree relatives exposed to passive smoking *(61)*.

VOLATILE SUBSTANCE ABUSE

Volatile substance abuse is the practice of inhaling fumes of volatile compounds to achieve a desired intoxicating effect. Acute and long-term neurological and short-term cardiac toxicity have been reported as a consequence of this relatively new practice. First tracked to California in the 1950s, by the mid-1960s, glue sniffing was popular among young people because of its accessibility, cost, and rapid effect. Since then, common household solvents and commercially bought solvents, gases, and fuels have been inhaled, including acetone, butane, propane, toluene, and nitrous oxides. The most common methods of use include "sniffing" fumes directly from a container, "huffing" from a drenched cloth placed over the face, and "bagging" from an enclosed bag placed over the head.

A survey in Great Britain found that use in some secondary school students was as high as 6% *(68)*. A recent study in the United States found 0.4% of students aged 12 to 17 yr abused inhalant substances *(69)*. A major risk factor for volatile substance abuse is low socioeconomic status. Given the low cost of these common substances, use for recreational means is likely to continue.

Association With Asthma

There is no direct reported association between asthma and inhalation of volatile substances. In a single study, Schickler *(70)* investigated possible PFT abnormalities in a cohort of 42 young solvent inhalers and 20 controls. There were no significant differences in FEV_1 or FVC values to suggest a variable obstructive defect, although increased residual volumes were seen in the substance abusers. Five of the volatile substance abusers did report acute wheezing after inhaling toluene, but no abnormalities suggestive of asthma could be demonstrated in them. Other reported pulmonary symptoms after volatile substance abuse include coughing, chronic rhinitis, and increased sputum production, as well as a case report of respiratory decompensation with pulmonary infiltrates after "fire-breathing" *(71,72)*. Currently, no consistent pattern can be identified linking volatile substance abuse to asthma. If volatile substance abuse becomes a more burdensome problem, then the establishment of an interaction with asthma may become possible.

HALLUCINOGENS

Hallucinogens are a general class of drugs that produce either alterations in perception of the environment or a dissociative state. Several drugs can cause this sensation, including certain designer amphetamines, volatile substances, anticholinergic drugs, and steroids. Each has unique neurohormonal actions and effects, but all are potentially hallucinogenic. Three recreationally abused drugs that produce this state in much lower concentrations are lysergic acid diethylamide (LSD), phencyclidine (PCP), and ketamine. PCP, or "angel dust," was marketed in the 1960s as a veterinary dissociative anesthetic with amnestic and analgesic properties, but its hallucinatory effects soon led to its ban. It has been ingested, smoked, and snorted illicitly since then and is abused primarily in inner cities and among young polysubstance abusers. Ketamine is still used in both human and veterinary medicine as a dissociative anesthetic, but diversion to illicit use has become an increasingly common problem. Compared to ketamine and PCP, LSD is more potent, easily synthesized, and readily available. LSD's actions are unclear, but speculation suggests that it may act on postsynaptic serotonin receptors, producing psychic sensations often described as depersonalization, with sensory hallucinations. All three can cause adverse psychological reactions, or "bad trips," but serious physiological side effects are uncommon.

Association With Asthma

There are no reports describing the onset of asthma after illicit PCP, ketamine, or LSD use or establishing a causal relationship between them. Ketamine is often used in status asthmaticus because of its favorable effects on airway SGaw. A previously described study on asthma deaths in Cook County, Illinois (8), noted that 2% of the young people with unexplained fatal asthma had positive toxicological screens for PCP. It is unclear, however, what role these intoxications may have played in the asthma-related death. No evidence to date has been found to support the notion that LSD, ketamine, or PCP causes or exacerbates asthma.

TREATMENT OF ASTHMA ASSOCIATED WITH RECREATIONAL DRUG ABUSE

A patient who presents to the emergency department with acute asthma symptoms or to a provider with subacute asthma and apparent recreational drug use should be treated in the same manner as other patients with asthma. Acute management, as described in the current asthma guidelines, initially includes administration of nebulized B_2-agonists with anticholinergics and either intravenous or oral corticosteroids. In patients who have been exposed to high doses of stimulants or hallucinogens, the acute asthma management may be difficult because of the profound psychomotor agitation that can occur. Drugs like haloperidol may be helpful in ameliorating some of these manifestations without depressing respiratory drive. Obviously, definitive treatment of patients who present with recurring flares of asthma after recreational drug use is abstinence from their drug habit. Similarly, passive tobacco smoke exposure should be avoided in children with asthma.

CONCLUSION

Case reports and small series describing the development of asthma after recreational drug abuse, particularly with cocaine, heroin, tobacco, and marijuana use, are increasingly prevalent. The evidence directly linking the association between asthma and drug use for the most part remains tenuous, but a real interaction probably exists in a subset of asthmatics (see Table 2). Airway irritants in the inhaled substances are able to trigger bronchospasm in many cases, but other mechanisms probably contribute for individual illicit substances, as well. Recreational drug use may be an important confounder in certain patients with asthma, and providers must be diligent in questioning patients with new-onset and difficult-to-control symptoms about potential drug use. Treatment includes standard asthma care and, most important, abstinence from their drug habit.

Table 2

Association Between Recreational Drugs of Abuse and Asthma

Drugs of abuse	*Strength of association*
Cocaine	+++
Amphetamines	+
Opioids	++
Marijuana	++
Tobacco	
Nicotine	?
Tobacco smoke	+++
Volatile substances abuse	+
Hallucinogens	?

++++, proven association; +++, many case reports/frequently reported; ++, several case reports/commonly reported; +, rare case reports; ?, no case reports/no known association.

REFERENCES

1. Carlisle MJ. Update: comparison of drug use in Australia and the United States in the 2001 National Household Surveys. *Drug Alcohol Rev* 2003; 22: 347–357.
2. Albertson TE, Gershwin ME, Eds. Pulmonary complications of recreational drug usage. *Clin Rev in Allergy Immunol* 1997; 15: 219–361.
3. Tashkin DP. Airway effects of marijuana, cocaine, and other inhaled illicit agents. *Curr Opin Pulm Med* 2001; 7: 43–61.
4. Barsky SH, Roth MD, Kleerup EC, et al. Histopathologic and molecular alterations in bronchial epithelium in habitual smokers of marijuana, cocaine, and/or tobacco. *J Natl Cancer Inst* 1998; 90: 1198–1205.
5. Waldbott GL. Asthma due to a local anesthetic. *JAMA* 1932; 99: 1942–1945.
6. Weiss KB, Gergen PG, Crain EF. The epidemiology of an emerging US public health concern. *Chest* 1992; 101: 362S–367S.
7. Greenberger PA, Miller TP, Lifschultz B. Circumstances surrounding deaths from asthma in Cook County, Illinois. *Allg Proc* 1993; 14: 321–326.
8. Levenson T, Greenberger PA, Donoghue ER, et al. Asthma deaths confounded by substance abuse. An assessment of asthma. *Chest* 1996; 110: 664–710.
9. Osborn HH, Tang M, Bradley K, et al. New-onset bronchospasm or recrudescence of asthma associated with cocaine abuse. *Acad Emerg Med* 1991: 20: 211–212.
10. Panacek EA, Jouriles NJ, Singer A, et al. Is unexplained bronchospasm associated with the use of cocaine? *Ann Emerg Med* 1991; 20: 211–212.
11. Rome LA, Lippmann ML, Dalsey WC, et al. Prevalence of cocaine use and its impact on asthma exacerbation in an urban population. *Chest* 2000; 117: 1324–1329.
12. Rubin RB, Neugarten J. Cocaine-associated asthma. *Am J Med* 1990; 88: 438–439.
13. Rebhun J. Association of asthma and freebase smoking. *Ann Allergy* 1988; 60: 339–342.
14. Rao AN, Polos PG, Walther FA. Crack abuse and asthma: a fatal combination. *NYS J Med* 1990; 90: 511–512.
15. Averbach M, Casey KK, Frank E. Near-fatal status asthmaticus induced by nasal insufflation of cocaine. *So Med J* 1996; 89: 340–341.
16. Meisels IS, Loke J. The pulmonary effects of free-base cocaine: a review. *Clev Clin J Med* 1993; 60: 325–329.
17. Dean NC, Clark HW, Doherty JJ, et al. Pulmonary function in heavy users of "freebase" cocaine. *Am Rev Respir Dis* 1988; 137S: 489.
18. Weiss RD, Goldenheim PD, Mirin SM, et al. Pulmonary dysfunction in cocaine smokers. *Am J Psychiatry* 1981; 138: 1110–1112.
19. Weiss RD, Tilles DS, Goldenheim PD, et al. Decreased single breath carbon monoxide diffusing capacity in cocaine freebase smokers. *Drug Alcohol Depend* 1987; 19: 271–276.

20. Susskind H, Weber DA, Vokow ND, et al. Increased lung permeability following long-term use of free-base cocaine. *Chest* 1991; 100: 903–909.
21. Itkonen J, Schnoll S, Glassroth J, et al. Pulmonary dysfunction in "freebase" cocaine users. *Arch Intern Med* 1984; 144: 2195–2197.
22. Tashkin DP, Kleerup EC, Koyal SN, et al. Acute effects of inhaled and IV cocaine on airway dynamics. *Chest* 1996; 110: 904–910.
23. Kissner DG, Lawrence WD, Selis JE, et al. Crack lung: pulmonary disease caused by cocaine abuse. *Am Rev Respir Dis* 1987; 136: 1250–1252.
24. Kikuchi Y, Okabe S, Tamura G, et al. Chemosensitivity and perception of dyspnea in patients with a history of near-fatal asthma. *N Engl J Med* 1994: 330: 1329–1334.
25. Zaas D, Brock M, Yang S, et al. An uncommon mimic of an acute asthma exacerbation. *Chest* 2002; 121: 1707–1709.
26. Dowling GP, McDonough ET, Bost RO. 'Eve' and 'Ecstasy'. A report of five deaths associated with the use of MDEA and MDMA. *JAMA* 1987: 257: 1615–1617.
27. Saito T, Yamanamoto I, Kusakabe T, et al. Determination of chronic methamphetamine abuse by hair analysis. *Forensic Sci Int* 2000; 112: 65–71.
28. Schmidt RA, Glenny RW, Godwin JD, et al. Panlobular emphysema in young intravenous Ritalin abusers. *Am Rev Respir Dis* 1991; 143: 649–656.
29. Sherman CB, Hudson LD, Pierson DJ. Severe precocious emphysema in intravenous methylphenidate (Ritalin) abusers. *Chest* 1987; 92: 1085–1087.
30. Del los Santos-Sartre S, Capote-Gil F, Gonzales-Castro A. Airway obstruction and heroin inhalation. *Lancet* 1986; 2: 1158.
31. Oliver RM. Bronchospasm and heroin inhalation. *Lancet* 1986; 1: 915.
32. Anderson K. Bronchospasm and intravenous street heroin. *Lancet* 1986; 1: 1208.
33. Hughes S, Calverley PMA. Heroin inhalation and asthma. *Br Med J* 1988; 297: 1611–1612.
34. Sapira JD. The narcotic addict as a medical patient. *Am J Med* 1968; 45: 555–587.
35. Ghodse AH, Wilson AF, Berke RA. Asthma in opiate addicts. *J Psychosom Res* 1987; 31: 41–44.
36. Cruz R, Davis M, O'Neill H, et al. Pulmonary manifestations of inhaled street drugs. *Heart Lung* 1998; 27: 297–305.
37. Brander PE, Tukianinen P. Acute eosinophilic pneumonia in a heroin smoker. *Eur Respir J* 1993; 6: 750–752.
38. Spiritus EM, Wilson AF, Berke RA. Lung scans in asymptomatic heroin addicts. *Am Rev Respir Dis* 1973; 108: 994–996.
39. Camargo G, Colp C. Pulmonary function studies in ex-heroin users. *Chest* 1975; 67: 331–334.
40. Overland ES, Nolan AJ, Hopewell PC. Alteration of pulmonary function in intravenous abusers. *Am J Med* 1980; 68: 231–237.
41. Krantz AJ, Hershow RC, Prachand N, et al. Heroin insufflation as a trigger for patients with life-threatening asthma. *Chest* 2003; 123: 510–517.
42. Eschenbacher WL, Bethel RA, Boushey HA, et al. Morphine sulfate inhibits bronchoconstriction in subjects with mild asthma whose responses are inhibited by atropine. *Am Rev Respir Dis* 1984: 130: 363–367.
43. Mestiri M, Lurie A, Frossard N, et al. Effect of inhaled morphine on the bronchial responsiveness to isocapnic hyperventilation in patients with allergic asthma. *Eur J Clin Pharm* 1991; 41: 621.
44. Field PL, Simmul R, Bell SC, et al. Evidence for opioid modulation and generation of prostaglandins in sulphur dioxide-induced bronchoconstriction. *Thorax* 1996; 51: 159–163.
45. Ulinski S, Palczynski C, Gorski P. Occupational rhinitis and bronchial asthma due to morphine: evidence from inhalational and nasal challenges. *Allergy* 1996; 51: 914–918.
46. Biagnini RE, Klincewicz SL, Henningsen GM. Antibodies to morphine in workers exposed to opiates at a narcotics' manufacturing facility and evidence for similar antibodies in heroin abusers. *Life Sci* 1993; 53: 99–105.
47. Tashkin DP, Coulson AH, Clark VA, et al. Respiratory symptoms and lung function in habitual, heavy smokers of marijuana alone, smokers of marijuana and tobacco, smokers of tobacco alone, and non-smokers. *Am Rev Respir Dis* 1987; 135: 209–215.
48. Bloom JW, Kaltenborn WT, Paoletti P, et al. Respiratory effects of non-tobacco cigarettes. *Br Med J* 1987; 295: 1516–1518.
49. Taylor DR, Poulton R, Moffitt TE, et al. The respiratory effects of cannabis dependence in young adults. *Addiction* 2000; 95: 1669–1677.

50. Tashkin DP, Shapiro FJ, Frank IM. Acute effects of smoked marijuana and Delta^9-tetrahydrocannabinol on specific airway conductance in asthmatic subjects. *Am Rev Respir Dis* 1974; 109: 420–428.
51. Tashkin DP, Simmons MS, Chang P, et al. Effects of smoked substance abuse on nonspecific airway hyperresponsiveness. *Am Rev Respir Dis* 1993; 147: 125–129.
52. Friedman H, Klein TW, Newton C, et al. Marijuana, receptors and immunomodulation. *Adv Exp Med Biol* 1995; 373: 103–113.
53. Spector SC, Klein TW, Newton C, et al. Marijuana effects on immunity: suppression of human natural killer cell activity of delta-9-tetrahydrocannibinol. *Int J Immunopharmacol* 1986; 8: 741–745.
54. US Center for Disease Control and Prevention. Tobacco use and usual source of cigarettes among high school students—United States, 1995 *MMWR Morbid Mortal Wkly Rep* 1996; 45: 413–418.
55. US Center for Disease Control and Prevention. Prevalence of cigarette use among 14 racial/ethnic population—United States, 1999-2001. *MMWR Morbid Mortal Wkly Rep* 2004; 53: 49–52.
56. American Thoracic Society. Cigarette smoking and health. *Am J Respir Crit Care Med* 1996; 153: 861–865.
57. Willers S, Svenonius E, Skarping G. Passive smoking and childhood asthma. *Allergy* 1991; 46: 330–334.
58. Cunningham J, Dockery DW, Speizer FE. Maternal smoking during pregnancy as a predictor of lung function in children. *Am J Epidemiol* 1994; 139: 1139–1152.
59. Weiss ST. Environmental risk factors in childhood asthma. *Clin Exp Allergy* 1998; 28: 29–34.
60. Annesi-Maesano I, Oryszczyn MP, Raherison C, et al. Increased prevalence of asthma and allied diseases among active adolescent tobacco smokers after controlling for passive smoking exposure. A cause for concern? *Clin Exp Allergy* 2004; 34: 1017–1023.
61. Jang A-S, Choi I-S, Lee S, et al. The effect of passive smoking on asthma symptoms, atopy, and airway hyperresponsiveness in schoolchildren. *J Korean Med Sci* 2004; 19: 214–217.
62. Janson C. The effect of passive smoking on respiratory health in children and adults. *Int J Turberc Lung Dis* 2004; 8: 510–516.
63. LeSon S, Gershwin ME. Risk factor for asthmatic patients requiring intubation. I. Observations in children. *J Asthma* 1995; 32: 285–294.
64. Eisner MD, Yelin EH, Henke J, et al. Environmental tobacco smoke and adult asthma. The impact of changing exposure status on health outcomes. *Am J Repir Crit Care Med* 1998; 158: 170–175.
65. Flodin U, Jonsson P, Ziegler J, et al. An epidemiologic study of bronchial asthma and smoking. *Epidemiology* 1995; 6: 503–505.
66. White JR, Froeb HF. Small-airways dysfunction in nonsmokers chronically exposed to tobacco smoke. *N Engl J Med* 1980; 302: 720–723.
67. Schwartz J, Timonen KL, Pekkanen J. Respiratory effects of environmental tobacco smoke in a panel study of asthmatic and symptomatic children. *Am J Respir Crit Care Med* 2000; 161: 802–806.
68. Chadwick O, Anderson R, Bland M, et al. Neuropsychological consequences of volatile substance abuse: a population based study of secondary school pupils. *Br Med J* 1989; 298: 1679–1683.
69. Wu LT, Pilowsky DJ, Schlenger WE. Inhalant abuse and dependence among adolescents in the United States. *J Am Acad Child Adolesc Psych* 2004; 43: 1206–1214.
70. Schickler KN, Lane EE, Seitz K, et al. Solvent abuse associated pulmonary abnormalities. *Concepts Alcohol Subst Abuse* 1984; 3: 75–81.
71. Meredith TJ, Ruprah M, Liddle A, et al. Diagnosis and treatment of acute poisoning with volatile substances. *Hum Toxicol* 1989; 8: 277–286.
72. Cartwright TR, Brown D, Brashear RE. Pulmonary infiltrates following butane 'fire breathing.' *Arch Int Med* 1983; 143: 2007–2008.

IV LIVING WITH ASTHMA

17 Self-Management in Asthma

Empowering the Patient

Arvind Kumar, MD, and M. Eric Gershwin, MD

KEY POINTS

- National and international consensus bodies have identified asthma education and guided self-management as essential components of efforts to empower patients and reduce asthma morbidity and mortality *(1–6)*.
- Asthma self-management cannot be achieved without appropriate asthma education *(7)*.
- Asthma self-management education improves outcomes in asthma *(7)*.
- Self-management requires effective communication among physician, patient, and those who care for the patient *(8)*.
- Self-management goals and programs must be individualized to the needs, desires, abilities, and socioeconomic situation of the patient.
- Each interaction with the patient can be an opportunity to deliver and reinforce self-management messages.
- Education or information must be combined with plans for self-management to be maximally effective *(9)*.
- Patient nonadherence is a complex and pervasive problem that requires assessment and efforts to manage the psychological issues related to asthma *(8)*.
- Asthma self-management started in asthma camps but has entered new venues, including schools, doctors' offices, emergency rooms, hospitals, HMO disease management groups, and communities.
- The Internet allows physicians and patients to gather information regarding asthma and self-management resources that is available at the local and national levels.

From: *Current Clinical Practice: Bronchial Asthma:*
A Guide for Practical Understanding and Treatment, 5th ed.
Edited by: M. E. Gershwin and T. E. Albertson © Humana Press Inc., Totowa, NJ

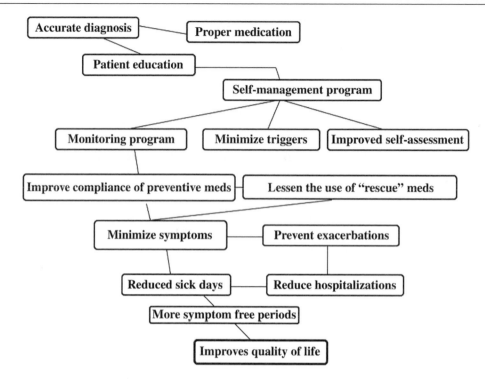

Fig. 1. Good asthma self-management programs can improve outcome.

INTRODUCTION

Asthma prevention or control depends on patients acquiring information about their disease and effectively incorporating this information into self-management skills to be applied over long periods of time. In many cases, patients with asthma and other chronic diseases do not perceive that working out a preventative strategy is worth the time and effort involved. Most individuals arrive at adequate coping procedures largely through a trial-and-error process. For severe asthma, this approach does not work well. This chapter focuses heavily on empowering the patient to take charge. With this in mind, let's begin with a cautionary tale of failure of asthma self-management (*see* Fig. 1).

Roger and Emmy are in their mid-30s and have been living together for the last 6 yr. Both developed asthma and allergic rhinitis in childhood, with symptoms linked initially to the pollen season. Emmy's attacks are still mainly seasonal, but Roger's have become year-round attacks, and their onset is associated with exposure to a variety of substances: pollens, dust, viral infections, aspirin, and wine are the ones he knows about.

Their medical histories are surprisingly similar. When their symptoms first appeared, they were each taken to their family doctors who, after a perfunctory examination, prescribed an oral antihistamine and theophylline. This tactic worked well enough, but the side effects of the medications were so distressing that they went on to consult allergists who conducted skin tests, found positive reactions to several different pollens, and started a course of immunization shots. The shots helped to some degree but were not continued long enough to desensitize them to the allergens. They disliked the process immensely—the injections, the necessity to appear at the allergist's office regularly, and the need to wait in the office after the shot had been given.

After high school, they both left home; Roger to attend college on the west coast and Emmy to pursue a musical career. They stopped the shots, but the hay fever and asthma symptoms persisted.

During college, Roger's asthma became much more persistent and severe, and he had to seek emergency treatment on three occasions, all at the time of the year when grass was pollinating. The college health service referred Roger to an allergist who, after reviewing his situation, put him on a regular schedule of theophylline—he doesn't remember the dosage—with an aerosol β-agonist backup for more acute episodes. Roger took the medication faithfully. He graduated from college, moved to Los Angeles, married his college sweetheart, and had the marriage fail under conditions of considerable stress and tension after 3 yr. During this period, Roger's asthma worsened. He broke with the opinion of his doctor and concluded that his asthma was psychogenic in origin and that he was nothing more than a slave to his medications. He abruptly stopped using them and, after the demise of his marriage, moved to northern California.

During this same period, Emmy noticed that her asthma was getting worse. She blamed this on constant travel, contending it brought her in contact with pollens to which she was sensitive. She too consulted an allergist who put her on antihistamines and aerosols. She had to have something because she played in and was lead singer in a bluegrass band, and without medication, she simply could not perform.

Emmy, too, wound up in northern California, became tired of her medication and its side effects, and gave up on it. Besides, it was costing her a lot of money she didn't have. She and Roger first met in the waiting room of an herbalist to whom they had gone for what they both believed would be more "organic" and less drastic and harmful treatment.

Now, 6 yr later, Roger is still considerably troubled by asthma. He observes the regimen prescribed by the herbalist, which, he believes, has been somewhat helpful. However, as he puts it, "Sometimes I do things that aren't too smart. Like, if there's a bottle of good red wine around, I may take a few hits of it. I know what'll happen, but I just can't resist."

Emmy, too, is still asthmatic. She now finds that she will sometimes lapse into asthma when she has a viral infection, but she is less bothered with pollens, in large measure because the area of northern California where she lives does not grow the plants to which she formerly reacted. That fact may also explain Roger's marginal improvement.

Last winter, Emmy was in bed with a severe cold and fever and moderate asthma symptoms. A friend who visited her during this episode asked if she was doing anything for it.

"Rest and teas," Emmy wheezed.

"Don't you want some Contac or something?" the friend asked. "I'd be glad to go out and get it for you just to help you breathe better."

"I'd die before I took any of that stuff," Emmy gasped.

This cautionary tale of failure in treatment probably typifies the experiences of many patients with asthma. It owes much to the breakdown of preventive strategies (either through ignorance of or neglect of them) combined with nonexistent or failed efforts to educate patients about the nature and care of their disease.

This cautionary tale was originally described in the second edition of this textbook in collaboration with Dr. Edwin Klingelhofer, and it is ironic that the tale is just as appropriate today as it was in 1986.

In fact, asthma has become a familiar disease to people throughout the world. It is a chronic inflammatory disorder of the respiratory tract that can be characterized by periods of apparent quiescence interrupted by periods of severe respiratory distress. In the United States, more than 20 million people, or 20 in 1000, report that they have asthma *(10)*. An early release of data from the 1997–2004 National Health Interview Surveys indicates that the prevalence of asthma in 2004 was 7.2% of the total American population *(11)*. The same report states that in 2004, 4.2% of the US population experienced an asthma attack in the previous 12 mo. In 2002, American children missed 14.7 million school days because of asthma, and adults missed 11.8 million work days because of this disease *(10)*. There were 13.9 million outpatient visits and 1.9 million emergency room visits for asthma in 2002. There were 484,000 asthma hospitalizations and 4261 deaths from asthma in that year as well. Direct and indirect costs of asthma in the United States are $14 billion annually *(12)*. Knowledge of mechanisms and treatment of asthma has advanced significantly in the last decade. Unfortunately, the prevalence of the disease has increased by 75% during the last 20 yr *(13)*. There has been no significant improvement the numbers of asthma patients who state that their activity is limited by asthma. Since 1995, rates of outpatient and emergency room visits for asthma have increased. Hospitalization and death rates have decreased overall but are still significant and are disproportionately high in blacks *(14)*. The potential to improve these statistics and the quality of life of patients with asthma has been recognized by various national and international groups and has prompted creation of multiple consensus statements on how to improve asthma care. Each of these guidelines emphasizes the critical role that patient education and self-management play in improving asthma care *(2–6,15)*. This chapter reviews the significance and history of asthma self-management, considers the barriers to effective self-management, discusses the various types of programs available, and identifies educational resources for clinicians and patients that can empower those with asthma to achieve better outcomes.

THE CONCEPT OF ASTHMA SELF-MANAGEMENT

"Self-management" was described by Creer in 1976, when he used this term in reference to teaching children with asthma how to actively manage their disease *(16)*. Since then, self-management has become a commonly used term when describing educational and management programs for patients with chronic disease *(17)*. Clearly, every patient with any disease practices some form and degree of self-management. One can argue that the patient who goes home and discards his or her medications, ignores any of his or her doctor's recommendations, and decides not to learn anything about his or her disease is practicing a form of self-management *(17)*. Of course, when the term is used today, it is implied that the goal is "optimal and positive" self-management. The term connotes improved understanding of one's disease, effective management of symptoms using a plan of action, medications, and appropriate psychological coping skills. A self-management program is a multifaceted plan of education and care that is supported by the physician but relies heavily on patient acceptance and involvement. Asthma self-management can be subdivided in different ways. One way to conceptualize asthma self-management is to identify tasks that are important in achieving optimal asthma outcomes. Table 1 includes goals common to many programs of self-management.

Table 1
Goals in Asthma Self-Management

1. Acquiring knowledge about asthma: definition, treatment, and triggers.
2. Accepting that one has a disease that may have a chronic, intermittent pattern.
3. Acquiring skills needed to take medications and to conduct self-monitoring, proper use of inhalers, peak-flow meters, and nebulizers.
4. Adhering to short- and long-term medication prescriptions.
5. Self-monitoring of symptoms or peak flows.
6. Adjusting medications when needed based on some form of asthma action plan: written or verbal action plans based on symptoms and/or peak flows.
7. Avoiding or removing triggers from the environment: tobacco smoke, cockroaches, and house dust mites.
8. Knowing when and how to seek medical advice/care in the setting of a partnership with the medical care team.
9. Accessing available social support mechanisms: parents, friends, doctors, nurses, counselors, teachers, and Internet support groups.
10. Establishing appropriate and useful coping mechanisms to address the psychological sequelae of living with a chronic disease.

Adapted from refs. *2–4, 8, 17, 18.*

SIGNIFICANCE OF ASTHMA SELF-MANAGEMENT

The continuing morbidity and mortality related to asthma is clear from the previous discussion. Although management guidelines have been created and kept updated, evidence suggests that the goals of these guidelines are not always being reached. In one study, 58% of patients with asthma were on medication regimens inconsistent with the guidelines published by the British Thoracic Society just 1 yr earlier *(19)*. Another study found that in the sample of previously hospitalized children with asthma, only 35% of patients that met National Asthma Education and Prevention Program (NAEPP) criteria for persistent asthma were receiving daily anti-inflammatory agents *(20)*. Explanations for falling short of guideline goals are multifactorial and involve issues of patient adherence, physician management patterns, and access to health care.

Several large American *(21)* and international *(22)* surveys have identified that problems exist in inadequate prescription of corticosteroids to patients with persistent asthma. For many, there is a lack of adequate access to regular medical care, particularly patients in minority groups *(23)*. Aside from these issues, there are also significant problems relating to a lack of adequate patient knowledge *(24)* about asthma management and lack of patient adherence *(25)* to prescribed medical regimens. Additionally, patients often underestimate *(22)* the severity of their asthma and may have difficulty recognizing early symptoms of worsening disease. Such problems may allow exacerbations to progress and often lead to unscheduled visits to the clinic and emergency room. In this setting, delay in seeking treatment may lead to fatal outcomes in some *(26)*. Self-management of asthma is important because it can improve outcomes related to some of these issues *(7)*.

Asthma self-management can improve outcomes, but it is not a panacea. Certainly it cannot resolve suboptimal prescription practices or provide universal access to asthma medical care. However, it can positively affect areas such as patient knowledge, patient adherence, and improved self-assessment of asthma severity. Asthma self-management can improve outcomes, and this has been documented in the literature. A recent Cochrane review of 36 randomized-control trials on the effectiveness of asthma self-management showed that education in asthma self-management involving self-monitoring, along with regular medical review and a written action plan, improves health outcomes for adults with asthma *(7)*. This study found that self-management education reduced hospitalizations, emergency room visits, unscheduled visits to the doctor, days off work or school, and nocturnal asthma frequency and also improved quality-of-life measures.

Ideally, asthma self-management allows the patient to minimize symptoms and medication side effects while maximizing understanding about the disease and a sense of control over one's life. In this way, such efforts can help reduce anxiety regarding the diagnosis, attacks, and medications *(27)*. Self-management is not intended to replace visits to and management by the physician, but it can often be helpful at times before medical advice is available. This is particularly important because even severe asthma attacks often develop gradually at home before direct medical care is available. Knowing how to handle asthma exacerbations at home may prevent symptoms from progressing *(28)*. Self-management also may allow the patient or caregiver to adjust the home environment to minimize the presence of asthma triggers *(29)*. By their very nature, these adjustments are made outside the medical setting and, therefore, require comprehension and management by the patient or his or her caregiver.

Self-management is necessary in every condition in which one is required to administer medications or treatment outside a medical facility. In asthma, patients may have periods without symptoms and others with severe symptoms. Rescue medications or oral corticosteroids may need to be started or increased during flares. On the other hand, preventive medications may need to be continued even during symptom-free periods for persistent asthma. Such variability in asthma symptoms makes the ability to take and adjust medications appropriately vital for optimal asthma care.

THE ISSUE OF NONADHERENCE

Adherence refers to the extent to which a patient follows medication and treatment plans formed in conjunction with the physician. Unfortunately, nonadherence is common and hinders efforts at asthma self-management and leads to poor outcomes. Compliance with medication in patients with asthma is estimated to be as low as 30% in some cases *(8)*. A complete analysis of the reasons for nonadherence is largely beyond the scope of this discussion. However, a useful overview of the problem is provided by Bender's classification of reasons for nonadherence. He divides these reasons into provider-related, treatment-related, and patient-related issues. Provider-related reasons include scheduling problems, lack of continuity of care, perceived clinician disinterest, and time constraints. Treatment-related barriers to adherence include complicated and prolonged medical regimens, costs of medications, adverse effects, and delayed onset of action. Patient-based barriers include suboptimal understanding of asthma and the need for treatment, lack of confidence in the provider, mild or severe asthma, low motivation toward behavioral change, and the presence of psychological problems. This last barrier can include fear of the disease, fear of treatment side effects, and fear of becoming dependent on medications, as well as anxiety and depression that may be associated with any chronic disease. The clinician cannot remove all of these barriers, but efforts to minimize them may yield rewards. These efforts must include frequent patient contact, use of multiple encounters for educational training, simplification of regimens when possible, and fostering improved communication between physician and patient.

ORIGINS AND TYPES OF ASTHMA SELF-MANAGEMENT PROGRAMS

Early Efforts Toward Self-Management: Asthma Camps

Before the late 1960s, asthma was managed via traditional modes of patient–physician interaction, including clinic visits and inpatient stays (30). Some asthma self-management programs during this time were inpatient residential care programs. Such programs have become increasingly less common in the current era of decreased insurance coverage of prolonged inpatient care. Many would argue that the origins of more modern asthma self-management programs are found in the 1970s, which saw the birth and growth of numerous outpatient asthma education programs directed at children (30). These were called "asthma camps." One of the first asthma camps was called Bronco Junction (31). In a supportive setting, children were given information about asthma and how to manage it by being encouraged to participate in normal camp activities. Numerous other asthma camp programs followed, each tailored to fit the social and cultural needs of the children involved. Open Airways was started in 1976 in New York and was the first program created specifically for minority children living in the inner city. Open Airways in modified forms is still used today in schools and communities and reduces asthma recidivism and decreases the cost of care (32). Over time, the programs have been subject to more critical and placebo-controlled, randomized evaluation regarding outcomes and effectiveness. Programs have demonstrated improved knowledge regarding asthma, fewer patient symptoms (32), and decreased urgent care visits (33). In the 1980s, curricula from several programs were distributed nationally via organizations, including the American Lung Association (Superstuff program) and Rohr pharmaceuticals (Winning Over Wheezing program). The University of California at Davis Asthma Network (UCAN) had its first asthma camp in 2004. In 1988, the Consortium on Children's Asthma Camps was established to act as a central coordinating body for camp programs sponsored by national asthma groups, including the American Lung Association; American Academy of Allergy, Asthma and Immunology (AAAAI); Allergy and Asthma Network Mothers of Asthmatics (AANMA); American Academy of Pediatrics; American College of Allergy, Asthma, and Immunology (ACAAI); and the American Thoracic Society. The consortium's Web site allows parents to easily identify camps in their state. California alone has 16 camps listed in various parts of the state. Today, millions of children attend these camps yearly. Per the consortium Web site, the goals of these camps are as follows:

1. Provide an enjoyable and safe camp experience for children with asthma, ages 8–15 yr.
2. Provide asthma education for children, parents, and medical personnel.
3. Promote improved self-care, self-image, and independence for children with asthma.
4. Facilitate future camp experiences in a regular nonspecialty camp.

School-Based Programs for Children With Asthma

Asthma camps provide education and support but are by their nature short-term. Without support and continued education outside the camp, gains are likely to be short-lived *(30)*. Recognition of these needs may have been important in the spread of self-management efforts beyond the camps. One place where educators may enjoy a captive-audience effect is in the schools. Many asthma self-management educational interventions and programs have been centered on schools. Asthma educational sessions conducted in inner-city schools in San Diego, CA, resulted in increased asthma knowledge, improved skills for peak flow meter and inhaler use, and a reduction in the severity of asthma symptoms *(34)*. A shortened Open Airways school intervention was effective in improving asthma knowledge *(35)*. Using a randomized controlled trial of a comprehensive school-based asthma intervention, Clark found decreased pediatric asthma symptoms and improved asthma management *(36)*. The Kunsberg School in Denver, CO, enrolls children with asthma and other chronic diseases into a daily program of school-based disease management and directly observed anti-inflammatory medication. This program has reduced asthma severity in inner-city children with asthma *(37)*. A video game used to educate fourth-graders improves asthma knowledge *(38)*. The NAEPP has a resolution for management of asthma at school, which includes recommendations for a written asthma action plan and rules allowing students to self-administer medications if appropriate *(39)*. Many of the national asthma organizations, including the AAAAI, ACAAI, and the National Heart, Lung, and Blood Institute (NHLBI), have educational materials available for use in the schools or by parents to enhance self-management. Much of this material is available online *(see* Table 2). The Asthma and Allergy Foundation of America (AAFA) has a program called Power Breathing designed for asthma education of adolescents and one for the parents of preschoolers called Wee Wheezers. The latter program has increased symptom-free days and improved parental sleep measures *(40)*.

Physician's Office and Home-Based Programs for Children and Adults With Asthma

Asthma self-management education is still an essential part of asthma management in the doctor's office. The interventions in the office may then be translated into efforts at the patient's home via knowledge gained and implementation of asthma action plans. In both adults and children, self-management educational programs in asthma improve lung function and self-efficacy and reduce morbidity and health care utilization *(41,42)*. Many self-management programs include education on the pathophysiology of asthma, triggers of asthma, description of medications used, training on symptom monitoring, training on inhaler technique, and discussion of exacerbation management.

Most consensus guidelines *(4–6)* and many self-management interventions also recommend a written asthma action plan, particularly in patients with more severe disease. The ideal is that the patient or caregiver will understand and be able to review medications to take when feeling well and will be able to adjust them when symptoms become more severe or if a trigger is encountered, before seeing the physician. Gibson's systematic review of the literature showed that comprehensive self-management education that included a written action plan and medical review improved outcomes *(7)*. He performed another analysis of robust trials looking at action plans themselves and found that individualized written action plans based on personal best peak flow, having two to four action points, and recommending both inhaled corticosteroids and oral corticosteroids for treatment of exacerbations consistently improved asthma

Table 2
Asthma Resources for Clinicians

Organization	Website
American Academy of Allergy, Asthma and Immunology (AAAAI)	http://www.aaaai.org/
American Academy of Pediatrics (AAP)	http://www.aap.org
American College of Allergy, Asthma, and Immunology (ACAAI)	http://www.acaii.org
American College of Chest Physicians (ACCP) Journal	http://www.chestjournal.org/
American Lung Association (ALA)	http://www.lungusa.org/site/pp.asp?c=dvLUK9O0E&b=23705
American Lung Association (ALA) Asthma Profiler	https://www.lungprofiler.nexcura.com/Secure/InterfaceSecure.asp?CB=26272
American Lung Association of Minnesota	http://www.alamn.org/InfoCenter/Provider/index.asp
American Thoracic Society statements	http://www.thoracic.org/statements/
Asthma and Allergy Foundation of America (AAFA)	http://www.aafa.org/display.cfm?id=4&sub=79&cont=353
Centers for Disease Control and Prevention DC National Center for Health Statistics Fast Facts	http://www.cdc.gov/nchs/fastats/asthma.htm
Global Initiative for Asthma (GINA)	http://www.ginasthma.com/
National Jewish Medical and Research Center (NJC)	http://asthma.nationaljewish.org/
National Heart, Lung, and Blood Institute/National Institutes of Health	http://www.nhlbi.nih.gov/health/prof/lung/index.htm#asthma
US Environmental Protection Agency: Asthma and Indoor Air Quality Resource	http://www.epa.gov/asthma/hcprofessionals.html
Up To Date[a]	http://www.uptodate.com/

[a]Subscription required.

health outcomes (18). This data analysis suggests that plans based on peak flows are equivalent to those based on symptoms. Asthma action plans are particularly important when the patient's treatment regimen is complex, when changes have been made to the plan, or if the patient has difficulty remembering what the plan of action is in different situations. Clearly, the type and complexity of the asthma action plan, just as the overall program of treatment, must be individualized to the patient's level of education, level of willingness to be involved in management decisions, and severity of disease. Importantly, a Cochrane review found that education alone about asthma is not effective in improving asthma outcomes, despite increases in patient knowledge (9). This makes it clear that education about the disease process must be accompanied by information on self-management plans and skills to be clinically and socially significant. Asthma action plans are a concrete and practical way of accomplishing this. Examples of asthma action plans are available on the Internet from the NAEPP (6), National Jewish Medical Center (43), and consumer sites, such as WebMD (44). There has been some debate regarding the common action plan practice of doubling inhaled steroid dose during exacerbations. Some have argued that it is not evidence-based. Certain studies have suggested it may not be beneficial *(45)*. However, others have suggested that increasing the dose by more than double may be useful *(46)*.

Some managed care settings also provide asthma education classes. One example is the Breathe Easier program in northern California Kaiser Permanente clinics. A similar program in a Colorado Kaiser clinic *(47)* revealed that it resulted in increased prescription of inhaled corticosteroids for children with moderate to severe asthma, which is consistent with asthma guidelines.

Several programs use technology to improve asthma care. The Health Buddy program *(48)* is a Web-based program that allows a child to assess and monitor his or her symptoms and quality of life and transmit this information from home to health care providers. This program improved peak-flow readings and self-management behavior. Computer-generated written plans are also used by some. Such efforts can reduce the time necessary to create written and individualized handouts for patients. This is important because physicians have consistently related that time pressure is often an issue in clinical practice. One example of a computerized action plan generator is available online for general use *(49)*. Finally, major asthma-related organizations (AAAAI, ACAAI, NHLBI, and AAFA) are excellent resources for educational materials, both printed and electronic, for use by patients and medical professionals at home and in the office (*see* Tables 2 and 3).

Emergency Room and Hospital Discharge Programs

When patients are treated and then discharged for asthma from hospitals and emergency rooms, a window of opportunity to instill self-management information and skills is opened. It is not surprising that many interventions have been attempted in such settings. A short self-management program during hospital admission reduced postdischarge morbidity and readmission for adult asthma patients in one study *(50)*. Another inpatient educational program reduced rehospitalization *(51)*. As one would suspect, scheduling follow-up appointments with a primary care doctor for a child seen in the emergency department for asthma improves follow-up *(52)*. One-hour education and skills development sessions performed in the emergency room on adult minority patients who frequently received asthma care in that setting decreased subsequent emergency visits *(53)*. Discharge planning after an asthma visit is emphasized by most consensus guidelines. As mentioned, the University of California, Davis, runs an asthma program known as UCAN, which consists of clinical care, educational interventions, and outreach. UCAN is an example of multidisciplinary disease management, which has been applied to asthma care at other institutions, including the National Jewish Medical Center in Colorado.

Community-Based and Other Programs

A variety of other innovative programs increase opportunities for effective asthma management. A lunchtime asthma educational program conducted by Bank One, Chicago, in 2001 improved outcomes in a pre-posttest design trial *(54)*. An intervention conducted in various community sites, such as churches, libraries, and senior centers, targeted Kaiser Permanente patients with asthma and other chronic diseases. Session topics included information on action plans, relaxation to manage symptoms, handling fear and anger, understanding medications, and communicating

Table 3
Asthma Resources for Patients

Organization	Website
Allergy & Asthma Network Mothers of Asthmatics(AANMA)	http://www.aanma.org/
American Academy of Allergy, Asthma and Immunology (AAAAI)	http://www.aaaai.org/patients.stm
American Academy of Pediatrics (AAP)	http://www.aap.org/healthtopics/asthma.cfm
American Association of Respiratory Care	http://www.yourlunghealth.org/
American College of Chest Physicians (ACCP)	http://www.chestnet.org/education/ patient/guides/asthma_control/
American Lung Association (ALA)	http://www.lungusa.org/site/pp.asp?c =dvLUK9O0E&b=33276
American Lung Association (ALA) Patient Profiler	https://www.lungprofiler.nexcura.com/ Secure/InterfaceSecure.asp?CB=26270
American Lung Association of Minnesota	http://www.alamn.org/InfoCenter/ PatientHome.asp
Asthma Action America	http://www.asthmaactionamerica.org/
Asthma and Allergy Foundation of America (AAFA)	http://www.aafa.org/display.cfm?id=8
Health Finder Service (US Department of Health and Human Services)	http://www.healthfinder.gov/scripts/ SearchContext.asp?topic=75
Kaiser Permanente Northern California	http://members.kaiserpermanente.org/ kpweb/asthma/entrypage.do?engine= Overture&KeywordGroup=Asthma& Keyword=asthma
Kids Health (for parents, teenagers, and kids)	http://kidshealth.org/index.html
Mayo Clinic	http://www.mayoclinic.com/invoke.cfm?id= DS00021
Medline Plus (National Library of Medicine and National Institute of Health)	http://www.nlm.nih.gov/medlineplus/ asthma.html
National Heart, Lung, and Blood Institute/ National Institute of Health	http://www.nhlbi.nih.gov/health/public/ lung/index.htm
National Jewish Medical and Research Center	http://asthma.nationaljewish.org/
U.S. Environmental Protection Agency— Asthma and Indoor Air Quality Resource	http://www.noattacks.org/
Up To Date Patient Information	http://www.patients.uptodate.com/ toc.asp?toc=allergy_and_asthma&title= Allergy%20and%20asthma
Virtual Children's Hospital (University of Iowa)	http://www.vh.org/pediatric/patient/ pediatrics/asthma/index.html
WebMD	http://my.webmd.com/medical_information/ condition_centers/asthma/default.htm?z=3 074_00000_1005_00_02

effectively with the health care team *(55)*. It, too, improved outcomes. Another program that improved use measures was in Hawaii and included a multidisciplinary, community-based program tailored to the cultural and social needs of the population *(56)*.

Disease Management Programs

Disease management (DM) refers to a multidisciplinary approach to managing several chronic diseases, including congestive heart failure, diabetes, and asthma. These programs involve data collection from pharmacy records, case management by nurses and physicians, self-management educational programs, and telephone service lines for patient questions. These programs have grown in number and size because they have decreased health care use and improved asthma outcomes. Blue Cross/Blue Shield has a DM program called CareFirst, an option for patients in their health plan. It provides educational materials, telephone support with a nurse, case management by a nurse who communicates with the primary physician, and online services. Kaiser Permanente, the National Jewish Medical Center, and other institutions either have their own DM program or purchase DM programs targeting similar goals.

Media and Governmental Efforts

A national initiative called Healthy People 2010 has asthma as a key component, and its asthma objectives are increasing the prevalence of formal patient education, including information regarding community and self-help resources *(57)*. This program identifies self-management education as an essential part of asthma management. Public television cartoon characters with asthma include Buster the bunny on the *Arthur* show and Dani, from *Sesame Street*. The NAEPP conducts the Nationwide Asthma Screening Program in cooperation with the AANMA and the AAFA. The Breathmobile, an asthma screening, education, and treatment program, is another effort to manage this growing problem.

CONCLUSION

Asthma is a growing problem in this nation and throughout the world. The economic and social burden created by this disease is undeniable. Although we have not reached all of the goals set forth by consensus guidelines, it is clear that efforts at self-management education can be fruitful in empowering patients and clinicians and improving outcomes. As health care providers, it is our task to seize the opportunity of each patient encounter to realize these possibilities.

REFERENCES

1. National Asthma Education and Prevention Program. Expert Panel Report: Guidelines for the Diagnosis and Management of Asthma Update on Selected Topics—2002. *J Allergy Clin Immunol* 2002; 110(5 Suppl): S141–S219.
2. Guidelines for the diagnosis and management of asthma. National Heart, Lung, and Blood Institute. National Asthma Education Program. Expert Panel Report. *J Allergy Clin Immunol* 1991; 88(3 Pt 2): 425–534.
3. International Consensus Report on Diagnosis and Management of Asthma. International Asthma Management Project. *Allergy* 1992; 47(13 Suppl): 1–61.
4. Guidelines for the management of asthma: a summary. British Thoracic Society and others. *Br Med J* 1993; 306(6880): 776–782.
5. National Heart, Lung, and Blood Institute. *Global Strategy for Asthma Management and Prevention. Global Initiative for Asthma.* National Institutes of Health, Bethesda MD, 1995.
6. National Heart, Lung, and Blood Institute. *Guidelines for the Diagnosis and Management of Asthma. National Asthma Education Program. Expert Panel Report 2.* National Institutes of Health, Bethesda MD, 1997.
7. Gibson PG, Powell H, Coughlan J, et al. Self-management education and regular practitioner review for adults with asthma. *Cochrane Database Syst Rev* 2003(1): CD001117.

8. Bender B, Milgrom H, Rand C. Nonadherence in asthmatic patients: is there a solution to the problem? *Ann Allergy Asthma Immunol* 1997; 79(3): 177–185; quiz 85–86.

9. Gibson PG, Powell H, Coughlan J, et al. Limited (information only) patient education programs for adults with asthma. *Cochrane Database Syst Rev* 2002(2): CD001005.

10. Lethbridge-Çejku M SJ, Bernade L. Summary health statistics for U.S. Adults: National Health Interview Survey, 2002. National Center for Health Statistics. *Vital Health Stat.* 2004; 1–15.

11. Schiller JS, Hao C, Barnes P. *Early Release of Selected Estimates Based on Data From the January-June 2004 National Health Interview Survey.* Centers for Disease Control and Prevention, Hyattsville, MD, 2004.

12. American Lung Association. Epidemiology and Statistics Unit, Best Practices and Program Services. *Trends Morbid Mortal,* Vol. 1, 2004.

13. Mannino DM, Homa DM, Pertowski CA, Ashizawa A. Centers for Disease Control. Surveillance for asthma—United States, 1960–1995, Surveillance summaries. *MMWR Morbid Mortal Wkly Rep* 1998; 47 (SS-1).

14. Mannino DM, Homa DM, Akinbami LJ, Moorman, JE. Centers for Disease Control. Surveillance for Asthma—United States, 1980–1999, Surveillance summaries. *MMWR Morbid Mortal Wkly Rep* 2002; 51: 1–13.

15. National Asthma Education and Prevention Program. Expert Panel Report: Guidelines for the Diagnosis and Management of Asthma Update on Selected Topics—2002. *J Allergy Clin Immunol* 2002; 110(5 Suppl): S141–S219.

16. Creer TL, Renne CM, Christian WP. Behavioral contributions to rehabilitation and childhood asthma. *Rehabil Lit* 1976; 37(8): 226–247.

17. Lorig KR, Holman H. Self-management education: history, definition, outcomes, and mechanisms. *Ann Behav Med* 2003; 26(1): 1–7.

18. Gibson PG, Powell H. Written action plans for asthma: an evidence-based review of the key components. *Thorax* 2004; 59(2): 94–99.

19. Roghmann MC, Sexton M. Adherence to asthma guidelines in general practices. *J Asthma* 1999; 36(4): 381–387.

20. Warman KL, Silver EJ, Stein RE. Asthma symptoms, morbidity, and antiinflammatory use in inner-city children. *Pediatrics* 2001; 108(2): 277–282.

21. Adams RJ, Fuhlbrigge A, Guilbert T, Lozano P, Martinez F. Inadequate use of asthma medication in the United States: results of the asthma in America national population survey. *J Allergy Clin Immunol* 2002; 110(1): 58–64.

22. Rabe KF, Adachi M, Lai CK, et al. Worldwide severity and control of asthma in children and adults: the global asthma insights and reality surveys. *J Allergy Clin Immunol* 2004; 114(1): 40–47.

23. Sin DD, Bell NR, Man SF. Effects of increased primary care access on process of care and health outcomes among patients with asthma who frequent emergency departments. *Am J Med* 2004; 117(7): 479–483.

24. Radeos MS, Leak LV, Lugo BP, et al. Risk factors for lack of asthma self-management knowledge among ED patients not on inhaled steroids. *Am J Emerg Med* 2001; 19(4): 253–259.

25. Williams LK, Pladevall M, Xi H, et al. Relationship between adherence to inhaled corticosteroids and poor outcomes among adults with asthma. *J Allergy Clin Immunol* 2004; 114(6): 1288–1293.

26. Tough SC, Green FH, Paul JE, Wigle DT, Butt JC. Sudden death from asthma in 108 children and young adults. *J Asthma* 1996; 33(3): 179–188.

27. Thoren C, Petermann F. Reviewing asthma and anxiety. *Respir Med* 2000; 94(5): 409–415.

28. Marks GB, Heslop W, Yates DH. Prehospital management of exacerbations of asthma: relation to patient and disease characteristics. *Respirology* 2000; 5(1): 45–50.

29. Cabana MD, Slish KK, Lewis TC, et al. Parental management of asthma triggers within a child's environment. *J Allergy Clin Immunol* 2004; 114(2): 352–357.

30. Robinson LD, Jr. Pediatric asthma self-management: current concepts. *J Natl Med Assoc* 1999; 91 (8 Suppl): 40S–44S.

31. Scherr MS. Camp Bronco Junction—second year of experience. *Ann Allergy* 1970; 28(9): 423–433.

32. Clark NM, Feldman CH, Freudenberg N, et al. Developing education for children with asthma through study of self-management behavior. *Health Educ Q* 1980; 7(4): 278–297.

33. Sorrells VD, Chung W, Schlumpberger JM. The impact of a summer asthma camp experience on asthma education and morbidity in children. *J Fam Pract* 1995; 41(5): 465–468.

34. Christiansen SC, Martin SB, Schleicher NC, et al. Evaluation of a school-based asthma education program for inner-city children. *J Allergy Clin Immunol* 1997; 100(5): 613–617.

35. Horner SD. Using the Open Airways curriculum to improve self-care for third grade children with asthma. *J Sch Health* 1998; 68(8): 329–333.
36. Clark NM, Brown R, Joseph CL, et al. Effects of a comprehensive school-based asthma program on symptoms, parent management, grades, and absenteeism. *Chest* 2004; 125(5): 1674–1679.
37. Anderson ME, Freas MR, Wallace AS, et al. Successful school-based intervention for inner-city children with persistent asthma. *J Asthma* 2004; 41(4): 445–453.
38. Yawn BP, Algatt-Bergstrom PJ, Yawn RA, et al. An in-school CD-ROM asthma education program. *J Sch Health* 2000; 70(4): 153–159.
39. NAEPP Resolution on Asthma Management at School. National Heart, Lung and Blood Institute website: http://www.nhlbi.nih.gov/public/lung/asthma/resolut.htm. Accessed 8/19/05.
40. Wilson SR, Latini D, Starr NJ, et al. Education of parents of infants and very young children with asthma: a developmental evaluation of the Wee Wheezers program. *J Asthma* 1996; 33(4): 239–254.
41. Guevara JP, Wolf FM, Grum CM, Clark NM. Effects of educational interventions for self management of asthma in children and adolescents: systematic review and meta-analysis. *Br Med J* 2003; 326(7402): 1308–1309.
42. Wolf FM, Guevara JP, Grum CM, Clark NM, Cates CJ. Educational interventions for asthma in children. *Cochrane Database Syst Rev* 2003(1): CD000326.
43. National Jewish Medical Center Web site asthma action plan. http://www.nationaljewish.org/disease-info/diseases/asthma/living/tools/action/index.aspx. Accessed 8/15/05.
44. WebMD sample asthma action plan. http://my.webmd.com/hw/health_guide_atoz/aa126229.asp. Accessed 8/15/05.
45. FitzGerald JM, Becker A, Sears MR, et al. Doubling the dose of budesonide versus maintenance treatment in asthma exacerbations. *Thorax* 2004; 59(7): 550–556.
46. Foresi A, Morelli MC, Catena E. Low-dose budesonide with the addition of an increased dose during exacerbations is effective in long-term asthma control. On behalf of the Italian Study Group. *Chest* 2000; 117(2): 440–446.
47. Lukacs SL, France EK, Baron AE, Crane LA. Effectiveness of an asthma management program for pediatric members of a large health maintenance organization. *Arch Pediatr Adolesc Med* 2002; 156(9): 872–876.
48. Guendelman S, Meade K, Benson M, Chen YQ, Samuels S. Improving asthma outcomes and self-management behaviors of inner-city children: a randomized trial of the Health Buddy interactive device and an asthma diary. *Arch Pediatr Adolesc Med* 2002; 156(2): 114–120.
49. South M. Asthma Action Plan Generator from Royal Children's Hospital, Melbourne, Australia. http://www.rch.org.au/clinicalguide/forms/asthmaPlanRequest.cfm. Accessed 8/15/05.
50. Osman LM, Calder C, Godden DJ, et al. A randomized trial of self-management planning for adult patients admitted to hospital with acute asthma. *Thorax* 2002; 57(10): 869–874.
51. Castro M, Zimmermann NA, Crocker S, et al. Asthma intervention program prevents readmissions in high healthcare users. *Am J Respir Crit Care Med* 2003; 168(9): 1095–1099.
52. Zorc JJ, Scarfone RJ, Li Y, et al. Scheduled follow-up after a pediatric emergency department visit for asthma: a randomized trial. *Pediatrics* 2003; 111(3): 495–502.
53. Kelso TM, Self TH, Rumbak MJ, et al. Educational and long-term therapeutic intervention in the ED: effect on outcomes in adult indigent minority asthmatics. *Am J Emerg Med* 1995; 13(6): 632–637.
54. Burton WN, Connerty CM, Schultz AB, Chen CY, Edington DW. Bank One's work site-based asthma disease management program. *J Occup Environ Med* 2001; 43(2): 75–82.
55. Lorig KR, Sobel DS, Ritter PL, Laurent D, Hobbs M. Effect of a self-management program on patients with chronic disease. *Eff Clin Pract* 2001; 4(6): 256–262.
56. Beckham S, Kaahaaina D, Voloch KA, Washburn A. A community-based asthma management program: effects on resource utilization and quality of life. *Hawaii Med J* 2004; 63(4): 121–126.
57. US Department of Health and Human Services. Respiratory diseases [Goal 24]. *Healthy People 2010, Vol II.* U.S. Government Printing Office, Washington, DC, 2000; 24: 1–27.

18 The Challenge of Asthma in Minority Populations

Albin B. Leong, MD

Contents

KEY POINTS

- Although asthma affects all races and ethnic groups, there is a significant disparity in asthma morbidity and mortality. Minority populations suffer disproportionately higher rates of fatalities, hospitalizations, and emergency department visits resulting from asthma. For example, non-Hispanic blacks have more than three times the death rate of non-Hispanic whites in the United States.
- Few studies have addressed ethnic differences in asthma in countries outside of the United States. International survey data have shown considerable variation in asthma prevalence in both children and adults among other countries, with higher prevalence in English-speaking countries, including the United Kingdom, Australia, New Zealand, and Ireland.
- In the United States, Puerto Ricans, blacks, and American Indians/Alaskan Natives have the highest current and lifetime asthma prevalence and asthma attack rate.
- Racial/ethnic designations may disguise important differences within groups. For example, Puerto Rican Americans have the highest Hispanic current, lifetime, and

From: *Current Clinical Practice: Bronchial Asthma:*
A Guide for Practical Understanding and Treatment, 5th ed.
Edited by: M. E. Gershwin and T. E. Albertson © Humana Press Inc., Totowa, NJ

asthma attack prevalence, which are comparable to, and exceed rates for, blacks. The larger numbers of Mexican Americans, who have a low prevalence, mask this difference. Hispanics have consequently been considered to have low asthma prevalence.

- Low socioeconomic status (SES) is an independent and significant factor for increased asthma morbidity and mortality for many minority groups. When controlling for SES, significant disparities in asthma morbidity and mortality generally remain for racial/ethnic minority populations.
- Barriers to care exist because of lower SES, with decreased access to care and inadequate care, including underprescription of inhaled corticosteroids, increased environmental exposures in urban settings, substandard living conditions, and increased psychosocial dysfunction and cultural differences.
- Comprehensive and individualized environmental intervention strategies can be effective in reducing allergen environmental burden in urban settings and reduce asthma morbidities.
- Asthma-susceptibility genes with different ethnic frequencies have been found, with the strongest evidence for 6p21 in European Americans, 11q21 in blacks, and 1p32 in Hispanic Americans. Questions remain regarding the degree of heterogeneity, gene–gene interactions, and gene–environment interactions for different racial/ethnic groups.
- Culturally competent strategies can be effective in helping to reduce the disparity in asthma health care and outcomes in racial/ethnic minorities.
- Reduction of asthma disparity in racial and ethnic minority groups is an important challenge and goal and a national priority.

INTRODUCTION

Minorities are individuals or groups of individuals especially qualified. The masses are the collection of people not specifically qualified.

—José Ortega y Gasset
Mirabeau and Politics (1927)

In the United States, minority groups are increasing in relative proportion of the population, especially Hispanics, Asians, and Pacific Islanders. Currently, according to the 2000 census, the US population is 72% non-Hispanic white, 12% black, 11% Hispanic, and 5% Asian and other. Hispanics are projected to pass blacks as the largest minority in the United States by 2005–2015. The United States is now the third largest Spanish-speaking country in the world. By 2050, "minorities" are projected to compose 47% of the US population. Whites are now a minority in 48 of the largest 100 cities in the United States and a minority in California, Hawaii, and the District of Columbia *(1)*.

Even as asthma has been an increasing problem, it is even greater among many minority groups in addition to low-income groups. Although asthma affects all races and ethnic groups, minority populations suffer significantly and disproportionately higher rates of fatalities, hospitalizations, and emergency department visits resulting from asthma. For example, blacks had almost four times more emergency room visits and more than three times more deaths owing to asthma than whites based on the latest 2002 data *(2)*. Thus, the issue of asthma in minorities is clearly important from multiple perspectives, including social, economical, and medical. The elimination of the disparity in asthma burden in minorities and those living in poverty has become a national priority. The National Institute of Allergy and Infectious Diseases, a component of the National Institutes of Health, has sought to resolve issues of health disparity in minorities through research support on asthma with particular focus on minority populations, such as with the National Cooperative Inner-City Asthma Study, Demonstration and Education Research Project, and studies on the genetic basis of asthma (3,4).

Thus, the burden and disparity of asthma in minorities presents a significant challenge. This chapter reviews data on asthma epidemiology among minorities and reviews the available information regarding possible reasons for the differences among ethnic groups, in addition to discussing strategies of intervention and culturally sensitive care. Different definitions of "minority" exist, including distinctions based on religion. For the purposes of this chapter, minority, in terms of race and ethnicity, refers to non-white US Office of Management and Budget classification of race. In addition to whites, these racial designations include blacks, Asian, Native Hawaiian or other Pacific Islander, and American Indian or Alaska native. In this chapter, ethnicity refers to Hispanic or Latino. The term "race/ethnicity" is used throughout this chapter, then, to refer to minority populations.

ASTHMA DIFFERENCES BETWEEN COUNTRIES

Worldwide asthma prevalence among children varies considerably. A range up to 15- to 20-fold differences among countries was found by the questionnaire survey study of the International Study of Asthma and Allergies in Childhood (ISAAC) (5,6). For example, for 13- to 14-yr-old children and the survey question on presence of "wheezing or whistling in the chest in the last 12 mo," there was a positive response range from as low as 2.1–4.4% in Albania, China, Greece, Georgia, Indonesia, Romania, and Russia, and up to 29.1–32.2% in the English-speaking countries of Australia, New Zealand, Republic of Ireland, and the United Kingdom. In general, prevalence data in this survey were higher in developed English-speaking countries and some Latin-American, non-English-speaking countries, including Costa Rica, Brazil, and Peru, and lower in Asia, Northern Africa, Eastern Europe, and the Eastern Mediterranean regions (see Figs. 1 and 2). Among the areas, however, there were differences. For example, within Latin America, lower prevalence of asthma was found in Argentina. More variation was noted among countries than within countries, although this may result from selection bias (6).

In contrast to much of Asia, several affluent Asian regions, such as Hong Kong, Singapore, and Japan, had relatively high asthma prevalence. A notable dissimilarity was seen between Hong Kong and Guangzhou (10.1 vs 2.0% 12-mo prevalence of wheezing), areas that are geographically and ethnically similar but differ in affluence.

There are many limitations in the ISAAC survey data including lack of a standard asthma definition and thus the use of asthma symptoms, such as "wheezing or whistling" and night cough, for example, in the questionnaire, validity of the questionnaire across cultures and languages, and limitations in the locations and numbers of areas surveyed within countries, as well as between countries, in addition to potential reporting differences. Nonetheless, these are the best data available. No specific data on prevalence based on ethnicity are available for the countries in this survey study. The ISSAC study authors postulate that the major differences among the countries likely result from environmental factors.

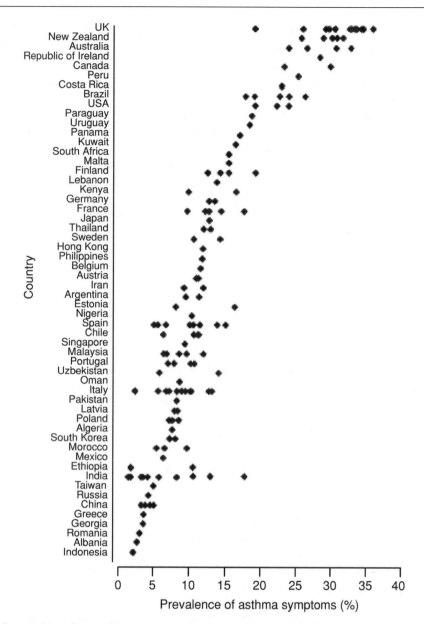

Fig. 1. International Study of Asthma and Allergies in Childhood (ISSAC): Current asthma prevalence (written questionnaire) for children aged 13–14 yr (1996). (Reprinted with permission from Elsevier. *See* ref. *5.*)

For adults, a smaller study, the European Community Respiratory Health Survey for 20- to 44-yr-olds primarily in Europe also reported higher prevalence in English-speaking countries, including the United Kingdom, Australia, New Zealand, and the Republic of Ireland, and lower in Eastern and Southern Europe. Overall agreement between the ISAAC and European Community Respiratory Health Survey study was noted *(7,8).*

International data on racial/ethnic population composition are imprecise, and classification categories vary from country to country. For example, a person of Pakistani

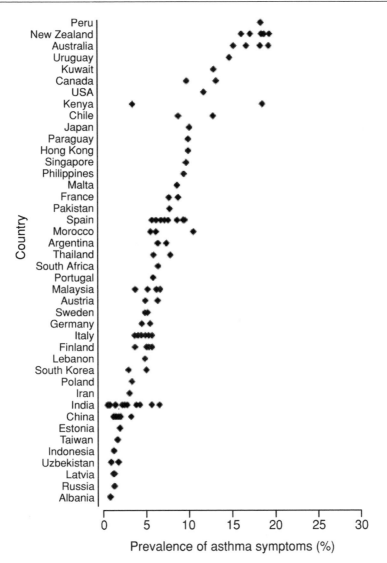

Fig. 2. International Study of Asthma and Allergies in Childhood (ISSAC): Current asthma prevalence (video questionnaire) for children aged 13–14 yr (1996). (Reprinted with permission from Elsevier. *See* ref. *5*.)

origin might be noted as either "black," "colored," or "South Asian" in the United Kingdom in contrast to "Asian" or possibly "white" in the United States.

There are limited data evaluating racial/ethnic differences in asthma outside the United States. A recent survey indicated that many, but not all, asthma trials in the United States include racial/ethnic data on study subjects, but this information is rarely obtained in clinical studies from Europe *(9)*. Because of racial/ethnic differences in asthma severity and prevalence, lack of inclusion of such data may confound clinical study results and comparisons. Some examples of the studies of minorities outside the United States are summarized.

In Sweden, Hjern et al. evaluated pediatric hospital admission data regarding social and ethnic factors. This study showed a lower prevalence of asthma admissions for children born outside of Western Europe, the United States, and Australia, as well as for children born in Sweden to mothers born in Eastern and Southern Europe. The authors suggested that ethnic differences in asthma prevalence may account for the differences. In this study, socioeconomic factors of social welfare, single-parent households, and maternal smoking during pregnancy for children less than 3 yr old also increased the risk for admission *(10)*.

An editorial and study regarding ethnic differences in asthma in the United Kingdom concluded that asthma and asthma admissions may be more common in South Asians (Indian subcontinent) but also that asthma may be underdiagnosed and undertreated in this population. Possible cultural barriers may exist, as dissimilar results were noted in asthma outcome for South Asians vs white Europeans despite similar medication and asthma education and self-management training. There was no reduction in hospitalizations and use of rescue corticosteroids in the South Asians compared with white Europeans, who did benefit. Possible effects, such as Westernized lifestyle and environment, as well as barriers, including cultural attitudes, communication problems, and possible health professional and patient interaction issues were cited as possible reasons in addition to potential intrinsic differences. The latter was considered unlikely based on lack of evidence *(11)*. Similar confounding variables for racial/ethnic minorities that have been studied or postulated in the United States are discussed in the section on Factors in Racial/Ethnic Differences of Asthma.

Similar to US data on American Indians and Alaska natives, a Canadian study showed an increased incidence in emergency (2.1 times higher) and office visits (1.6 times higher) for asthma among aboriginals compared with nonaboriginals in a retrospective cohort study in Alberta, Canada. Specialty care (55% less) and spirometry use (66% less) were lower, however, suggesting barriers in access to quality care *(12)*.

Differences have been noted in mortality asthma admission rate for Maoris and Pacific Islander children compared to whites in New Zealand. However, the differences were not believed to result from prevalence, genetic, or socioeconomic factors but rather differences in medical management, especially prescribing patterns by medical practitioners *(13)*. Differences in prescribing practices for minorities in the United States have been noted and are discussed in "Factors in Racial/Ethnic Differences of Asthma."

Recent reports from various countries involving different age and racial/ethnic groups have shown conflicting results in changes in asthma prevalence. Some countries have reported decreases, including Rome, Italy, Saskatchewan, Canada, Melbourne, Australia, and Mexico. Others have reported increases, including Saudi Arabia, south Australia, and Patras, Greece. Because of differences in asthma case definitions, survey techniques, the survey time periods, and population characteristics studied, these and other studies are not easily comparable *(14)*.

NATIONAL CENTER FOR HEALTH STATISTICS: ASTHMA PREVALENCE, HEALTH CARE USE, AND MORTALITY, 2000–2001, 2002

Race/Ethnic Differences Within the United States

In the United States, ethnic differences have been noted in national survey data, with significant differences in morbidity and mortality. Before 2002, limited data on ethnic differences in asthma was available for US data other than for non-Hispanic whites, non-Hispanic blacks, and Hispanics. In the Centers for Disease Control and

Table 1
Estimated Annual Prevalence of Self-Reported Asthma (1980–1996) or an Episode of Asthma
or Asthma Attacks (1997–1999) during the Preceding 12 mo, by Race, Sex, and Age Group
(National Health Interview Survey—United States, 1980–1999)[a,b]

	1980	1985	1990	1995	1996	1997	1998	1999
	Self-reported asthma prevalence during the preceding 12 mo					Episode of asthma or asthma attack during the preceding 12 mo		
Race[c]								
White	31.4	37.0	41.5	54.5	53.6	40.5	37.5	37.6
Black	33.1	38.6	45.8	64.8	65.5	45.4	46.7	42.7
Other	19.9[d]	12.8[d]	40.2	44.4	43.2	34.7	33.7	38.9
Sex[c]								
Male	30.5	33.8	39.1	48.6	43.0	33.0	31.7	31.6
Female	31.9	38.9	44.2	61.1	65.5	47.9	44.4	44.5
Age Group (yr)								
0–4	23.0	36.7	44.0	60.5	40.1	41.2	46.4	42.1
5–14	45.1	50.9	63.7	82.0	69.8	60.0	57.8	56.4
15–34	30.0	36.1	37.3	57.8	67.2	44.2	37.5	42.2
35–64	29.9	30.8	38.4	50.1	46.2	37.0	35.7	33.4
≥65	31.9	38.6	36.3	39.4	45.5	27.3	28.7	22.1
Total[c]	31.4	36.6	41.9	55.2	54.6	40.7	39.2	38.4

[a]Per 1000 population.
[b]All relative standard errors are <30%, unless otherwise indicated.
[c]Age-adjusted to 2000 US population.
[d]Relative standard error of the estimate is 30–50%: the estimate is unreliable.
(Adapted from ref. 15.)

Prevention surveillance for asthma in the United States, covering 1980–1999, significant racial disparity for asthma in morbidity and mortality between blacks and whites was evident. In this report, race data were indicated by white, black, and "other." Compared with the roughly similar differences in asthma prevalence, disproportionally higher rates of asthma emergency department visits were noted for blacks compared with whites. In addition, alarmingly higher rates of asthma hospitalizations and deaths persisted for both blacks and "other" compared with whites during this time period. The relative death rate for blacks compared with whites remained greater than 200% during this period, ranging from 214% in 1980 to 274% in 1999 (see Tables 1–4). Concerning these differences, the Centers for Disease Control and Prevention stated, "The continued presence of substantial racial disparities in these asthma endpoints highlights the need for continued surveillance and targeted interventions" (15).

By 2002, more specific racial/ethnic data became available. The most recent available National Health Interview Survey (NHIS) in the United States again indicated substantial ethnic differences in prevalence, health use, and mortality (see Tables 5 and 6) (2,16).

In this most recent national data set, greater lifetime prevalence of asthma was noted in non-Hispanic blacks (138/1000), 24% higher compared with non-Hispanic whites (111/1000), and 66% higher than Hispanics (83/1000). American Indians were almost as high as non-Hispanic blacks (133/1000). However, a difference within Hispanics in

Table 2

Estimated Annual Rate of Emergency Department Visits for Asthma as the First-Listed
Diagnosis, by Race, Sex, and Age Group (National Hospital Ambulatory Medical Care
Survey—United States, 1992–1999)[a,b]

	1992	1995	1996	1997	1998	1999
Race[c]						
White	43.7	46.9	54.6	57.7	58.2	59.4
Black	143.2	226.4	188.7	171.2	183.7	174.3
Other	49.3[d]	56.2[d]	56.2[d]	—[e]	45.8[d]	38.4
Sex[c]						
Male	51.7	54.4	71.9	59.5	66.7	68.6
Female	61.5	85.9	72.0	81.8	82.3	77.2
Age Group (yr)						
0–4	153.0	131.2	172.6	177.8	170.2	141.8
5–14	80.6	85.8	94.4	88.6	113.8	98.5
15–34	55.3	72.7	84.6	86.5	86.4	81.3
35–64	41.0	66.5	52.7	49.4	49.8	58.1
≥65	28.0	28.7	25.8	28.3	30.9	35.5
Total[c]	56.8	70.7	72.4	71.2	75.1	73.3

[a]Per 1000 population.
[b]All relative standard errors are <30%, unless otherwise indicated.
[c]Age-adjusted to 2000 US population.
[d]Relative standard error of the estimate is 30–50%: the estimate is unreliable.
[e]Relative standard error of the estimate exceeds 50%.
(Adapted from ref. *15*.)

Table 3

Estimated Annual Rate of Hospitalization for Asthma as the First-Listed Diagnosis, by Race,
Sex, and Age Group (National Hospital Discharge Survey—United States, 1980–1999)[a,b]

	1980	1985	1990	1995	1996	1997	1998	1999
Race[c]								
White	15.6	15.8	12.6	11.8	10.9	11.9	10.1	10.6
Black	27.0	31.1	38.3	40.7	38.2	34.4	32.5	35.6
Other	—[d]	29.9	22.5	22.4	26.6	29.4	21.4	31.5
Sex[c]								
Male	17.4	17.4	15.6	16.1	14.8	15.3	12.5	14.1
Female	20.3	22.2	22.1	22.4	20.6	20.4	18.4	20.6
Age Group (yr)								
0–4	37.3	47.8	55.6	62.6	60.2	63.9	47.3	55.4
5–14	18.1	17.3	18.5	25.0	21.3	24.1	19.6	21.5
15–34	8.5	9.7	9.4	10.2	9.4	9.1	7.3	10.1
35–64	18.9	18.6	15.5	15.0	15.2	13.7	13.9	13.4
≥65	32.8	34.4	33.0	23.5	17.7	19.3	17.8	21.1
Total[c]	19.0	19.7	19.2	19.5	17.9	18.1	15.7	17.6

[a]Per 1000 population.
[b]All relative standard errors are <30%, unless otherwise indicated.
[c]Age-adjusted to 2000 US population.
[d]Relative standard error of the estimate exceeds 50%.
(Adapted from ref. *15*.)

Table 4
Annual Rate of Deaths with Asthma as the Underlying Cause of Death Diagnosis, by Race, Sex, and Age Group (Underlying Cause of Death Data Set—United States, 1980–1999)[a,b]

	1980[c]	1985	1990	1995	1996	1997	1998	1999[d]
Race[e]								
White	12.9	15.6	17.5	18.8	18.1	17.4	17.0	14.2
Black	27.6	34.8	40.9	46.2	48.0	42.5	44.7	38.7
Other	13.5	16.9	23.6	23.3	27.6	26.6	22.7	20.4
Sex[e]								
Male	14.7	15.9	17.8	17.9	17.7	16.6	16.5	13.1
Female	14.4	19.2	22.1	25.1	25.0	23.7	23.3	20.4
Age Group (yr)								
0–4	1.8	1.5	2.0	1.8	2.3	1.9	2.1	1.7
5–14	1.9	2.9	3.2	4.0	4.6	3.4	3.8	3.6
15–34	3.0	4.2	5.0	6.7	6.5	6.1	6.4	5.9
35–64	14.0	17.7	18.8	20.6	20.3	19.0	17.8	15.8
≥65	61.8	72.5	87.0	90.8	90.3	86.7	86.9	69.9
Total[e]	14.4	17.7	20.2	21.9	21.8	20.6	20.3	17.2

[a]Per 1 million population.

[b]All relative standard errors are <30%.

[c]Code 493 from World Health Organization. Manual of the international statistical classification of diseases, injuries, and causes of death. Ninth revision Geneva, Switzerland: World Health Organization. 1977.

[d]Codes J45–J46 from World Health Organization. Manual of the international statistical classification of diseases, injuries, and causes of death. Tenth revision Geneva, Switzerland: World Health Organization. 1999.

[e]Age-adjusted to the 2000 US population.

(Adapted from ref. 15.)

the United States was noted. Puerto Ricans had the highest overall rate (196/1000) among Hispanics—indeed among all ethnic groups—in comparison with Mexicans, who had the lowest rate (61/1000). Thus, group racial/ethnic categorization of "Hispanics" would have obscured these prominent differences (see Fig. 3).

Current asthma prevalence revealed a similar greater prevalence in racial/ethnic minorities. Puerto Ricans were 80% higher, whereas non-Hispanic blacks and American Indians were 30% higher compared with non-Hispanic whites. On the other hand, Mexicans were 50% less than non-Hispanic whites. Overall Hispanic rates again masked the significant difference for Puerto Ricans (see Fig. 4).

Higher asthma-attack rates were found among minorities, often greater in proportion to prevalence data. American Indians were approx 10% higher, non-Hispanic blacks approx 30% higher, and Puerto Ricans 100% higher compared with non-Hispanic whites. The lowest rate was found among Mexicans, who were approx 50% lower than non-Hispanic whites (see Fig. 5).

Because of less race/ethnic data for health care use, little specific data is available for outpatient health care use. Blacks, however, were noted with disproportionately higher rates of asthma morbidity. Blacks experienced the significantly higher rates of 380% greater for asthma emergency department visits and 225% greater for hospitalizations, compared with whites (see Figs. 6 and 7). Disturbingly, the trend of more than 200% more asthma deaths of blacks compared with whites has continued based on the latest national data from 2002 (Fig. 8; ref. 2).

Table 5

US Rates for Current Asthma and Asthma Attack Prevalence (2001), Health Care Utilization (2000), and Mortality (2000)[a]

	Lifetime asthma prevalence (per 1000)	Current asthma prevalence (per 1000)	Asthma attack prevalence (per 1000)	Outpatient visits (per 10,000)	Emergency room visits (per 1000)	Hospital (per 10,000)	Mortality (per 100,000)
Race							
Non-Hispanic white	116	75	44	—	—		1.3
Non-Hispanic black	121	83	54	—	—		4.0
Hispanic	92	58	34	—	—		1.5
White (including Hispanic)[a]	—	—	—	366	59	10	
Black (including Hispanic)[a]	—	—	—	515	133	32	
Sex							
Female	117	83	50	397	75	19	1.8
Male	108	63	36	354	58	15	1.3
Age							
0–17 yr	126	87	57	649	104	30	0.3
18 yr and older	109	69	38	285	54	12	2.1
Total	114	73	43	379	67	17	1.6

[a]Age adjusted for the 2000 population. Data for health care outcomes is not available for Hispanic ethnicity. Data for white and black race for these outcomes include persons of Hispanic ethnicity (Adapted from ref. 16.)

Table 6
US Rates for Current Asthma and Asthma Prevalence, Health Care Utilization, and Mortality (2002)

	Lifetime asthma prevalence (per 1000)	Current asthma prevalence (per 1000)	Asthma attack prevalence (per 1000)	Outpatient visits (per 10,000)	Emergency room visits (per 1000)	Hospital (per 10,000)	Mortality (per 100,000)
Race							
Non-Hispanic white	111	72	42				1.2
Non-Hispanic black	138	95	55				3.7
Total Hispanic	83	49	31				1.4
Puerto Rican	196	131	85				
Mexican	61	36	20				
Non-Hispanic American Indian	133	99	47				
White				493	45	11	
Black				482	217	36	
Sex							
Female	116	81	49	585	69	19	1.7
Male	106	62	36	384	65	14	1.2
Age							
18 yr and older	106	68	37	181	24	13	1.9
0–17 yr	122	83	58	687	100	27	0.3
Total	111	72	43	492	67	17	1.5

Age adjusted for the 2000 population. Data for white and black race for these outcomes include persons of Hispanic ethnicity (Adapted from ref. 2.)

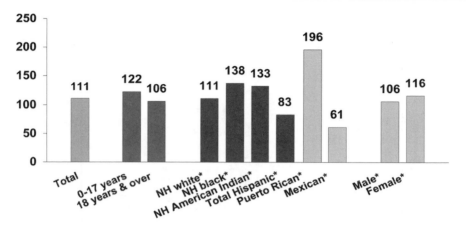

Fig. 3. Prevalence of lifetime asthma diagnosis per 1000 population, 2002. *Age adjusted to 2000 population. (Adapted from ref. 2.)

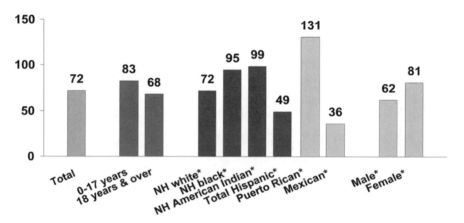

Fig. 4. Current asthma prevalence per 1000 population, 2002. *Age adjusted to 2000 population. NH, non-Hispanic. (Adapted from ref. 2.)

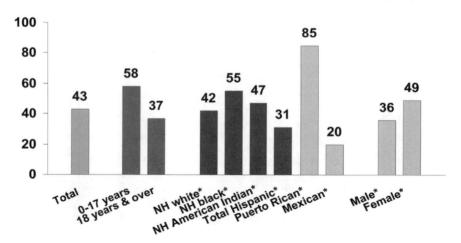

Fig. 5. Asthma attack prevalence per 1000 population, 2002. *Age adjusted to 2000 population. NH, non-Hispanic. (Adapted from ref. 2.)

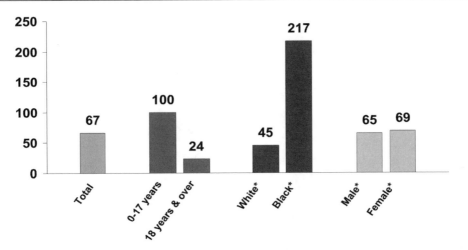

Fig. 6. Asthma emergency department visits per 10,000 population, 2002. Hispanic ethnicity not available; estimates for racial categories include both Hispanic and non-Hispanic persons. *Age adjusted to 2000 population. (Adapted from ref. 2.)

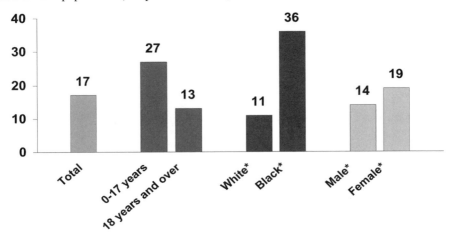

Fig. 7. Asthma hospitalizations per 10,000 population, 2002. Hispanic ethnicity not available; estimates for racial categories include both Hispanic and non-Hispanic persons. *Age adjusted to 2000 population. (Adapted from ref. 2.)

SPECIFIC ETHNIC DATA: ASTHMA IN CALIFORNIA

The 2001 California Health Interview Survey (CHIS) was a recent large study to assess the health and access to health care in California. It is the largest health survey ever conducted in any state and one of the largest surveys ever conducted in the United States. CHIS randomly selected a total of 55,428 households from every county in California, with interviews available in six languages. It covered a range of health concerns, including health status and conditions, health-related behaviors, health insurance coverage, and access to health care services. More specific ethnic data were collected in this survey, which is the largest, most complete database on specific asthma rates among different ethnic groups. Data from this survey included prevalence, access to care, emergency department use, hospitalizations, and frequent asthma symptoms. Statistically significant differences were frequently noted.

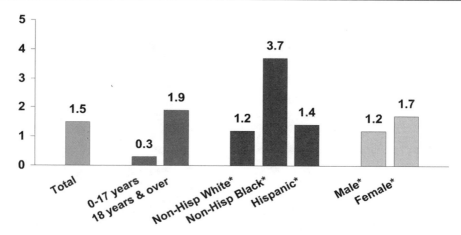

Fig. 8. Asthma deaths per 100,000 population, 2002. *Age adjusted to 2000 population. (Adapted from ref. 2.)

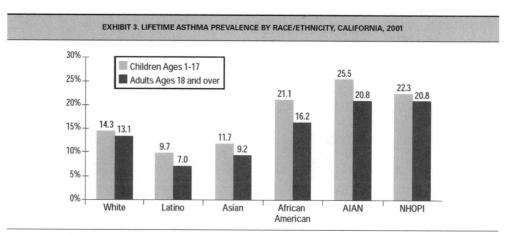

Fig. 9. Lifetime asthma prevalence by race/ethnicity in California, 2001 (Adapted with permission from ref. 17.)

Lifetime asthma prevalence was statistically significantly higher among blacks (21.1% of children ages 1–17 yr and 16.2% of adults) and even greater for American Indians and Alaska Natives (25.5% of children, 20.8% of adults) compared with whites, Latinos, and Asians. Although higher rates were noted in Native Hawaiian and other Pacific Islanders (22.3% of children and 20.8% of adults), these differences were not statistically significant compared with whites (*see* Fig. 9).

Although Latinos had lower rates in the CHIS *(18)*, there are significant differences among Latino ethnic groups, expanding on the US data regarding Puerto Ricans and Mexicans in the National Center for Health Statistics (NCHS) report noted above (ref. 2; Figs. 3–5). Puerto Ricans (18.9% prevalence for all ages) and South Americans (12.7%) were noted, with significantly higher prevalence in comparison with other Latino subgroups, including Mexicans, Salvadorans, Guatemalans, and Central Americans (*see* Fig. 10). The increased prevalence among Puerto Ricans was also indicated by the Behavioral Risk Factor Surveillance System survey, with the highest lifetime prevalence

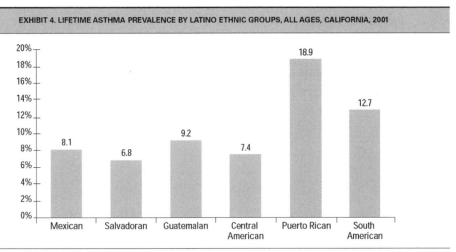

EXHIBIT 4. LIFETIME ASTHMA PREVALENCE BY LATINO ETHNIC GROUPS, ALL AGES, CALIFORNIA, 2001

Source: 2001 California Health Interview Survey

Fig. 10. Lifetime asthma prevalence by Latino ethnic groups, all ages in California, 2001. (Adapted with permission from ref. *17*.)

of 15.9% in Puerto Rico among the United States, District of Columbia, Guam, Puerto Rico, and the Virgin Islands. (Louisiana had the lowest prevalence of 8.0% in this survey) *(15)*. Furthermore, the Genetics of Asthma in Latino Americans Study revealed that Puerto Ricans with asthma have lower lung function and lower responsiveness to β-2 agonist bronchodilators, as well as earlier onset of asthma and greater health care use *(18)*. The overall low prevalence of asthma among Latinos in California is believed to most likely result from the fact that 75% of Latinos in California are of Mexican heritage. Thus, both the CHIS and the NCHS reports indicate that overall Hispanic data masks important differences among the Hispanic groups.

Similarly, heterogeneous differences were seen among Asian American subgroups in California. Japanese and Filipinos had significantly higher prevalence compared with Chinese, Vietnamese, Koreans, Cambodians, or South Asians (*see* Fig. 11).

The authors of this University of California Los Angeles study cautioned that several issues may affect the data on prevalence among the different ethnic subgroups. The variations may result from differences in the likelihood of a diagnosis of asthma rather than actual asthma prevalence. These include potential differences in financial or geographic access to health care, parents' health care-seeking behaviors, and physician practice patterns. Thus, populations with higher poverty, no insurance, or underinsurance may have underestimated prevalence rates. The authors also pointed out that recent immigrants have significant barriers to care because of the additional issues of language, acculturation, and immigration status. Because proportions of the newer immigrants to California are higher among some of the Latino and Asian American populations, the potential for underdiagnosis and lower understanding of asthma when diagnosed is greater.

Racial and ethnic differences were also seen in use of the emergency room for asthma. Black and Latino adults and Latino children were noted with statistically significant higher rates of emergency room use compared with whites (*see* Fig. 12). There were also increased trends noted in hospitalizations, but the differences were not statistically significant. Thus, the 2001 CHIS revealed a significant disparity in asthma burden in

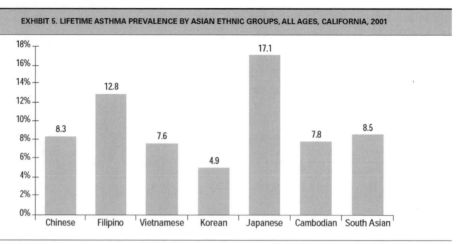

Source: 2001 California Health Interview Survey

Fig. 11. Lifetime asthma prevalence by Asian ethnic groups, all ages in California, 2001. (Adapted with permission from ref. *17*.)

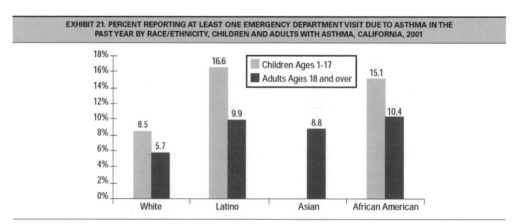

Note: The numbers of American Indian and Alaska Natives and Native Hawaiians   Source: 2001 California Health Interview Survey
        and other Pacific Islanders were too small to produce a reliable estimate
        of emergency department visits for adults or children. The number of
        Asian children was too small to produce a reliable estimate.

Fig. 12. Percent reporting at least one emergency department visit owing to asthma in the past year by race/ethnicity, children and adults with asthma in California, 2001. (Adapted with permission from ref. *17*.)

racial/ethnic minority groups, especially among American Indian/Alaska Natives, blacks, Native Hawaiian and other Pacific Islanders, Puerto Ricans, and South Americans *(17)*.

FACTORS IN ASTHMA RACIAL/ETHNIC DISPARITIES

Underuse of inhaled corticosteroids (ICS) in racial/ethnic minorities has been noted in several studies. A prospective, Multicenter Airway Research Collaboration emergency room study evaluated racial/ethnic differences in asthma severity and management in children. This study found similar acute severity, emergency department (ED) management care, and course, including similar hospitalization rates and rate of persistent symptoms and relapse 2 wk after discharge, for blacks, Hispanics, and whites. However, despite a history of more severe chronic asthma in minorities, including past hospitalizations and ED rates, the prescription rate of ICS was similar, rather than increased, for minority patients leaving the ED. The authors noted that other outpatient studies have shown similar deficits in preventive asthma prescription use among patients who have asthma and are members of minority groups. This is important because minorities often use the ED as a point of care. Data are limited about whether this deficit of ICS use in minorities results from discrepancies in prescribing or lack of filling the prescription. This study indicated that lack of prescribing was prevalent by ED physicians. The explanation for this pattern is unclear and may relate to assumption for chronic care by the primary care provider, unfamiliarity with controller medications, and/or perceptions of cost (19).

In a similar prospective study in adults by the Multicenter Airway Research Collaboration, significant racial/ethnic differences were seen in Hispanics and blacks with greater chronic asthma severity and lower initial peak expiratory flow rate at presentation to the ED and worse postdischarge outcomes. Similar ED management was noted for different racial/ethnic groups. Socioeconomic status accounted for much of the differences in the severity of asthma severity. However, after adjustment for sociodemographic factors, persistent differences were noted in asthma hospitalization, with Hispanics and blacks more than twice as likely to be admitted to hospital compared with whites in this adult study in contrast to the pediatric study. As in the pediatric study, ED discharge medication prescription of controller medications did not differ, despite the increased chronic severity in Hispanics and blacks (20).

Allergy has been previously noted as a major risk factor for asthma. Racial/ethnic differences in allergic disease experience exist for both children and adults. For example, in a large study of adults, Asians have a higher risk of atopic conditions (including asthma with hay fever) compared with whites, whereas blacks have greater nonatopic asthma. This difference for Asians has also been noted in the United Kingdom and Australia. Study data suggest that nongenetic conditions, such as social and/or environmental factors and possibly acculturation, may be important in determining risk of asthma and atopy in different immigrating groups (14,21).

The importance of environmental factors has been further suggested in considering the possible reason for increased prevalence of asthma noted in a recent analysis of US-born compared to Mexican-born Mexican Americans (7% [SE 0.5] vs 3% [SE 0.3]) in the Third National Health and Nutrition Examination Survey, 1988-1994 (NHANES III) and the NHIS for 1997–2001 (8.1% [0.4] vs 2.5% [0.2]). Residency duration in the United States was also associated with increased asthma prevalence, further implicating possible gene–environmental interactions as a risk factor for asthma (22).

There is also an outpatient clinic prescription discrepancy for different racial/ethnic groups. Controlling for multiple measures of sociodemographic variables, a cross-sectional study of different health plans found worse asthma status, based on direct parent report, and less use of preventive asthma medications for black and Latino compared with white children. This difference occurred within the same managed Medicaid populations so that financial access to health care was equal, including prescription coverage. In this study, the disparity in preventive medication use was also found even when severity of asthma status was adjusted. Processes of asthma care, such as use of preventive visits and specialists, written management plans, having no pets or smokers in the home, and ratings of providers and asthma care, were equal or better for minority compared with white children. Nonfinancial barriers to use of preventive therapy exist for minorities and were seen in this study in each of the five health plans in three different states. Other studies have also found persistent racial/ethnic disparities in asthma care in adults within the same managed care. Thus, these and other studies indicate that targeting and increasing the use of preventive medications in minority populations would be important in helping to reduce racial/ethnic disparity in asthma (23).

Many studies have indicated that low socioeconomic status (SES) is an independent and important variable for poor asthma management and outcomes (19,20,24,25). SES as a variable is complex. It has been suggested that SES be conceptualized as a chronic, multidimensional rather than an acute, one-dimensional state (19). Comparing studies based on SES and various corrections for asthma risk factors is often difficult because of the different measures used. For example, annual household income, average lifetime income, poverty status, type of insurance and Medicaid status, parental education, single-parent family, number of children, urban residence, presence of health behaviors (such as presence of smokers and lack of prenatal care), and patient variables (such as allergy, obesity, history of bronchiolitis, and prematurity) are among the various variables often used but not comparable among studies. In addition, underdiagnosis of asthma, differences in perception of and response to symptoms, lower ratings of health care, and lower response rates in studies of impoverished and minority populations are limitations of studies in these populations (23,24,26,27).

Low socioeconomic level and race/ethnicity are intertwined and intricate variables. There are conflicting results on increased asthma prevalence in minorities when adjusted for SES. A few studies have suggested that SES differences may even account for most, if not all, of the race-/ethnicity-associated differences in asthma. For example, Weitzman et al. previously evaluated national data from the 1981 NHIS and found that the increased prevalence of asthma in black children and poor children was accounted for by several social and environmental characteristics, such as maternal smoking, low birth-weight, large family, smaller home size, and young maternal age (28). In another example, in a cross-sectional analysis in Boston, income, area of residence, and level of education accounted for a large proportion of the increased prevalence differences for blacks and Hispanics, although the incidence of Hispanics was small in this study (29).

On the other hand, many other studies have shown a still increased prevalence when socioeconomic factors are controlled. In addition, other studies, discussed in Chapter 1, have shown that *higher* SES may be a risk factor for asthma owing to the "hygiene hypothesis." Low SES and asthma have been associated in a number of studies within the United States and outside the United States. These studies, when controlling for various measures of SES, have shown still increased prevalence for black and Hispanic children for multiple asthma morbidities. These include higher prevalence, more severe symptoms, suboptimal asthma care, increased emergency department use, and increased hospitalizations (19–21,23,24,26,30).

Some studies have indicated that low SES is an independent variable of race/ethnicity with regard to asthma mortality. However, the effect of race/ethnicity is greater than that of SES. Grant et al. evaluated this from the National Center for Health Statistics for 1991–1996. For both blacks and whites, lower asthma mortality occurs when socioeconomic status and educational level increase. However, mortality among blacks is still greater than it is in whites in all socioeconomic levels. Thus, for example, for persons aged 5–34 yr during 1991–1996, the mortality rate among blacks compared to whites in the highest quintile for median income was nearly 400% greater, 1.29 vs 0.26/100,000, and almost 200% greater in the lowest quintile for median income, 1.52 vs 0.51, for blacks compared with whites. Also, there was a racial disparity despite comparable education. Mortality rates from asthma were greater for blacks vs whites throughout educational levels, with a rate of 1.50 vs 0.26/100,000 in the highest quintile and 1.86 vs 0.48 for the lowest quintile for educational level. In addition to increased mortality, epidemiological data indicate that after correction for socioeconomic and environmental factors, racial/ethnic differences still remain for asthma hospitalizations (25).

For many minorities, coexistent low SES is an important comorbidity affecting asthma outcomes. Several factors that are increased with low SES contribute to this burden. These include decreased access to health care, including lack of insurance, limited access to health care providers, lack of transportation to health care facilities, poor access to support groups, and inability to afford medications.

All racial/ethnic groups have lower rates of employment-based insurance and higher uninsured rates compared with non-Latino whites. Latinos have the highest uninsured rates. Low education and income, as well as lack of citizenship, are significant contributing factors for Latinos. There is a range among Asian Americans and Pacific Islanders in education, income, immigration status, and insurance. First- and second-generation Koreans and Southeast Asians have poor health insurance coverage. As a result of low income, low rates of job-based insurance, and declines in Medicaid coverage, almost one in four nonelderly blacks is not insured. Data are limited on American Indians and Alaskan Natives, but these groups do encounter limited coverage by Indian Health Service and low rates of job-based insurance coverage. Thus, many minorities face barriers to health care because of lack of insurance, which contributes to the disparity in health status (31).

Another effect of low SES is inadequate medical care, including underdiagnosis or improper diagnosis, primary care physicians who are less well trained, lack of asthma severity recognition, and underprescription of controller medications. There are also increased contributing factors including obesity, low birth-weight, prematurity, and increased upper respiratory tract infections for those living in poverty. Inadequate asthma education has also been found, including lack of understanding of pathophysiology, lack of appreciation about the importance of early intervention, overuse and inappropriate use of asthma medications, and poor adherence to treatment plans. Low levels of literacy and education also affect understanding and adherence.

Attitude correlates strongly with adherence, such as belief in the benefits and less fear of adverse effects of ICS. However, modifiable barriers, such as knowledge, communication, depression, self-efficacy, and support did not affect the race/ethnicity effect on adherence in a recent study on adults with asthma. Instead, immutable factors, such as income, education, having commercial insurance, and recent symptoms, affected adherence. This study has implications for understanding barriers to adherence for providers and health care delivery systems (32).

Furthermore, for families living in poverty, psychosocial dysfunction of patient and family have been noted, including increased depression, mood and anxiety disorders, hopelessness and despair, stress from exposure to crime and violence, and illicit drug use. Mental health problems of caretakers and children have been associated with increased asthma hospitalizations and symptoms. Lack of social support occurs with single-parent families, young mothers, social isolation of caregivers, and lack of child care resources. In addition, there is increased exposure to indoor and outdoor environmental exacerbants, including allergens, such as cockroaches, molds, dust mites, and air pollution and environmental tobacco smoke (ETS). Finally, deprived living conditions exist with overcrowded living conditions, substandard housing, and dilapidated physical environment. Indeed, studies have indicated that asthma status and severity had no difference in measurements of quality of life in young urban children, indicating that other factors, such as the social and emotional milieu, are important in understanding the adaptation and functioning to a chronic disease, such as asthma, within the context of low SES. Thus, numerous coexisting factors further affect and complicate the burden of asthma in racial/ethnic minorities (24,33–36).

INTERVENTION STRATEGIES

As a result of the environmental exposures in urban settings, inner-city inhabitants with asthma are exposed to multiple indoor allergens and irritants, such as cockroach, fungi, dust mites, rat, mice, cat and dog danders, and ETS. It has been demonstrated that most inner-city children with moderate to severe asthma are sensitized to multiple indoor allergens. The Inner-City Asthma Study Group evaluated a multifaceted, home-based, environmental 1-yr intervention for urban children with asthma. The intervention was individualized and comprehensive. A successful reduction in allergen burden was achieved, which included an approach based on social learning theory. This reduction was remarkable, in contrast to previous studies, which often targeted only one allergen or environmental factor, such as cockroach or ETS. The success of this study's approach emphasizes the importance of the intervention strategy, especially in such a high-risk population. Furthermore, the reductions achieved were associated with reduced asthma morbidity. Affected outcomes included improvements with decreases of asthma morbidities, including days of symptoms, unscheduled asthma-related visits, disruption of caretaker's plans, caretaker's and child's lost sleep, and school days missed. Continued improvement, compared to the control group, was noted in days of symptoms and caretaker sleep loss in the follow-up year after intervention (37).

Thus, environmental risk factor reduction can be a successful strategy to reduce asthma complications in high-risk, inner-city patients, who are mostly minorities, with asthma. In addition, the National Cooperative Inner-City Asthma Study multifaceted intervention program has been analyzed to be cost-effective when compared with usual care (38).

Other intervention strategies and models have been evaluated, especially in urban, low-income minorities. Improvement in diagnosis has resulted from use of a novel asthma questionnaire to detect presence of asthma in a multicultural inner-city population (39). Improvements in access to specialty care, including ongoing access and provision of comprehensive asthma care plans, have resulted in reduced acute care, hospitalizations, and increased preventative care with possible cost reductions. Another strategy involves acute care. Standardization and centralization of acute asthma care have resulted in reduced length of stay in EDs and hospitals. Facilitation of transition from acute to outpatient care for optimal preventive care has resulted in reduced ED and inpatient readmission rates.

Strategies for improving patient and family education (such as the Inner-City Asthma Study group), and involving coordination of care, assistance with allergen reduction, and/or monitoring of self-management care practices have resulted in fewer symptomatic days, reduced hospitalizations, possible reduction of acute care visits, and improved environmental control measures. Community-based interventions to affect behavior changes and improved asthma management, as well as improved education, have been successful in reaching high-risk, low-income minority populations and affecting asthma management with potential reduction in acute care rates in more active participants *(24,40)*.

Finally, culturally competent strategies can be effective in helping to reduce the disparity of asthma in racial/ethnic groups. This is discussed in the section entitled, Culturally Competent Care.

GENETICS

Research by the Collaborative Study for the Genetics of Asthma has shown heterogeneity or different frequencies of polymorphisms in asthma gene markers among ethnic groups. These differences may contribute to susceptibility on a genetic basis to asthma among different race/ethnic groups. Asthma-susceptibility genes with different ethnic frequencies have been found, with the strongest evidence for 6p21 in European Americans, 11q21 in Blacks, and 1p32 in Hispanic Americans. Also, allergic response markers on chromosomes 10p, 11q, 17q, and 20p with complex gene interactions have been identified, although ethnic variability is unclear. However, this work is preliminary and different studies have often yielded conflicting data. Questions remain regarding the degree of heterogeneity, gene–gene interactions, and gene–environment interactions for different race/ethnic groups *(41–43)*.

Recent research in pharmocogenetics has shown differences that may help explain asthma differences among minority populations. For example, blacks have been noted with diminished T-lymphocyte response to glucocorticoids *(44)*. Between Puerto Ricans and Mexicans, pharmacogenetic differences in response to albuterol have been shown *(45)*. Thus, genetic polymorphisms in drug receptors may help explain phenotypic differences in asthma variability among different racial/ethnic populations *(46)*.

CULTURALLY COMPETENT CARE

In addition to such factors as SES, many racial/ethnic minority populations face unique health care barriers. These include language and communication, limited access to understandable information, different customs, taboos, folk beliefs, religious concepts, and varied responsibility for health care. Because effective communication, understanding, and, therefore, treatment can be affected, these factors are often associated with poorer health outcomes. To help overcome these factors, health care delivery systems and providers must avoid medical ethnocentrism and develop awareness, understanding, and acceptance of racial and ethnic differences to be more effective health care providers for diverse populations.

Developing an appreciation of such factors as different perceptions and beliefs of, for example, the role of foods and supplements, illness, disease, healing, curing, death, and who is responsible for medical decisions, is an important step in developing an effective medical partnership with a patient and family. Appropriate and sensitive attitudes, behaviors, and policies are vital for effective, cross-culturally appropriate, and effective healthcare delivery. Some examples of asthma-specific culturally competent care are mentioned. Further details are available in the review by George and general information in numerous textbooks on this topic (47,48, and selected books in culturally competent care).

An example of a health care barrier is communication not only because of language but also the specific expressions used for the condition being assessed. For example, the language and perception of and response to breathlessness and its management vary among racial/ethnic groups. Some of the differences are summarized in Table 7. For example, in a study evaluating description of airway obstruction by induced bronchoconstriction, blacks reported symptoms of breathing discomfort with upper airway descriptors. A Puerto Rican relative may be noted to fan or blow on a patient in the belief of providing oxygen or relief of dyspnea. A tea from alligators' tail, snails, or *Savila* plant leaf may also be offered to improve or heal asthma-related dyspnea in the cultural context of a Puerto Rican family. Having a clear, understandable, and a culturally sensitive dialog between patient and health care provider is required for more effective symptom assessment, monitoring, and management (48,49).

Many cultures use medicinal teas and herb supplements. Awareness and asking about these may elicit information about different patients' beliefs. This may lead to a better acceptance and understanding of the role of prescription medications. In addition, effective communication may elicit information on potentially harmful therapies being used, such as use of ginseng, which can cause bronchoconstriction, or royal jelly (bee saliva and pollen), which can lead to anaphylaxis in patients with bee allergies.

Awareness of religious beliefs, such as possible abstinence of oral and inhaled medications during the fasting month of Ramadan for Muslims, may help the provider and patient arrive at a more effective, alternative treatment program. In addition, there are several cultural beliefs regarding body function, such as the "hot–cold" theory of health and disease and the "cleansing model" of body function. The cleansing model believes in the role of sputum production, coughing, sneezing, and rhinorrhea as natural cleansing mechanisms. Consequently, believers feel that agents that may decrease mucous drainage, such as ICS and antihistamines, may be counterproductive. Asians, Islamic, East Asians, and Latinos perceive asthma as a "cold" disease. Puerto Rican mothers have been reported to dress their children and heat their homes warmly in an attempt to treat this "cold" disease. In addition, other home-based remedies commonly used in Puerto Rican communities for asthma exacerbations might include rubbing the chest and back, use of Vicks VapoRub® or alcanfor (camphor rubs), having the child rest and kept calm, the administration of fluids, and prayer (50). Awareness of the belief in this humoral, "hot–cold," theory may then help the provider to avoid use of an inhaler with a "cold" blue casing and prescribe one with a "warm" orange casing instead. Thus, sensitivity to the issues of alternative health viewpoints should improve understanding and communication and allow for a more culturally consistent and acceptable medical care plan.

A recent systematic review of the effectiveness of interventions designed to improve the quality of healthcare in racial or ethnic minorities showed evidence that such interventions are effective (51). A specific prospective cohort study in childhood asthma in five health plans revealed that certain policies could predict higher quality of care for children with asthma in managed Medicaid. Improvements were noted in decreased underprescription of preventive medication, parental ratings of care, and asthma physical status. The policies

Table 7
Dyspnea: Description and Symptom Management in Different Racial/Ethnic Groups

- African Americans: Descriptors—tight throat, scared-agitated, voice tight, itchy throat, tough breath; "difficulty catching breath"; acceptance of oxygen and/or opiates to control dyspnea if explained (fear of addiction is strong).
- American Indian: Calmly offer reassurance and inquire about the character of dyspnea. Listen for such subtleties of expression as, "The air is heavy; the air's not right," which may be complaints of dyspnea.
- Arab Americans: (*Deeket nafas*) Panic attached to being unable to breathe. Tend to hyperventilate. Need careful coaching about meaning of oxygenation, associated with severity and urgency of situation. May panic more.
- Brazilians: (*Falta de ar*—lack of air) Attributed to both emotional and physical causes. Generally accept oxygen.
- Cambodians: Anxious if cannot breathe. Some Khmer have died from sudden unexpected nocturnal death syndrome (SUNDS), inability to breathe plus cardiac symptoms.
- Central Americans: Anxious when dyspneic. Use of oxygen or other "high-tech" interventions viewed as sign of increasing gravity of illness.
- Chinese Americans: Caused by too much Yin. Some patients will treat with hot soups/broths and wear warm clothes.
- Columbians: To be without air or unable to breathe. *Quedarse sin aire* or *no poder respirar* are common expressions of dyspnea. Patient/relatives may be anxious when this happens. Oxygen accepted and expected when this occurs.
- Cubans: (*Corto de aire*—short of breath) May become expressive during dyspnea. Understand numerical scale. Easy acceptance of oxygen. Nonpharmacological methods for controlling dyspnea useful.
- Ethiopians and Eritreans: Will hyperventilate and panic. Family members also panic and hover over the sick person. Will use oxygen; however, need reassurance because using oxygen and any other major intervention is associated with gravity of disease. Also explain to family members the necessity for oxygen, because their panic increases patient's anxiety level.
- Filipinos: (*Hindi makahinga*—can't breathe) Get frantic when dyspneic. Will hyperventilate. Will use oxygen after some explanation. Some will be more anxious about using oxygen, associating its use with increasing gravity of disease.
- Gypsies: Prone to excitement and hyperventilation. Use of oxygen usually accepted but general fear of anesthesia (referred to as "little death"). Oxygen mask may be mistaken for anesthesia.
- Haitians: A primary respiratory ailment is *oppression*, a term used to describe asthma but includes more than asthma. Describes a state of anxiety and hyperventilation instead of asthma. *Oppression* considered a "cold" state, as are many respiratory conditions. Patient will say *M ap toufe* or *mwen pa ka respire*. Oxygen should be offered only when absolutely necessary because use of oxygen is associated with seriousness of disease.
- Hmong: Lung disease common among older Hmong, and considerable lung disease is noted in opium smokers. This is accepted as part of life, and rarely complained about.
- Iranians: Will be anxious during this time. Will accept medication of any nature and oxygen to control the state and to relieve accompanying fear. Give hope to patient and family that symptom of dyspnea can be controlled to a degree.
- Japanese Americans: Can't breathe. Will accept oxygen.
- Koreans: *Soomi cham-nida* means shortness of breath or dyspnea. Will be worried and try to breathe faster and deeper; oxygen may not be welcomed because of fear of progressive disease or worsening of condition.
- Mexican-Americans: Tendency to feel that something is wrong if oxygen required.

(Continued)

Table 7 (*Continued*)

- Puerto Ricans: *Asfixiado*—word describing shortness of breath. Fanning or blowing into patient believed to provide oxygen or relieve dyspnea. Tea from alligator's tail, snails, or *Savila* (plant leaf) believed to improve/heal dyspnea-related illnesses, such as asthma and congestive heart failure.
- Russians: *Odishka* (dyspnea) May get anxious because of language barrier. Will accept oxygen.
- Samoans: *Fa'afaufau* (fah ah fow)/*fa'asuati* (fah ah soo ah tee)—trouble with breathing. Oxygen can be given after explanation of procedure. Shortness of breath may cause anxiety.
- South Asians: *Sans Ukhma* describes breathlessness. May get anxious and hyperventilate because dyspnea is also considered sign of death. Will accept oxygen with some explanation. Must be approached calmly. Some may use home remedies, such as licorice and ginger tea.
- Vietnamese: *Khôtho* —difficulty in breathing. Patient's family will report more than patient. Will get anxious and begin to hyperventilate. Offer oxygen and reassure.
- West Indians: Viewed as serious medical condition, generally associated with asthma, for which conventional medical help will be sought. Will accept use of oxygen and opioids to control dyspnea and, if asked, will express discomfort experienced in breathing, using words to describe discomfort level.
- Whites: Descriptors—deep breaths, light headed, out of air, aware of breathing, hurts to breathe.

Adapted from refs. *48* and *49*.

included promotions of cultural competence, asthma reports to clinicians, and access and continuity. Cultural-competence policies evaluated in this study included recruitment of ethnically diverse or bilingual nurses and providers, attempts to minimize cultural barriers through printed materials, provision of cross-cultural or diversity training, and training in communication skills. In addition, communication-related practices, such as access to interpreters and low-literacy health education materials, were also assessed *(52)*.

Thus, culturally competent strategies can be effective in helping to reduce the disparity in asthma health care and outcomes in racial/ethnic minorities. These strategies must include improvement over barriers to effective communication, understanding and acceptance of patients' health beliefs, and more effective approaches to improvement in treatment adherence.

CONCLUSIONS

There are disparities in the health and health care of minorities. One of the goals of the Department of Health and Human Services' national health agenda, *Healthy People 2010*, is the reduction and elimination of health disparities in asthma through: "critical new understanding of approaches to treating minority and economically disadvantaged populations" *(3,4)*.

The reasons for racial/ethnic differences in increased asthma morbidity and mortality are complex. Furthermore, the association of racial/ethnic minorities with low SES is intricate. The associated risk factors of low SES contribute to asthma morbidity and mortality. They include limited access to medical care, inadequate care, increased comorbid conditions, inadequate asthma education, low level of literacy, lack of social support, increased environmental triggers, poor living conditions, and psychosocial dysfunction. Additional factors may include asthma genome differences and potential differences in gene–gene–environment interactions, such as with infections and allergens, which may vary among racial/ethnic groups. Other reasons for disparity in asthma outcomes include language and cultural differences and consequent miscommunication, mistrust, and less effective care. Also, unintentional or conscious racism by providers may contribute to disparities in asthma health care *(19,53)*.

These asthma disparities have significant direct and indirect economic, as well as societal, costs and represent an important challenge. Research on the effects of specific genotypes, gene–environment interactions, environmental exposures, health care quality improvement, symptom perception and adherence, different responses to therapy, and culturally competent care will undoubtedly lead to better understanding and treatment for different racial/ethnic minority groups. Understanding the reasons for these disparities may and should lead to more specific recommendations for improved prevention, disease modification, greater specificity in treatment with pharmocogenetics, and improved management of all persons with asthma. A comprehensive approach by government, researchers, health care providers and organizations, pharmaceutical companies, community and racial/ethnic organizations, and patients is necessary to be successful in overcoming the disproportional burden of asthma. Improved health care access, culturally appropriate communication and interventions, adequate education and empowerment, and improvement of living conditions within the context of a supportive community environment can lead to meeting the challenge and goal of reduction of the asthma disparity suffered by racial and ethnic minorities, as well as low-income and uninsured groups.

ACKNOWLEDGMENT

The author thanks Ms. Yvonne Sargent, medical librarian Assistant.

REFERENCES

1. Population Resource Center. Available at: http://www.prcdc.org/summaries/changingnation/changingnation.html. Last accessed January 1, 2005.
2. Asthma Prevalence, Health Care Use and Mortality, 2002. Available at: http://www.cdc.gov/nchs/products/pubs/pubd/hestats/asthma/asthma.htm. Last accessed December 30, 2004.
3. Action against asthma. A strategic plan for the Department of Health and Human Services. May 2000. Available at: http://aspe.hhs.gov/sp/asthma/. Last accessed January 1, 2005.
4. Department of Health and Human Services. Coordination of Federal Asthma Activities. Available at: http://www.nhlbi.nih.gov/resources/docs/asth01rpt.htm. Last accessed January 8, 2005.
5. Worldwide variation in prevalence of symptoms of asthma, allergic rhinoconjunctivitis, and atopic eczema: ISAAC. The International Study of Asthma and Allergies in Childhood (ISAAC) Steering Committee. *Lancet* 1998; 351: 1225–1232.
6. Worldwide variations in the prevalence of asthma symptoms: the International Study of Asthma and Allergies in Childhood (ISAAC). *Eur Respir J* 1998; 12: 315–335.
7. Variations in the prevalence of respiratory symptoms, self-reported asthma attacks, and use of asthma medication in the European Community Respiratory Health Survey (ECRHS). *Eur Respir J* 1996: 9: 687–695.
8. Pearce N, Sunyer J, Cheng S, et al., on behalf of the ISSAC Steering Committee and the European Community-Respiratory Health Survey. Comparison of asthma prevalence in the ISAAC and the ECRHS. *Eur Respir J* 2000; 16: 420–426.
9. Sheikh A, Panesar SS, LassersonT, Netuveli G. Recruitment of ethnic minorities to asthma studies. *Thorax* 2004; 59: 634.

10. Hjern A, Haglund B, Bremberg S, Ringbäck-Weitoft G. Social adversity, migration and hospital admissions for childhood asthma in Sweden. *Acta Paediatr* 1999; 88: 1107–1112.

11. Partridge MR. In what way may race, ethnicity or culture influence asthma outcomes? *Thorax* 2000; 55: 175–176.

12. Sin DD, Wells H, Svenson LW, Paul Man SF. Asthma and COPD among aboriginals in Alberta, Canada. *Chest* 2002; 121: 1841–1846.

13. Mitchell EA. Racial inequalities in childhood asthma. *Soc Sci Med* 1991; 32: 831–836.

14. Shafazand S, Cokice G. Asthma. The epidemic has ended, or has it? *Chest* 2004; 125: 1969–1970.

15. Mannino DM, Homa DM, Akinbami LJ, et al. Surveillance for asthma—United States, 1980–1999. *MMWR Surveill Summ* 2002; 51 (SS1): 1–13.

16. Asthma Prevalence, Health Care Use and Mortality, 2000–2001. Available at: http://www.cdc.gov/nchs/products/pubs/pubd/hestats/asthma/asthma.htm. Last accessed October 1, 2004.

17. Meng YY, Babey SH, Malcolm E, Brown ER, Chawla N. *Asthma in California: Findings from the 2001 California Health Interview Survey*. UCLA Center for Health Policy Research, Los Angeles, 2003.

18. Burchard EG, Avila PC, Nazario S, et al. Genetics of Asthma in Latino Americans (GALA) Study. Lower bronchodilator responsiveness in Puerto Rican than in Mexican subjects with asthma. *Am J Respir Crit Care Med* 2004; 169: 386–392.

19. Boudreaux ED, Emond SD, Clark S, Camargo Jr CA, on behalf of the Multicenter Airway Research Collaboration Investigators. Race/ethnicity and asthma among children presenting to the emergency department: Differences in disease severity and management. *Pediatrics* 2003; 111: e615–e621.

20. Boudreaux ED, Emond SD, Clark S, Camargo Jr CA. Acute asthma among adults presenting to the emergency department. The role of race/ethnicity and socioeconomic status. *Chest* 2003; 124: 801–812.

21. Chen JT, Krieger N, Van Den Eeden SK, Quesenberry CP. Different slopes for different folks: Socioeconomic and racial/ethnic disparities in asthma and hay fever among 173,859 U.S. men and women. *Environ Health Perspect* 2002; 10 (suppl 2): 211–216.

22. Holguin F, Mannino DM, Antó J, et al. Country of birth as a risk factor for asthma among Mexican Americans. *Am J Respir Crit Care Med* 2005; 171: 103–108.

23. Lieu TA, Lozano P, Finkelstein JA, et al. Racial/ethnic variation in asthma status and management practices among children in managed Medicaid. *Pediatrics* 2002; 109: 857–865.

24. Jones CA, Clement LT. Inner city asthma. In: Leung DYM, Sampson HA, Geha RS, Szefler SJ, eds. *Pediatric allergy. Principles and practice*. Mosby, St. Louis, MO, 2003, pp. 392–404.

25. Grant EN, Lyttle CS, Weiss KB. The relation of socioeconomic factors and racial/ethnic differences in US asthma mortality. *Am J Public Health* 2000; 90: 1923–1925.

26. Miller JE. The effects of race/ethnicity and income on early childhood asthma prevalence and health care use. *Am J Public Health* 2000; 90: 428–430.

27. Yeatts K, Davis KJ, Sotir M, Herger C, Shy C. Who gets diagnosed with asthma? Frequent wheeze among adolescents with and without a diagnosis of asthma. *Pediatrics* 2003; 11: 1046–1054.

28. Weitzman M, Gortmaker S, Sobol A. Racial, social, and environmental risks for childhood asthma. *Am J Dis Child* 1990; 144: 1189–1194.

29. Litonjua AA, Carey VJ, Weiss ST, Gold DR. Race, socioeconomic factors, and area of residence are associated with asthma prevalence. *Pediatr Pulmonol* 1999; 28: 394–401.

30. Weitzman M, Byrd RS, Auinger P. Black and white middle class children who have private health insurance in the United States. *Pediatrics* 1999; 104: 151–157.

31. Brown ER, Ojeda VD, Wyn R, Levan R. *Racial and ethnic disparities in access to health insurance and health care*. UCLA Center for Health Policy Research, Los Angeles, CA, 2000.

32. Apter AJ, Boston RC, George M, et al. Modifiable barriers to adherence to inhaled steroids among adults with asthma: It's not just black and white. *J Allergy Clin Immunol* 2003; 111: 1219–1226.

33. Montalto D, Bruzzese J-M, Moskaleva G, Higgins-D'Alessandro A, Webber MP. Quality of life in young urban children: Does asthma make a difference? *J Asthma* 2004; 41: 497–505.

34. Bach PB, Pham HH, Schrag D, Tate RC, Hargraves JL. Primary care physicians who treat blacks and whites. *N Engl J Med* 2004; 351: 575–584.

35. Mortimer KM, Neas LM, Dockery DW, Redline S, Tager IB. The effect of air pollution on inner-city children with asthma. *Eur Respir J* 2002; 19: 699–705.

36. Weil CM, Wade SL, Bauman LJ, et al. The relationship between psychosocial factors and asthma morbidity in inner-city children with asthma. *Pediatrics* 1999; 104: 1274–1280.

37. Morgan WJ, Crain EF, Gruchalla RS, et al., for the Inner-City Asthma Study Group. Results of a home-based environmental intervention among urban children with asthma. *N Engl J Med* 2004; 351: 1068–1080.

38. Sullivan SD, Weiss KB, Lynn H, et al., for the National Cooperative Inner-City Asthma Study Investigators. The cost–effectiveness of an inner-city asthma intervention for children. *J Allergy Clin Immunol* 2002; 110: 576–581.
39. Galant SP, Crawford LJR, Morphew T, Jones CA, Bassin S. Predictive value of a cross-cultural asthma case-detection tool in an elementary school population. *Pediatrics* 2004; 114: e307–e316.
40. Fisher EB, Strunk RC, Sussman LK, Sykes RK, Walker WS. Community organization to reduce the need for acute care for asthma among African American children in low-income neighborhoods: The Neighborhood Asthma Coalition. *Pediatrics* 2004; 114: 116–123.
41. Lester LA, Rich SS, Blumenthal MN, et al., and the Collaborative Study on the Genetics of Asthma. Ethnic differences in asthma and associated phenotypes: Collaborative Study on the Genetics of Asthma. *J Allergy Clin Immunol* 2001; 108: 357–362.
42. Blumenthal MN, Langefeld CD, Beaty TH, et al. A genome-wide search for allergic (atopy) genes in three ethnic groups: Collaborative Study on the Genetics of Asthma. *Human Genet* 2004; 114: 157–164.
43. Xu J, Meyers DA, Ober C, et al., and the Collaborative Study on the Genetics of Asthma. Genome wide screen and identification of gene-gene interactions for asthma-susceptibility loci in there U.S. populations: Collaborative Study on the Genetics of Asthma. *Am J Human Genet* 2001; 68: 1437–1446.
44. Federico MJ, Covar RA, Brown EE, Leung DYM, Spahn JD. Racial differences in T-lymphocyte response to glucocorticoids. *Chest* 2005; 127: 571–578.
45. Choudhry S, Ung N, Avila PC, et al. Pharmacogenetic differences in response to albuterol between Puerto Ricans and Mexicans with asthma. *Am J Respir Crit Care Med* 2005; 171: 563–570.
46. Evans DAP, McLeod HL, Pritchard S, Tariq M, Mobarek A. Interethnic variability in human drug responses. *Drug Metab Dispos* 2001; 29: 606–610.
47. George M. The challenge of culturally competent health care: Applications for asthma. *Heart Lung* 2001; 30: 392–400.
48. Lipson JG, Dibble SL, Minarik PA. *Culture and nursing care: A pocket guide.* UCSF Nursing Press, San Francisco, 1996.
49. Hardie GE, Janson S, Gold W, Carrieri-Kohlman V, Boushey HA. Ethnic differences: Word descriptors used by African-American and white asthma patients during induced bronchoconstriction. *Chest* 2000; 117: 935–943.
50. Pachter LM, Cloutier MM, Bernstein BA. Ethnomedical (folk) remedies for childhood asthma in a mainland Puerto Rican community. *Arch Pediatr Adolesc Med* 1995; 149: 982–988.
51. Beach MC, Cooper LA, Robinson KA, et al. *Strategies for Improving Minority Healthcare Quality. Evidence Report/Technology Assessment No. 90* (Prepared by the Johns Hopkins University Evidenced-based Practice Center, Baltimore, MD). Agency for Healthcare Research and Quality, Rockville, MD, January 2004. AHRQ Publication No. 04-E008-02.
52. Lieu TA, Finkelstein JA, Lozano P, et al. Cultural competence policies and other predictors of asthma care quality for Medicaid-insured children. *Pediatrics* 2004; 114: e102–e110.
53. Epstein A, Ayanian J. Racial disparities in medical care. *N Engl J Med* 2001; 344: 1471–1472.

SELECTED BOOKS ON CULTURALLY COMPETENT CARE

1. Helman CG. *Culture, Health and Illness*, 4th ed. Butterworth Heinemann, Oxford, UK, 2000.
2. Purnell LD, Paulanka BJ, eds. *Transcultural Health Care. A Culturally Competent Approach*, 2nd ed. FA Davis, Philadelphia, 2003.
3. Spector RE. *Cultural Diversity in Health and Illness*, 6th ed. Pearson Education, Upper Saddle River, NJ, 2004.

WEBSITES

- http://www.niaid.nih.gov/factsheets/asthma.htm
  Fact sheet on "Asthma: A concern for minority populations" by the National Institute of Allergy and Infectious Diseases, a component of the National Institutes of Health (NIH), outlining specific components of its basic, clinical and intervention programs on asthma concerning minorities.

- http://www.medlineplus.gov/esp/
  MEDLINEplus: NIH's National Library of Medicine (NLM) offers MEDLINEplus, the Spanish-language companion health Web site to NLM's MEDLINE, which provides authoritative, full-text medical resources.
- http://www.cdc.gov/asthma/spanish/sp_faqs.htm
  Center for Disease Control and Prevention Asthma website and direct link to "Basic Asthma Facts" in Spanish.
- http://www.healthfinder.gov/espanol/
  Healthfinder en Español: This Spanish-language Web site helps consumers access reliable information quickly and easily on the Internet.
- http://www.sunyit.edu/library/html/culturedmed/foreign/
  Foreign language health materials compilation by the SUNY Institute of Technology.
- http://medstat.med.utah.edu/24languages
  The 24 Languages Project, funded by the NLM, in partnership with the Utah Department of Health and many others, to improve access to health materials in multiple languages.
- http://www.healthtranslations.vic.gov.au/
  This is the web link for the Health Translations Online Directory from the Department of Health Resources, State Government of Victoria, Australia, which allows both health care providers and patients a web-based translated health information base in 58 languages. For example, there are 20 links for "asthma" in Vietnamese.
- http://www.omhrc.gov/
  Office of Minority Health Resource Center (OMHRC): The OMHRC serves as a national resource and referral service on minority health. The center collects and distributes information including print and electronic publications for professionals and consumers. OMHRC provides access to minority health experts from across the country and technical and capacity-building assistance for community-based organizations and AIDS service organizations.
- http://www.hhs.gov/ocr/lep/
  Office for Civil Rights: The US Department of Health and Human Services Office for Civil Rights drafted written policy guidance to assist health and social services providers in ensuring that persons with limited English skills can effectively access critical health and social services.

19 Asthma and the Law

Charles Bond, JD

CONTENTS

KEY POINTS

- Air pollution—indoors and outdoors—can create suffering for patients with asthma. To help protect individuals with respiratory problems, govenments at all levels have enacted clean air laws regulating everything from car emissions to tobacco smoke. Courts have also provided remedies for asthmatic victims of air pollution. Notably, part of the justification for a recent tobacco settlement was to pay for the care of patients with asthma whose condition was caused or exacerbated by smoking or second-hand smoke.
- Improper or out-of-date asthma treatment can lead to malpractice claim. The standard of care is becoming a national standard based on the level of care that would be rendered by a specialist in the same or similar circumstances. Therefore, it is important for physicians to keep up with the literature and disease management protocols. Because many problems arise from patients not receiving or not understanding medical instructions, documented, informed consent is extremely important.
- Asthma can be an expensive disease for physicians bearing financial risks under a management care contract. Accordingly, when negotiating medical care contracts, the asthma should be separately calculated and negotiated. Whenever physicians gain financially by rendering less care under a management care contract, there is a potential ethical dilemma. This dilemma can be resolved for asthma patients by prescribing appropriate disease management measures, which may entail short-term costs, especially pharmaceutical expenses, but in the end, will save money on the overall cost of the patients care. This chapter outlines available measures if health maintenance organization authorizers will not authorize the appropriate cure.

From: *Current Clinical Practice: Bronchial Asthma:*
A Guide for Practical Understanding and Treatment, 5th ed.
Edited by: M. E. Gershwin and T. E. Albertson © Humana Press Inc., Totowa, NJ

- This chapter also discusses policies, especially those involving drug testing, and the need to harmonize those policies with the privacy rights of patients with asthma.
- The Americans with Disabilities Act or the Federal Rehabilitation Act will protect individuals with asthma (especially those with severe cases) from job discrimination, and will ensure their access to insurance, although there is currently still a strong conflict regarding insurance access.
- Finally, this chapter offers legal information for physicians who must render expert opinions regarding the scope of an asthmatic's disability or its cause.

INTRODUCTION

This chapter raises and highlights some of the legal issues associated with asthma, from the perspective of both patients and the physician. As with all medical conditions, especially those defined as disabilities, the possible topics are so numerous that complete treatises could and have been written on such subjects. Therefore, the author has chosen to focus on only a few specific legal issues pertaining to asthma. No direct law has been enacted or has been made by the courts that is applicable solely to asthma. However, because asthma would likely be considered a disability, this chapter focuses on some of the key legal issues associated with all disabilities, including discrimination, access to health service, insurance coverage, denials of claims for medical treatment, and actions for professional liability. Moreover, it is important to note that, although federal law may cover many of the legal issues, state law may apply and often is more stringent than federal law, and it may provide additional remedies on the same subject. Therefore, anyone with particular legal questions should consult a local health care lawyer who is familiar with particular state laws regarding disabilities, such as asthma. For further information, the reader is encouraged to review the Web site of The National Conference of State Legislatures, which allows visitors to search for information on current state asthma-related bills and laws: www.ncsl.org/programs/esnr/asthma.cfm.

THE INCREASING INSTANCE OF ASTHMA AND ITS LEGAL IMPLICATIONS FOR ENVIRONMENTAL LAW

With asthma rates growing, the legal implications of the disease are widespread. Asthma is viewed as a barometer of our environmental health. It presents physical symptoms that reflect how clean our air and the surrounding environment may be at any given time. As a result, numerous laws at the state and local levels are being passed to help ensure a clean breathing environment for individuals who may suffer from asthma or severe allergies.

In the work environment, there are much stricter Occupational Safety and Health Administration regulations to prevent job-related asthma. Public buildings, even apartment dwellings, are being subjected to tighter ventilation and air-filtering requirements. Air polluters, such as oil refineries and others, have to pay asthma sufferers for major accidents or long-term polluting activities. Recently, indoor air quality (especially related to mold, which is a known cause of asthma) has also been the subject of increased attention from courts and government agencies. For more information and updates on the subject, consult the Environmental Protection Agency's Web site at: www.epa.gov/iaq/index.html. The heightened awareness of asthma and its personal and social costs is improving the quality of the environment for those who do not suffer from the disease, as well as for those who do.

SUCCESSFUL MANAGEMENT OF ASTHMA
AND PREVENTION OF MALPRACTICE

As the medical standards for managing asthma improve, the standard of care for asthma diagnosis and treatment is being elevated. Although this means better treatment for patients, it also means that physicians throughout the country are expected to adhere to the accepted improving standards. The law provides that:

In performing professional services for patients, physicians have the duty to have that degree of learning and skill ordinarily possessed by reputable physicians practicing in the same or similar locality and under similar circumstances. It is furthermore the duty of the physician to use reasonable diligence and his best judgment in the exercise of his skill and the application of learning, in an effort to accomplish the purpose for which the physician is employed. A failure to fulfill any such duties is negligence.

—*Judicial Council of California Civil Jury Instructions (CACI) 501,*
Mathew Bender & Co. (2005).

Although the standard of care references the locality where the physician practices, a failure by local physicians to adhere to national and accepted standards is not an excuse for malpractice. Furthermore, primary care physicians who attempt to care for and manage asthma will be held to the same standards as allergists or rheumatologists. As national standards emerge for disease management, it will be the responsibility for all physicians who are treating asthma patients to be up to date regarding those standards. This does not mean that practitioners must accept every new proposed treatment, only those who have become accepted in practice or recommended by leading national standard setting academies, associations, or organizations. The law provides that:

A [physician] is not necessarily negligent just because [he/she] chooses one medically accepted method of treatment... and it turns out that another medically accepted method would have been a better choice. (CACI, 506, Matthew Bender & Co. [2005]).

Physicians should be aware that if they do not follow mainstream and standard procedures, they are more likely to be second- guessed by experts at trial.

Recently, as asthma management has improved and the standard of care has become better defined, the number of claims for failure to diagnose or promptly treat asthma has increased. Particularly, there has been an increase in the number of claims alleging failure to properly instruct the patients and their families how to handle asthma emergencies. Physicians undertaking asthma care, therefore, should consider using instruction sheets and should always document patient instructions in the chart. Emergency rooms and other departments that receive asthma patients must be current in their methods of recognizing and treating problems. In short, the practice of good medicine will lead to fewer malpractice claims.

ASTHMA MANAGEMENT AND MEDICAL ECONOMICS

Treating asthma emergencies can be expensive. No only do patients with blocked airways require expensive emergency room treatment but also, if help is not provided in time, there can be serious complications, including brain damage, leading to costly long-term deficits and high levels of care. In this age of managed care, health insurers and managed care organizations, including physicians' medical groups and independent physician associations, can be forced to bear the cost of care and treatment, depending on their contracts with health care organizations. Physicians who contract for the care of patients with asthma or patients with potential asthma—whether they be primary care physicians or specialists—should expressly negotiate a clause in their contracts singling out the asthma risk and ensuring that it is both identified and properly reinsured through stop-loss insurance.

HMO authorizers may try to limit or impede the physicians' aggressive management of asthma to save short-term costs, particularly pharmaceutical costs. Successful management of the disease not only means treatment of patients but also, under managed care or capitation, it means controlling an important economic risk in the patient population. In this instance, good medicine equals good disease management, which, in turn, equals good economics. Patients are entitled to appropriate care, and physicians are ethically and in most states legally bound to advocate appropriate care for patients, even if HMO authorizers say, "No." Physicians must appeal and take all steps possible to convince medical directors to provide appropriate care. If medical directors refuse to authorize appropriate care, physicians should write letters to the medical director setting their concerns and stating clearly that any adverse consequences of the medical decisions made by medical directors will be the responsibility of the director. Some physicians who have failed to gain authorization have gone so far as to report medical directors to the state licensing board for violation of the state Medical Practice Act. If the HMO tries to retaliate against the treating physician for advocating good patient care, the doctor may have statutory and common-law protection, depending on the state in which he practices. Medical associations throughout the country will often help their members in such situations.

From the patient's perspective, asthma can be difficult to diagnosis. Unfortunately, physicians often miss the diagnosis, particularly if they are in a rushed managed care environment. Patients who suspect that they have asthma but do not receive close medical supervision should contact the American Lung Association.

PATIENTS WITH ASTHMA AND PRIVACY

The US Constitution, as well as state constitutions, such as California's, guarantee an individual's right to privacy as a part of the "penumbral" or understood rights under the Constitution. California's constitution expressly guarantees the right of privacy to all its citizens. Notwithstanding these constitutional guaranties, the abuse of drugs has led to widespread practice of drug testing on the job, in sports, and in other venues. Under many circumstances, especially where motor skills are required or competition is involved, drug testing has been allowed by the courts. Readers may recall that an Olympic swimmer from the United States was deprived of his medal because he tested positive on a drug test after having taken drugs for his asthma.

One practical legal problem faced by patients with asthma is the increasing ban on inhalers, especially in schools. As a result, many children and young people must leave their inhaler with the school nurse or some other school official, risking an attack without the medication at hand. Research reveals no reports of death as a result of these policies, but there have been many frightening close calls. Obviously, we will see legal activity in the future to balance the rights of patients with asthma with our drug and drug testing policies.

PATIENTS AND THE AMERICANS WITH DISABILITIES ACT

Research reveals no case in the country that has yet held that asthma is a disability as defined in the Americans With Disabilities Act (ADA). The statutory definition of a disability, however, appears to apply to asthma. Under the ADA, a person is considered to be disabled and protected if:

- He or she has a record of having, or is regarded as having, a physical or medical impairment, and
- That impairment substantially limits one or more of the person's major life activities.

A "physical or medical impairment" is defined as any physiological disorder or condition, cosmetic disfigurement, or anatomical loss affecting one or more of several body systems, or any mental or psychological disorder. Such conditions as chronic fatigue syndrome, depression, diabetes, epilepsy, heart disease, high blood pressure, hypersensitivity to substances (such as cigarette smoke), learning disorders, mental retardation, migraine headaches, schizophrenia, shortness, stress disorders, and obesity are disabilities. Logically, asthma would similarly be considered to be a disability when other elements of the definition of disability are met.

The impairment must also affect one or more of the affected person's "major life activities," which are the activities that the average person can perform with minimal or no difficulty on a daily basis. Such activities would include caring for oneself, eating, drinking, walking, speaking, breathing, learning, hearing, and working, among others. Moreover, these activities must not simply be restricted or limited, but rather the person's impairment must "substantially limit" performance of "major life activities." Therefore, the ADA applies only to those impairments that are permanent or chronic or that have long-term effects; temporary, nonchronic impairment with short duration and little or no permanent impact would not be covered by the ADA. There is, however, no absolute and truly objective method for applying this requirement of the law.

The Equal Employment Opportunity Commission, which is the federal governmental agency empowered to enforce the disability discrimination laws, emphasizes that each case must be evaluated on its own merits. The episodic nature of asthma would not be a bar to its being classified as a disability, because the onset is unexpected, unanticipated, and not under the control of the individual. Even though the disability may be medically controlled, it still falls within the zone of protection of the ADA. The ADA and the Federal Rehabilitation Act provide protection for persons with disabilities against discrimination in the workplace. Under the ADA, equal job opportunity is guaranteed and the employer must make reasonable accommodations to ensure that the disabled person can take the job if he or she is otherwise qualified. Much has been written about the ADA and its effect on employers. From physicians' and patients' points of view, it is important to simply be aware that asthma should not limit the employability of an individual except under conditions that may trigger attacks.

The ADA also protects the rights of patients with asthma to health care services. As with all public accommodations, Title 3 of the ADA prohibits discrimination in the delivery of healthcare, requires the removal of any barriers to receiving health care, and mandates that construction and alterations consider the disabilities of patients. Building codes are increasingly strict regarding air filtration, and physicians specializing in rheumatology and asthma treatment should pay attention to the environmental accommodations that they make to their patients with asthma.

The ADA and the Federal Rehabilitation Act may also affect physicians who are contracting for managed care. As noted, physicians should negotiate special arrangements for patients with asthma to avoid assuming unsupportable financial risks. The language of those provisions as they relate to asthma and other patients with disabilities should be carefully worded, so as not to be construed as discriminatory, i.e., a refusal by the doctors to provide access to medical care for these individuals. Healthcare providers are prohibited from withholding medical benefits treatment services for patients with disabilities, so arrangements for such patients should be anticipated during contract negotiations.

There now exists a conflict in the laws regarding whether insurance companies are required to provide coverage as a public accommodation without discrimination to the disabled. The Sixth Circuit, in its opinion in *Parker v. Metropolitan Life Insurance Company*, clearly states that places that do not have physical boundaries, which would include insurance-benefit plans, are not to be considered public accommodations and are not subject to Title 3 of the ADA. Other case law, however, from other Circuits, holds that insurance is a public accommodation.

Employees may also be held liable for ADA violations if they deny insurance benefits to their employees based on disability. The discrimination must be showed to be disparate treatment. In sum, the ADA and the Federal Rehabilitation Act—and corresponding state laws protecting the disabled—may help patients gain access to care, access to insurance, and access to employment with reasonable accommodations to ensure a helpful working environment for them. Physicians may be called on to advocate for their patients to obtain the benefits of these laws, and they are encouraged to do so.

CONCLUSION

Asthma, like many life-threatening conditions, is a disability that has achieved legal attention. Patients are generally protected from discrimination by federal and state laws, and physicians are required to treat the ailment. Under managed care contracts, physicians should not assume the financial risk of catastrophic asthma treatment. That risk should be separately negotiated and separately insured with stop-loss insurance. Fortunately, disease management models are dealing with the ever-increasing number of patients with asthma. These disease management techniques should be used carefully to ensure better, more-timely, and less-costly treatment. In turn, the economic risk, under managed care, will be lowered. Part of the disease management for asthma includes use of drugs that may result in positive drug testing of patients with asthma. Protection of their privacy rights constitutes a medicolegal challenge that will be resolved in the courts in the coming years.

ACKNOWLEDGMENTS

The author thanks Torris Dorros, Esq., and Sophie Cohen, Esq., LL.M. for their assistance in the preparation of this chapter.

Index

6049